Neuroendocrine Tumors: A Multidisciplinary Approach

Frontiers of Hormone Research

Vol. 44

Series Editor

Ezio Ghigo Turin

Co-Editors

Federica Guaraldi Turin
Andrea Benso Turin

Neuroendocrine Tumors: A Multidisciplinary Approach

Volume Editors

Mauro Papotti Turin
Wouter W. de Herder Rotterdam

51 figures, 26 in color, and 27 tables, 2015

KARGER Basel · Freiburg · Paris · London · New York · Chennai · New Delhi · Bangkok · Beijing · Shanghai · Tokyo · Kuala Lumpur · Singapore · Sydney

Frontiers of Hormone Research

Founded 1972 by Tj.B. van Wimersma Greidanus, Utrecht
Continued by Ashley B. Grossman, Oxford (1996–2013)

Mauro Papotti, MD
Department of Pathology
University of Turin
Ospedale San Luigi
Orbassano, Turin, Italy

Wouter W. de Herder, MD, PhD
Department of Internal Medicine,
Sector of Endocrinology
Erasmus MC
Rotterdam, The Netherlands

Library of Congress Cataloging-in-Publication Data

Neuroendocrine tumors (Papotti)
Neuroendocrine tumors : a multidisciplinary approach / volume editors, Mauro Papotti, Wouter W. de Herder.
p. ; cm. -- (Frontiers of hormone research, ISSN 0301-3073 ; vol. 44)
Includes bibliographical references and indexes.
ISBN 978-3-318-02772-3 (hard cover : alk. paper) -- ISBN 978-3-318-02773-0 (electronic version)
I. Papotti, Mauro, editor. II. Herder, Wouter W. de, editor. III. Title. IV. Series: Frontiers of hormone research ; v. 44. 0301-3073
[DNLM: 1. Neuroendocrine Tumors--diagnosis. 2. Neuroendocrine Tumors--therapy. W1 FR946F v.44 2015 / QZ 380]
RC280.E55
616.99'437--dc23

2015021100

Bibliographic Indices. This publication is listed in bibliographic services, including Current Contents® and PubMed/MEDLINE.

Disclaimer. The statements, opinions and data contained in this publication are solely those of the individual authors and contributors and not of the publisher and the editor(s). The appearance of advertisements in the book is not a warranty, endorsement, or approval of the products or services advertised or of their effectiveness, quality or safety. The publisher and the editor(s) disclaim responsibility for any injury to persons or property resulting from any ideas, methods, instructions or products referred to in the content or advertisements.

Drug Dosage. The authors and the publisher have exerted every effort to ensure that drug selection and dosage set forth in this text are in accord with current recommendations and practice at the time of publication. However, in view of ongoing research, changes in government regulations, and the constant flow of information relating to drug therapy and drug reactions, the reader is urged to check the package insert for each drug for any change in indications and dosage and for added warnings and precautions. This is particularly important when the recommended agent is a new and/or infrequently employed drug.

www.karger.com
Printed in Germany on acid-free and non-aging paper (ISO 9706) by Kraft Druck GmbH, Ettlingen
ISSN 0301–3073
e-ISSN 1662–3762
ISBN 978–3–318–02772–3
e-ISBN 978–3–318–02773–0

KARGER 125 YEARS

Contents

Preface

Over 100 years ago the term carcinoid ('Karzinoide Tumoren des Dünndarmes', Siegfried Oberndorfer) entered the medical literature to describe a rare and peculiar type of epithelial neoplasm, apparently restricted to the intestine, characterized by a solid, trabecular or nested (organoid rather than glandular) histology and a less aggressive biological behavior [1]. Since then a large body of literature has expanded the concept of carcinoid, defining a wide spectrum of peculiar tumors, potentially affecting all organs and apparatuses, sharing common biological properties (i.e. signs of neuroendocrine, NE, differentiation), while presenting pathognomonic epidemiological, hormonal, pathological, radiological and, above all, clinical features and outcomes [2–7].

The more generalist term neuroendocrine neoplasm (NEN) was recommended in the latest WHO classification [4]. In the field of gastroenteropancreatic tumors, only two entities are now recognized, NE tumor and NE carcinoma, subclassified according to tumor grade and stage [4], although the acronym NET (neuroendocrine tumor) still remains the most popular in the medical community (the WHO classification itself recognizes NEN and NET as synonyms). This is not the case for pulmonary NETs, which still maintain the original nomenclature of the single different entities described over the years, including typical and atypical carcinoids, as well as small and large cell (NE) carcinomas [8], while the use of terms applied to the single tumor entities in the past (i.e. malignant carcinoid or well-differentiated neuroendocrine carcinoma) are discouraged for being potentially confusing.

Despite the extensive multidisciplinary studies on these rare tumors, several management (i.e. diagnostic work-up and the therapeutic strategies) controversies and gray areas still exist. Several impediments were identified 6 years ago at a National Cancer Institute summit in the USA, which have hampered or slowed down the development of valid solutions for NET care [9]. These include the poor understanding of NE cell and tumor biology and tumorigenesis mechanisms, the heterogeneous application of pathological classifications (including grading and staging), the incomplete knowledge of specific therapeutic targets as well as of complications and side effects in terms of morbidity and mortality, the limited availability of in vitro and in vivo models for research, and the paucity of relevant prognostic and predictive factors in NETs. Solutions to some of these impediments have begun to emerge and progress has been made in recent years. Nevertheless, the above difficulties support the opportunity of gathering experts from different fields of the involved medical disciplines and from centers of excellence for the cure of NETs to update the current knowledge on diagnosis and treatment, to highlight the most relevant controversial issues and, above all, to offer tentative or established answers.

The reason for undertaking such an adventure in the field of NET/NENs is primarily linked to the increasing evidence that these tumors are not as rare as they have been considered so far [9–12]. In addition, because of their widespread occurrence in the body, their partial biological and clinical similarities, and their unpredictable behavior, it seems that an organic and uniform approach to these diseases is necessary. This does not mean to interfere with the various specialists, in terms of their competence or entitlement to manage single affected patients, but rather to offer the chance of comparing the various diagnostic and therapeutic strategies for the management of NETs arising from the different organs, and realizing an advantage from it (indeed, irrespective of the site of origin and clinical background, these tumors share many biological properties and features).

General Design of the Current Volume

The current volume has been designed around four main areas of interest, with the aim of presenting the most important achievements in the management of NETs. Gastroenteropancreatic NETs will form the core of the volume, but pulmonary and thymic counterparts will also be discussed.

In the first interest area, NE tumors will be approached with regard to the clinical syndromes and symptoms that characterize this tumor type, and also to the relevant role of laboratory medicine for their definition. The chapters dedicated to imaging procedures will help to clarify the major controversies in NET recognition by computed tomography, ultrasonography and nuclear medicine imaging, as well as endoscopic techniques. In the following chapters, the pathology and genetics of NETs will be discussed, with an update on the major controversies related to NET nomenclature, classification, genetic, epigenetic, immunological and gene-expression profiles. Finally, a large part of the volume will be devoted to NET treatment.

Surgery represents the gold-standard approach for patient cure, and should be performed whenever possible. The various (traditional and new) currently available surgical approaches will be presented, concluding with a chapter dedicated to organ transplantation and debulking procedures, both of which are part of the surgical strategy for NETs management.

The volume will close with a session dedicated to currently available medical treatments (i.e. targeted, symptomatic and chemotherapy) for the various types of NETs, followed by radionuclear therapy modalities and, finally, new perspectives and novel biotherapy and immunotherapy options.

Rigorous classification, timely diagnosis and a high standard of surgical and medical treatment are mandatory to achieve the best results at the right time in patients affected by NETs. We hope this volume will be a valid tool for the broader scientific community dealing with the diagnosis and management of NETs.

Mauro Papotti, Turin
Wouter W. de Herder, Rotterdam
Ezio Ghigo, Turin
Federica Guaraldi, Turin

References

1 Oberndorfer S: Karzinoide Tumoren des Dünndarms. Frank Z Pathol 1907;1:426–429.
2 Kaltsas GA, Besser GM, Grossman AB: The diagnosis and medical management of advanced neuroendocrine tumors. Endocr Rev 2004;25:458–511.
3 van Eeden S, Offerhaus JA: Historical, current and future perspectives on GEP endocrine tumors. Virchows Arch 2006;448:1–6.
4 Bosman FT, Carneiro F, Hruban RH, Theise ND (eds): World Health Organization Classification of Tumours: Pathology and Genetics of Tumors of the Digestive System. Lyon, IARC Press, 2010, pp 13–14.
5 Modlin IM, Oberg K, Chung DC, Jensen RT, de Herder WW, Thakker RV, Caplin M, Delle Fave G, Kaltsas GA, Krenning EP, Moss SF, Nilsson O, Rindi G, Salazar R, Ruszniewski P, Sundin A: Gastroenteropancreatic neuroendocrine tumours. Lancet Oncol 2008;9:61–72.
6 Oberg K: Gastrointestinal neuroendocrine tumors. Ann Oncol 2010;21(S7):vii72–vii80.
7 Cives M, Strosberg J: An Update on Gastroentero-pancreatic Neuroendocrine Tumors. Oncology 2014;28:749–756.
8 Travis WD, Brambilla E, Muller-Hermelink HK, Harris CC (eds): World Health Organization Classification of Tumours: Pathology and Genetics: Tumours of the Lung, Pleura, Thymus and Heart. Lyon, IARC Press, 2004, pp 19–21.
9 Modlin IM, Moss SF, Chung DC, Jensen RT, Snyderwine E: Priorities for improving the management of GEP NETs. J Natl Cancer Inst 2008;100:1282–1289.
10 Yao J, Hassan M, Phan A, Dagohoy C, Leary C, Mares JE, Abdalla EK, Fleming JB, Vauthey JN, Rashid A, Evans DB: One hundred years after 'carcinoid': epidemiology of and prognostic factors for NET in 35,825 cases in the United States. J Clin Oncol 2008;26:3063–3072.
11 Modlin IM, Gustafsson BI, Pavel M, Svejda B, Lawrence B, Kidd M: A nomogram to assess small intestinal NET (carcinoid) survival. Neuroendocrinology 2010;92:143–157.
12 Hallet J, How Lim Law C, Cukier M, Saskin R, Liu N, Singh S: Exploring the rising incidence of neuroendocrine tumors: a population-based analysis of epidemiology, metastatic presentation, and outcomes. Cancer 2015;121:589–597.

Papotti M, de Herder WW (eds): Neuroendocrine Tumors: A Multidisciplinary Approach.
Front Horm Res. Basel, Karger, 2015, vol 44, pp 1–23 (DOI: 10.1159/000381970)

Epidemiology of Neuroendocrine Tumors

Merav Fraenkel[a] • Antongiulio Faggiano[b] • Gerlof D. Valk[c]

[a]Endocrinology Unit, Soroka University Medical Center and The Faculty of Health Sciences, Ben-Gurion University of the Negev, Beer Sheva, Israel; [b]Department of Molecular and Clinical Endocrinology and Metabolism, Federico II University of Naples, Napoli, Italy; [c]Department of Internal Medicine, University Medical Center Utrecht, Utrecht, The Netherlands

Abstract

Formerly named carcinoids, neuroendocrine tumors originate from diffuse endocrine cells, can involve any part of the gastrointestinal tract, endocrine pancreas and bronchopulmonary (BP) tree, and have a wide range of malignant potential. This chapter summarizes the data available on the epidemiology of neuroendocrine neoplasia (NEN) from around the world, including the relative frequency according to organ of origin, annual incidence rates (IR) and trends in IR at the various anatomic sites, age and stage at presentation, racial and gender differences in IR and 5-year survival rates. Over time, changes have been made in the classification and registration of NEN, both in the same registry and across the globe, thus confounding the possibility to draw conclusions as to the true rise in IR of NEN that is observed all over the world. BP NEN has become the most common site in many western countries, while NEN of the rectum is more common in the Far East. In some countries, appendiceal NEN is the most common site in females. When compared to adenocarcinoma of the same location, the prognosis of NEN patients is better. Five-year survival rates are highest for NEN originating in the rectum and appendix, but lower in small intestinal and pancreatic NEN. Future research is needed to understand the contribution of genetic and environmental factors to NEN epidemiology.

Neuroendocrine tumors (NETs) originate from diffuse neuroendocrine cells that are dispersed throughout the body, predominantly in the gastrointestinal tract, islets of Langerhans in the pancreas and the bronchopulmonary (BP) system. Neuroendocrine cells are unique in their capability to synthesize and secrete neuropeptides and hormones, leading to characteristic hormonal syndromes. NETs are comprised of cells that on immunohistochemistry may be identified by specific neuroendocrine markers, such as synaptophysin and chromogranin A. NETs are a heterogeneous group of tumors causing unique clinical syndromes and/or local symptoms, but, not uncommonly, may also be asymptomatic and discovered as an incidental finding [1].

NETs of the gastrointestinal tract were originally described by Oberndorfer in 1907, who coined the name 'Karzinoide' to describe submucosal tumors in the small bowel which followed an indolent course when compared to adenocarcinoma. The first description of BP NETs was made by Laennec about 100 years earlier [1].

Histologic Classification of Neuroendocrine Tumors

Major changes have been made in the classification of NETs throughout the years. The most widely accepted is the WHO classification, which is based on the histologic grade (according to the Ki-67 and mitotic index) and degree of differentiation (well vs. poorly differentiated) [2]. This new classification argues against the use of the term 'carcinoid' combined with the organ from which this tumor originated, as this may be misleading and does not reflect the diversity of malignant potential that these tumors may carry. The most recent WHO 2010 system renders all NETs as neoplasms with a malignant potential and calls for the use of the term neuroendocrine neoplasia (NEN) [3, 4]. This is in contrast to the older paradigm assuming these are rare, slow-growing tumors with an indolent behavior. Unfortunately, this new terminology of NEN has not yet been fully accepted around the world. Moreover, some publications still classify NEN according to the embryonic source of the organ. These complexities in classification and grading are further accentuated in the terminology of BP NEN. The most recent WHO classification of BP NEN, published in 2004, mainly relies on morphology, with the aid of mitotic count and assessment of the presence of necrosis, and divides BP NEN into 4 subtypes [3–5]. A grading system based on the Ki-67 index for BP NEN has recently been introduced but has not been officially accepted yet [6].

Coding Systems of Neuroendocrine Tumors

Most, but not all, national and local cancer registries used the International Classification of Disease for Oncology (ICD-O) coding system to collect data on the epidemiology of these NEN. This coding system has been updated periodically and, therefore, early reports are often incompatible with more recent data. The latest ICD-O-3, used for the coding of NEN, is presented in table 1. The first 4 digits designate the histologic diagnosis and the fifth digit, designated as 'behavior code', reports the biologic behavior according to the following: 0 = benign, 1 = borderline malignancy, 2 = in situ, 3 = malignant (http://seer.cancer.gov/behavrecode/). In addition, the anatomic site of the tumor is recorded.

Table 1. ICD-O codes for NETs

NET histology	ICD code
Carcinoid tumor	8240
Enterochromaffin cell carcinoid	8241
Goblet cell carcinoid	8243
Composite carcinoid	8244
Adenocarcinoid	8245
Neuroendocrine carcinoma	8246
Apudoma	8248
AC	8249
Stromal carcinoid	9091
Islet cell carcinoma	8150
Insulinoma	8151
Glucagonoma	8152
Gastrinoma	8153
Mixed islet cell/exocrine adenocarcinoma	8154
VIPoma	8155
Somatostatinoma	8156
Enteroglucagonoma	8157
Small cell neuroendocrine carcinoma of the lung	8002, 8040–8045
Large cell neuroendocrine carcinoma of the lung	8013
Small cell carcinoma, not otherwise specified	8041
Oat cell carcinoma	8042
Small cell carcinoma, fusiform cell	8043
Small cell carcinoma, intermediate cell	8044
Combined small cell carcinoma	8045
Adenocarcinoma with neuroendocrine differentiation	8574

Anatomic Sites of Neuroendocrine Neoplasia

NEN occur most commonly in the BP tree and digestive system. Most published reports on the epidemiology of NEN were dedicated to the incidence rates (IR) of NEN of the gastrointestinal tract with and without the pancreas (gastroenteropancreatic, GEP, NET). BP NEN were included in a few reports and in some a wider range of anatomic sites of NEN were covered. In this chapter, the epidemiology of GEP and BP NEN will be covered.

Limitations in the Interpretation of Data on Neuroendocrine Neoplasia Epidemiology

Classification and Coding

Variations in the coding and classification of NEN over time and in different geographical locations pose a major limitation in understanding the precise epidemiology of these malignancies, especially when trying to illustrate trends in incidence with time and when comparing IR from different countries. Some publications from

Table 2. Method employed by each country for the identification of NET patients for national/regional registry (only those reporting IR)

Country	Method of patient identification for national/regional registry	First author and year
USA (SEER database)[1]	Various editions of ICD-O codes	Modlin [27], 2003; Maggard [46], 2004; Modlin [52], 2007; Halfdanarson [53], 2008; Hauso [21], 2008; Yao [29], 2008; Lawrence [19], 2011; Tsikitis [49], 2012
Norway	Physicians and pathology departments reporting to national registry with checks by the Cancer Registry of Norway	Hauso [21], 2008
UK	Regional registries based on ICD-O codes	Ellis [20], 2010
Switzerland (Vaud)	Voluntary agreement between recording medical institutions and the registry; unclear how patients are identified	Levi [33], 2000
Sweden	National registry based on ICD-7 codes	Hemminki [31], 2001
Italy (Tuscany)	Regional cancer registry based on ICD-O codes	Caldarella [34], 2011
Austria	Registry based on reports from 40/41 pathology departments, WHO 2000	Niederle [15], 2010
France (Burgundy)	Data collected by cancer registry staff using multiple databases: pathology laboratories, university hospitals, local hospitals, private surgeons, oncologists, gastroenterologists, general practitioners, and monthly reviews of death certificates	Lepage [35, 51], 2004, 2006
Japan	Questionnaire to heads of departments about number of patients with GEP NET	Ito [7], 2015
Australia	Regional cancer registry; invasive neuroendocrine cancers, based on ICD-O-3	Luke [30], 2010
Taiwan	Taiwan Cancer Registry based on ICD-O-3 codes	Tsai [24], 2013

[1] Surveillance, epidemiology and end results.

national, regional and institutional cancer registries or registries dedicated to NET patients did not clearly define which classification was used for inclusion and/or relied on the diagnosis given by the treating physician/institution [7–12]. There are a few more recent publications on the epidemiology of NEN that used the 2000 WHO classification, only one of which reports IR, and a report from China published in 2012 that used the 2010 WHO classification [13–18] (table 2).

Malignant Potential

As mentioned above, ICD-O diagnosis codes also comment on the malignant potential of the tumor, where a '3' in the place of the fifth digit designates the tumor as malignant. Early on, most NEN were designated as benign unless there were clinically evident distant metastases, and were therefore not registered in cancer registries. Over time and in different parts of the world, data on NEN epidemiology inconsistently included either only malignant, or malignant and benign tumors. With time the understanding that all NEN have various rates of malignant potential served as the basis for including more and more of these neoplasia in NET cancer registries. For example, until 1986 'carcinoid' tumors were reported to the Surveillance Epidemiology and End Results (SEER) database only if they were considered malignant, while after this year all of these tumors were considered malignant and were therefore reported to SEER. These differences in registration policy may explain some of the rise in the incidence of NEN around the world [19–24].

Incidental versus Clinically Significant NEN

It is well accepted that there is a discrepancy between the IR of clinically apparent NEN and of the same tumors when they are reported from autopsy series. One such large autopsy series from Sweden between 1959 and 1969 reported an annual IR of 8.4/100,000 for various NEN (carcinoid), which is much higher than that reported in clinical series from the same period [25–27]. This discrepancy emphasizes the fact that many NEN may remain asymptomatic throughout life without having an apparent clinical significance. Nowadays, with the rising use of various imaging techniques (CT, MRI, EUS and others) for different indications, there is also a rise in the diagnosis of 'incidental NET' [28]. This should not always be attributed to a true rise in the incidence of a certain tumor type, but rather represents the growing number of asymptomatic incidental tumors that may not have clinical significance.

Sources of Information on Neuroendocrine Tumor Epidemiology

National Cancer Registries

National population-based cancer registries are the most important and informative sources for assessing NEN epidemiology. The USA National Cancer Institute (NCI) SEER database is the largest and most well-known national cancer registry. This database was preceded by the End Results Group (ERG) from 1950 to 1969 and the Third National Cancer Survey (TNCS) between 1969 and 1971. Initiated in 1973, the SEER program gradually expanded to cover larger parts of the US population. As of now, the most recent SEER 17, created in 2000, represents approximately 15% of the US population and includes data on 5,553,822 cancer patients diagnosed between 1973 and 2007, of which 49,012 were NEN cases. Based on the SEER data, the annual IR of various NEN were calculated and published numerous times [19, 26, 27, 29].

Other national cancer registries reporting NEN incidence originate from European countries, Taiwan, Japan and South Australia [7, 20, 21, 24, 30–32; for a more detailed review see 23]. IR are reported for all NEN by some or for all 'carcinoids', while others report on incidence by anatomic site. The report by Ito et al. [7] on IR of NEN in Japan claims to represent the national IR, although they are not based on a national cancer registry.

Another important source for the epidemiology on NEN are national registries dedicated to NET patients that are not population based, like those from Germany, France, Spain, Italy, Brazil and recently also from Korea. Unfortunately, these types of registries are unable to report on IR of NEN [8–10, 13, 14, 16, 17].

Regional and Institutional NEN Registries

In addition to national registries, regional registries in Europe and the USA, including Vaud in Switzerland, Tuscany in Italy, Burgundy in France, Girona in Spain and different regions within the USA (Olmstead county in Minnesota, Utah, Florida), have published data on NEN epidemiology [33–36; for more details see 23]. Last but not least, some of our information on NEN epidemiology relies on reports from large single institutions that serve as tertiary referral centers for patients with NEN. Data of this type are available from China, Taiwan, Australia and India [11, 12, 18, 37]. For clarity and simplicity, all IR are reported in this chapter as the number of new cases per 100,000 population per year.

Second Primary Malignancy in Patients with NEN

Multiple reports from institutional series and national cancer registries have reported on the association between NEN and second primary malignancies (SPM). This association was previously reviewed by Habal et al. [38] in 2000 and data from some more recent reports are summarized in table 3. Reports were not homogenous in several aspects, including in terms of the study population (PM vs. clinical series) and also the type of NEN, including all 'carcinoids', NEN of the gastrointestinal tract, GEP NEN, BP NEN or only small intestinal (SI) NENs. In addition, some studies reported on SPM that were diagnosed before, with and after the diagnosis of NEN, while others were limited to SPM that were diagnosed only after the diagnosis of NEN.

The frequency of SPM from institutional series is in the range of 13–46%, and most second malignancies were found in the gastrointestinal tract [11, 25, 37–39]. Rates of SPM from national series are in the range of 3.63–29% [27, 40–42] (table 3).

Rates of SPM in patients with SI NENs were reported separately by two national cancer registries. One, based on the SEER 17 data, found that 29% of patients with SI NET had SPM [41]. Zar et al. [42] reported in 2008 that, compared to patients in the Swedish cancer registry, those with SI NET had a standardized incidence ratio for SPM of 2.3–6.3.

Kamp et al. [43] reported SPM in 13.7% of 459 GEP NET patients treated in a tertiary referral center in the Netherlands. When compared to the general population in the Dutch National Cancer Registry, cancer rates in GEP NET patients were less than expected for cancer occurring before NET, more than expected for synchronous tumors, and as expected for metachronous tumors.

Table 3. Rates of SPM in various NET series

First author and [ref #], year	Patients, n	Type of series	Years	Country	Type of NEN	Second malignancy, %	Common sites	Comments
Kamp [43], 2012	459	Tertiary referral center	2000–2009	The Netherlands	GEP NEN	13.7	Breast, colorectal, melanoma, prostate	5.4% before NEN, 2.8% synchronous, 6.3% after NEN
Malik [11], 2013	107	Tertiary referral center	1998–2011	Canberra Hospital, Australia	G1 and G2 GEP NEN	33.6	GI (~33%)	
Cote [44], 2006	1,882	National	1988–2000	SEER, USA	BP NEN	NA	SIR for breast 1.8 SIR for prostate 2.8	SIR was increased only in the first 5 years from the Dx of 3P NEN
Modlin [27], 2003	13,715	National	1950–1999	ERG, TNCS and SEER, USA	Carcinoid	22.4	N/A	
Amin [41], 2012	8,331	National	1973–2007	SEER, USA	SI NEN	29.0	Prostate, breast, colon, lung	67% diagnosed before SI NEN and 33% after. % both pre and post
Zar [42], 2008	3,741	National	1960–2000	Swedish Cancer Registry, Sweden	SI NEN	SIR of 2.3–6.3	Melanoma, skin, endocrine, prostate	
Tsai [24], 2013	1,350	National	1996–2006	Taiwan	All NEN	3.63	Colon, lung, liver, breast	Those with cancer before NEN or within 3 months Dx of NEN were excluded. No difference in primary site of NEN and rate of SPM. SPM were more common with age >70 years
Li [37], 2008	228	Institutional	1970–2005	Taiwan	Carcinoid	14	GI (52%), lung, genitourinary	% was highest among SI NEN, followed by stomach and lung
Prommegger [39], 2004	96	Institutional	1987–2002	Innsbruck, Austria	All NEN	14.6	GI, genitourinary	36% synchronous, 57% metachronous

SIR = Standardized incidence ratio; GI = gastrointestinal; Dx = diagnosis.

Lately, a shift has been noted from the paradigm that the most common SPMs in NET patients are localized to the gastrointestinal tract, with an increasing occurrence of skin (melanoma), breast and prostate tumors as common SPM [40–44].

Taking all these data into consideration, it seems that SPM do occur more commonly in NET patients but the exact rates and distribution have not been fully elucidated. This association is partially explained by the extensive clinical work-up and follow-up in patients with a diagnosis of NET, referred to as surveillance bias. Other possible explanations can be related to common genetic factors, sex steroid milieu or environmental exposures that predispose for both tumors. Finally, this may reflect the tumorigenic properties of the various neuroendocrine peptides and growth factors secreted by neuroendocrine cells [27, 41].

Stomach

Gastric NEN (GNEN) are classified as type I, associated with achlorhydria of atrophic gastritis, type II, associated with hypergastrinemia as part of Zollinger-Ellison syndrome in multiple endocrine neoplasia type 1 (MEN1), type III, 'sporadic' with a high malignant potential, and recently also type IV, with poorly differentiated histology. Type I are the most common, comprising 70–80% of cases, followed by type III, comprising 14–20%, while types II and IV are rare [45]. Registration of GNEN by different cancer registries is variable, some documenting malignant tumors only, while others document benign and malignant tumors. In the SEER database, up to 1986 only GNEN that were designated as malignant (behavior code 3) on pathology reports were registered.

The relative frequency of gastric NENs (GNENs) among all GEP NETs is in the range of 3.7–14.6% [11, 13, 14, 17–21, 24, 26, 27, 30, 36, 46], and even up to 30% in a report of an institutional series from India [12] (table 4). Interestingly, a recent report from Austria found GNENs to be the most common site of all GEP NETs, with the majority being benign [15].

The earliest reports on the IR of GNENs from Europe and the USA, from as early as the 1970s, were in the range of 0.01–0.07 [20, 26, 33, 46, 47]. With time, IR in Europe, the USA, Australia and Taiwan increased, and in the 1990s, IR were as high as 0.1–0.15 (fig. 1). The increase in IR within the previous 4 decades is in the range of 11- to 16-fold in the USA and UK, and a more mild increase over shorter time periods has been documented in Norway, Switzerland, Australia and Taiwan [19–21, 24, 30, 31, 33, 34, 36, 46, 47]. There are several possible explanations for the rise in IR of GNENs, including to some extent a true rise in incidence, changes in the registration and classification of GNENs, increased use of gastroscopy and raised awareness of histologic diagnosis. There is a temporal association between the rise in IR of GNENs and the rising prescription of proton pump inhibitors, but causality between the two has not yet been proven [48].

Table 4. The relative frequency of the various anatomic sites for NEN in national/regional/institutional NEN registries

a All GEP NEN

First author and year	Country	Type of registry	Years	Comment	Site 1	% of all GEP NENS	Site 2	% of all GEP NENS	Site 3	% of all GEP NENS	Site 4	% of all GEP NENS
Alsina [36], 2011	Girona Province, Spain	Regional	1994–2004	BP NEN were the most common but these were mainly SCLC	Appendix	38	Pancreas	19	SI	18	Colorectum	16.9
Amarapurkar [12], 2010	Single center in Mumbai, India	Institutional registry	2000–2007		Stomach	30	Pancreas	23	Duodenum	18.9	Liver	13
Malik [11], 2013	Canberra Hospital, Australia	Institutional registry	1998–2011		SI	32	Rectum	22	Pancreas	11	UKP	9
Wang [18], 2012	The First Affiliated Hospital, Sun Yat-sen University, China	Institutional registry	1995–2012		Pancreas	34.8	Rectum	20.2	Stomach	14	Duodenum	7.3
Ellis [20], 2010[1]	UK (NCR)	National	2000–2006	Male	SI		Appendix		Colon		Stomach	
			2000–2006	Female	Appendix		SI		Colon		Stomach	
Cho [13], 2012	Pathology reports from 29 university and general hospitals, Korea	National database	2000–2009		Rectum	48	Stomach	14.6	Pancreas	8.7	Colon	7.9

Table 4. Continued
b All NEN

First author and year	Country	Type of registry	Years	Comment	Site 1	% of all NENS	Site 2	% of all NENS	Site 3	% of all NENS	Site 4	% of all NENS
Caldarella [34], 2011	Tuscan Cancer Registry, Italy	Regional	1985–2005		Lung	25.6	SI	23.5	Appendix	10.9	Colon	10.3
Hauso [21], 2008	Norway (NCR)	National	1993–2004		SI	26	BP	21	Colon	8	Rectum	7
	USA (SEER)	National	1993–2004	White	Lung	31.9	SI	17.7	Rectum	12.3	Colon	7.4
	USA (SEER)	National	1993–2004	Black	Rectum	27	SI	21	Lung	18.3	Colon	7.9
Hemminki [31], 2001	Swedish family cancer database	National	1983–1998	Male	SI	44.5	Appendix	16.3	Colon	9.4	Lung	8.2
		National	1983–1998	Female	Appendix	27.9	SI	26.9	Colon	13.4	Lung	9.6
Quaedvlieg [32], 2001	The Netherlands Cancer Registry (NCR)	National	1989–1996		Appendix		Lung		SI		Colorectum	
Yao [29], 2008	USA (SEER)	National	2000–2004	White	Lung		Rectum		SI		Stomach	
		National	2000–2004	Black	Rectum	27	SI	22	Lung	18	Colon	8
Tsai [24], 2013	Taiwan Cancer Registry	National	1996–2008		Rectum	25.4	Lung	20	Stomach	7.4	Pancreas	6
Levi [33], 2000	Vaud, Switzerland	Regional	1974–1997		Colorectum		SI		Lung		Stomach	
Luke [30], 2010	South Australia Cancer Registry	Regional	1980–2006		Lung	26	Colon including appendix	23	SI	20.6	UKP	15

NCR = National cancer registry; SCLC = small cell lung carcinoma; UKP = unknown primary.
[1] Pancreas was not included.

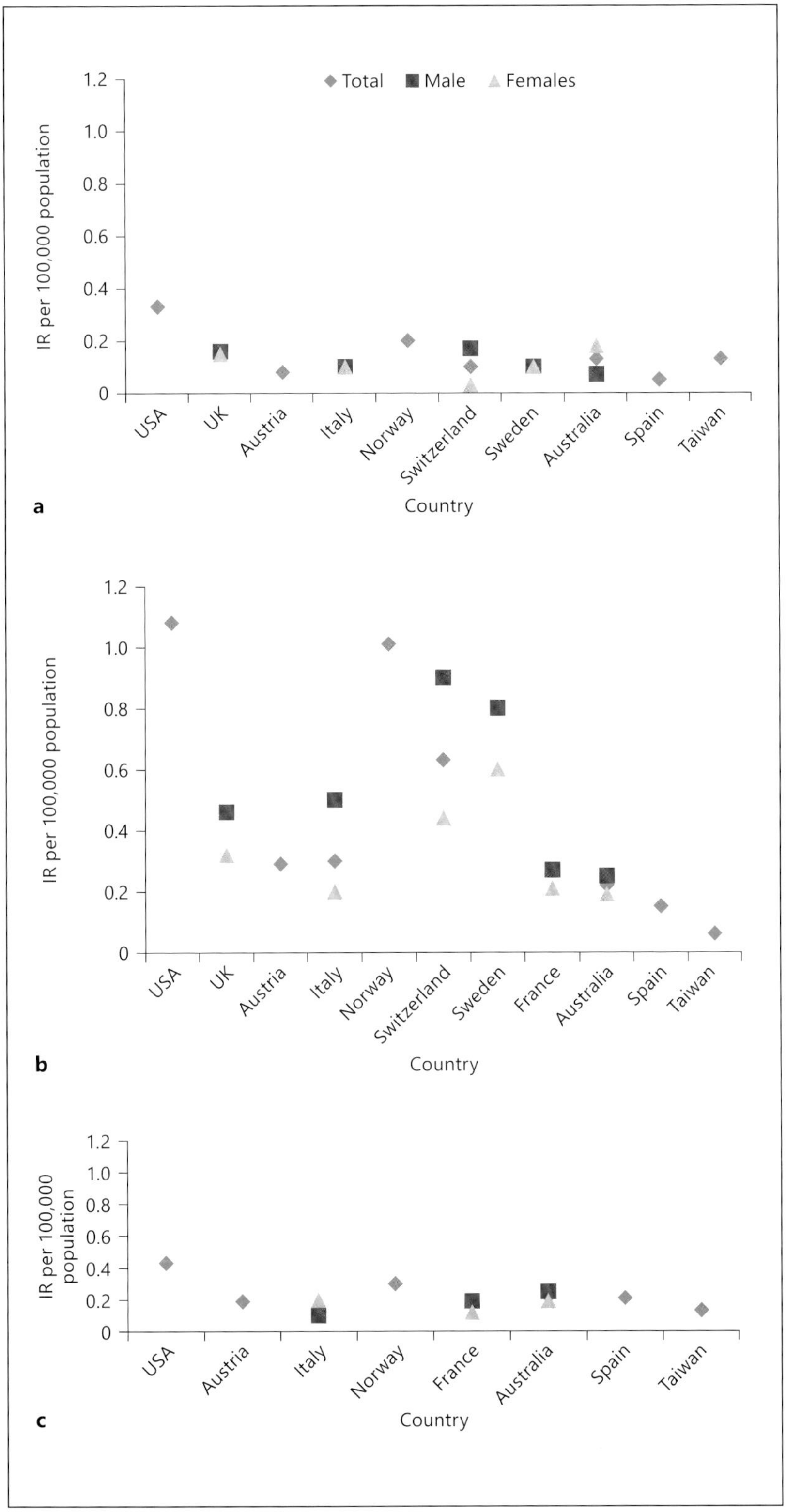

1

(*For figure 1d–f and legend see next page.*)

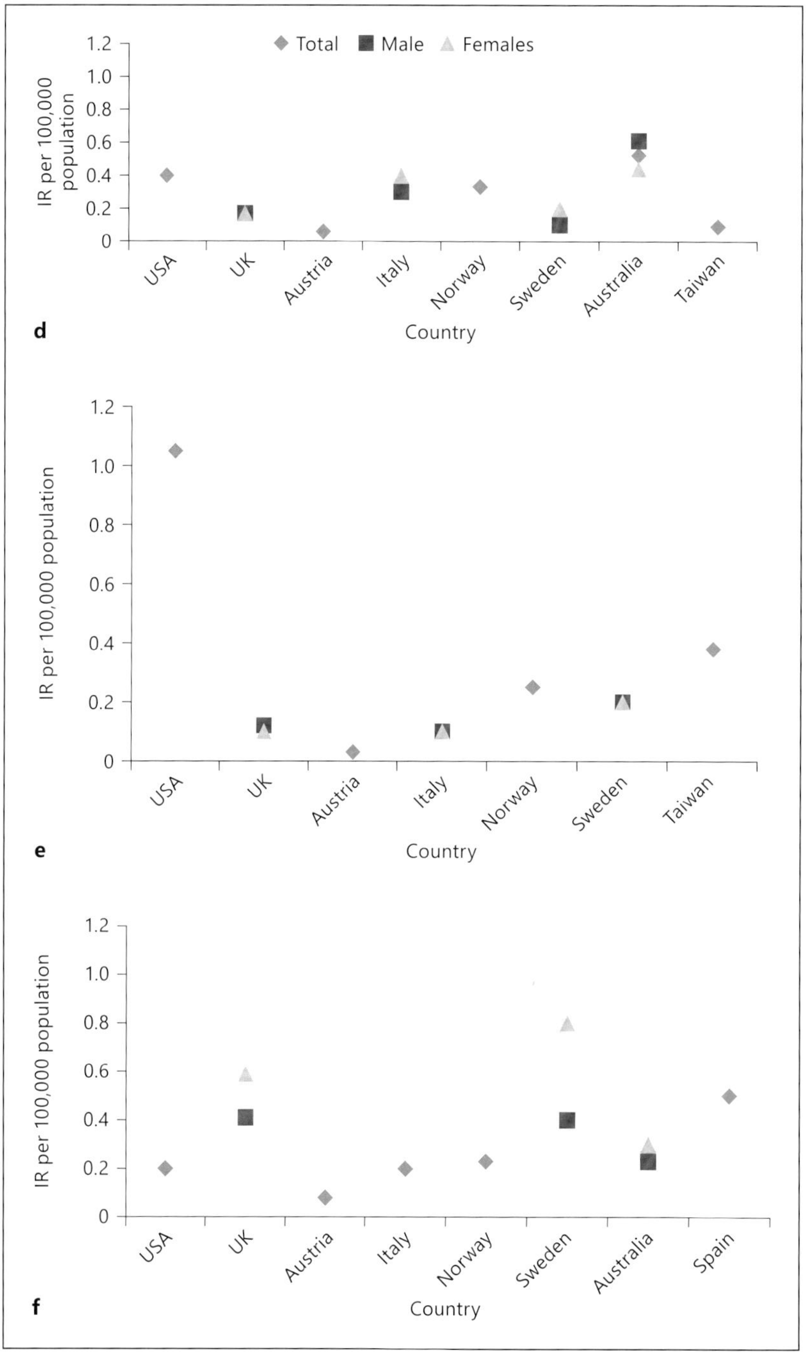

Fig. 1. Most recent IR in various countries for six types of NET: gastric (**a**), SI (**b**), pancreatic (**c**), colon (**d**), rectal (**e**) and appendiceal (**f**). Data for the various countries are from the following time periods: USA, 2003–2007 [19]; UK, 2000–2006 [20]; Austria, 2004–2005 [15]; Italy (Tuscany), 1985–2005 [34]; Norway, 2000–2004 [21]; Switzerland (Vaud), 1986–1997 [33]; Sweden, 1983–1998 [31]; France (Burgundy), 1976–1999 [35]; Australia (South Australia), 2000–2006 [30]; Taiwan, 2008 [24]; Spain (Girona), 1994–2004 [36].

There are no consistent gender differences in IR of GNENs [14, 16, 29–31, 33, 34, 49]. In the USA, the IR of GNENs is highest in the black population [27, 29, 47]. The mean age at presentation for GNENs in Europe and the USA is 60–67 years [16, 29, 31, 37, 49]. Most patients with GNEN present with local disease [14, 29, 46, 47]. In the USA, the 5-year survival of GNEN improved with time between 1973 and 2007 to reach a rate of 64%, while, according to other reports from the same SEER database, higher 5-year survival rates of 75–82% were recorded over the same time periods [19, 21, 46, 47, 49]. This rather low survival rate may reflect the inclusion of a larger proportion of malignant versus benign GNEN in the SEER database. Five-year survival rates were reported in other parts of the world; some were national cancer registries: 45% between 1993 and 2004 in Norway, 61% in Spain and 46% in the Taiwan cancer registry (1996–2008), while others were regional: 63.5% in Tuscany, Italy (1985–2005) and 66.4% in South Australia (1980–2006), and 100% in an institutional series from Taiwan (1970–2005) [14, 21, 24, 30, 34, 37]. In a report summarizing the 5-year survival of malignant GNEN from 12 European countries between the years 1985 and 1994, the rate was low at 45.6%, with the best prognosis in northern European countries [50]. The wide variation in 5-year survival rates of patients with GNEN may be due to geographic changes in the classification, diagnosis and management of these tumors.

Small Intestine

In some parts of Europe and in the USA, SI NENs were the most common among GEP NEN for some time, comprising 39% of malignant GEP NENs in the UK between 2000 and 2006, and 18.6% of all NENs in the pan SEER registry between 1973 and 2007 (table 4) [19, 20, 27]. This was the most common site in some series covering all NEN, such as the NRC from Norway and the Swedish family database [21, 31]. In the Netherlands, Switzerland and Germany SI NENs were the second most common GEP NENs [9, 32, 33]. Interestingly, in eastern Asia, SI NEN are relatively rare compared to western countries [7, 12, 13, 17, 18, 24, 37]. Similarly, SI NEN were only the third most common site for NEN in a registry from South Australia [30]. Among the different locations of SI NEN, the ileum is the most common site.

Annual age-adjusted IR of SI NEN are available from several countries in Europe [15, 20, 21, 31, 33–36, 51], Australia [30] and Taiwan [24], and have been published multiple times from the US SEER database [19, 26, 27, 29, 46, 49, 52], encompassing various periods between the years 1960 and 2008 [for a review see 23]. In Europe and the USA, IR of SI NEN are among the highest compared to other GEP NEN. In contrast to this, in eastern Asia, including Japan and Taiwan, IR are lower than other GEP NEN [7, 24]. There are large variations in the absolute IR of SI NEN in different parts of the world: in the USA, IR were more than twice as high as those in the UK over the same period (2000–2006): 1.08 in the US SEER database and only 0.46 and 0.32 in males and females in the UK [19, 20]. IR in Norway (2000–2004) were similar to those in the USA

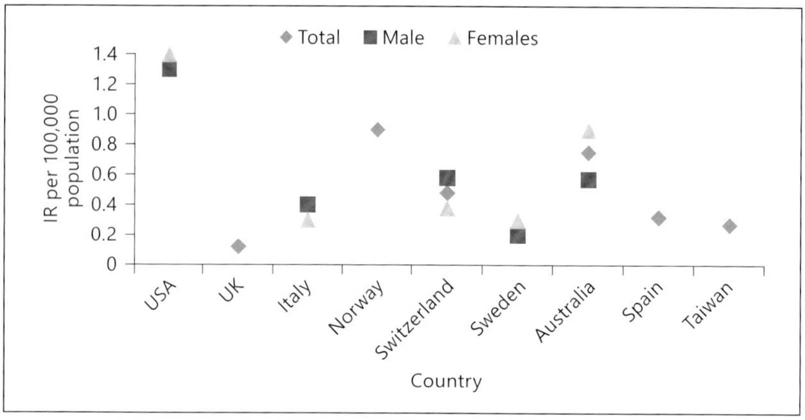

Fig. 2. Most recent IR in various countries for typical and atypical BP NEN. Data for the various countries are from the following time periods: USA, 2000–2004 [29]; UK, 1983–1994 [57]; Italy (Tuscany), 1985–2005 [34]; Norway, 2000–2004 [21]; Switzerland (Vaud), 1986–1997 [33]; Sweden, 1983–1998 [31]; Australia (South Australia), 2000–2006 [30]; Taiwan, 2008 [24]; Spain (Girona), 1994–2004 [36].

at 1.01, with lower IR reported over similar time frames in Austria (0.29) and Australia (0.72), and significantly lower rates reported in Taiwan (0.06) [15, 21, 24, 30] (fig. 2).

As for most other NEN, there is a clear increase in the IR of SI NEN with time: 3.8- and 1.8-fold in men and women, respectively, in the UK between 1971 and 2006, and a nearly 3-fold increase in IR from 1973 to 2007 (0.38 to 1.08, respectively) in the USA [19, 20]. This trend of increase in IR is observed to a more modest extent in many other registries throughout the world [21, 24, 30, 31, 35].

The IR of SI NEN start to rise at the age of 40 years, reaching a peak in the 8th decade of life [19, 20, 31, 32]. The mean age at diagnosis is between 59 and 65 years [9, 29, 31, 37, 46, 49], with most (58–71%) patients presenting with regional or distant spread [15, 27, 29, 52]. In most countries, SI NEN are more common in males [20, 21, 24, 27, 30, 31, 33, 34, 51]. The US SEER database points to major racial differences, with IR that are highest in African Americans compared to whites (both males and females) [21, 27, 29, 52]. Early reports from the 1970s on 5-year survival rates of SI NETs from the ERG and TNCS US databases were as low as 52% [26]. Since then, 5-year survival rates in the USA increased very mildly between 1973 and 2007, in the range of 62–71% [19, 52]. Based on the same SEER population, Tsikitis et al. [49] reported 5-year survival rates of 86.2% as of 2008. Data on 5-year survival rates seem to be lower in Norway, France and Taiwan (59, 56 and 48%, respectively) and higher in Italy, Spain and Australia (72, 89 and 74%, respectively) [14, 21, 24, 30, 34, 51]. In a report by the EUROCARE working group, 5-year survival rates of malignant SI NETs were in the range of 55–64% among 19 centers in 12 European countries, being lowest in eastern European countries [50].

In summary, SI NEN are among the most common GEP NEN in the western world, and are much less common in the Far East. The basis for these geographic changes is probably both due to genetic and environmental factors. Having said that, in all parts of the world there is a gradual rise in the IR of SI NEN, which again raises some questions of whether there is a true rise in the occurrence of these tumors, or if the trend only reflects increased awareness and diagnostic ability.

Pancreas

Data on the epidemiology of pancreatic NEN (PNEN) is limited. PNEN have an IR in several population studies of <1%, and in autopsy series PNEN are found in 0.07–10% of cases [24, 27, 30, 53]. Not uncommonly today, PNEN have become an incidental finding on imaging or surgery done for another indication, in the absence of a functioning endocrine syndrome or local symptoms suggesting this type of tumor [28].

PNEN are classified according to the cell of origin in the pancreatic islet. Functioning tumors secrete hormones that may lead to a clinical syndrome such as gastrinoma, insulinoma and, rarely, VIPoma, somatostatinomas and glucagonomas. Nonfunctioning tumors are more common than functioning ones. Among the functioning PNEN, insulinomas are the most common, followed by gastrinomas. VIPoma and glucagonomas are very rare [53].

The relative frequency of PNEN varies in different types of NET registries (see table 4): in institutional and national registries from Spain, Italy, China and Germany, the pancreas was the most common site among GEP NEN [9, 14, 16, 18], while in France, Girona province in Spain and in a single institution in Seoul, South Korea, and in Mumbai, India, they were the second most common tumor [10, 12, 17, 36]. In Australia, Taiwan and the pan-SEER population database, PNEN were much less common among all NEN or GEP NEN [19, 24, 27, 29, 30].

Absolute IR of PNEN are low in many parts of the world, but have been rising over the last decades. IR from Australia and the SEER database in the 1970s and 1980s were in the range of 0.1–0.2, whereas in more recent years the rates from Europe, Australia and the USA have been higher, peaking at an IR of 0.43 in the SEER 2003–2007 database [15, 19, 21, 29, 30, 34–36, 54]. Much higher IR of PNEN have been reported by a series from Japan (1.27), while much lower IR were reported from Taiwan (0.13) in 2006 [7, 24] (fig. 1). IR of PNEN increased by 1.5- to 3-fold over a range of 1–4 decades in the USA, Australia, Japan and some European countries [7, 19, 21, 29, 30], while in Taiwan they increased about 6-fold within only 1 decade [24]. As alluded to earlier, part of the increase in incidence around the world may be attributed to the rise in diagnosis of incidental PNEN which were not diagnosed in the past when clinically asymptomatic.

IR of PNEN peak between the 6th and 8th decades of life and the median age at presentation is 60 years [9, 16, 29, 32, 54]. Pancreatic NENs are slightly more common in males and in the USA, and they are slightly more common in African Americans compared to whites [21, 29, 30, 35, 54]. The majority of patients with pancreatic NETs

(77–86%) have regional or distant spread at presentation [14, 15, 29, 32, 54]. Patients with MEN1 have a 35–75% chance of developing a clinically manifest PNEN. In MEN1 patients, PNEN occur at a younger age, tend to be multiple and are usually diagnosed at an earlier stage because of periodic screening [55].

When compared with other GEP NEN, PNEN exhibited the lowest 5-year survival in the pan-SEER 1973–2007 period (27–37.6%). Similarly, 5-year survival rates were the lowest for PNEN in Australia and Taiwan [19, 21, 24, 29, 30, 54]. Survival is worse in patients presenting with advanced stage, and better in patients with functioning pancreatic NETs [53]. Higher 5-year survival rates have been reported from other countries and regions in Europe, including Norway, Spain, Burgundy in France and from Tuscany in Italy, in the range of 43–78% [14, 21, 34, 35]. The EUROCARE study group found 5-year survival rates of malignant PNEN to be higher in northern Europe (49%) compared to eastern European countries (8.5%) [50].

Colorectum

Different series have described NEN of the large intestine either separately as colon and rectal NEN, or grouped together as 'colorectal NEN'. To make things more complicated, some registries included appendiceal NEN as part of colon NEN [34]; in this review NEN of the appendix will be discussed separately.

Overall, colorectal NEN IR were reported from Burgundy, France, between 1976 and 1999, with an incidence of 0.19 in men and 0.12 in women, and were much higher in Vaud, Switzerland, from a similar time period (1974–1997): 0.7 in males and 1.74 in females, where they were the most common site of all NEN (table 4; fig. 1) [33, 35]. These gender differences in the IR of colorectal NEN from Vaud can be explained by the fact that this registry included appendiceal NEN as part of the colorectum. Between 1974 and 1997, the incidence remained high without change in Swiss women, but more than doubled in Swiss men, from 0.45 to 0.98. In Japan, the IR of hindgut carcinoid, which includes the colon and rectum, was the highest compared to other GEP NETs, with an IR of 1.26 in the year 2005, and rose to 2.12 in 2010 [7]. The EUROCARE study group reported 5-year survival rates for colorectal NETs from 12 European countries between the years 1975 and 2000 in the range of 49.9–67%, with the lowest rates in eastern and highest in western European countries [50].

Colon (Rectum Excluded)

All parts of the colon may be involved by NEN, from the cecum to the sigmoid, with a predominance of right-sided tumors. Colon NEN (CNEN) are the third most common NEN in Sweden, the UK and Norway, comprising 8–13.4% of all NEN [20, 21, 31], and are even less common in other parts of the world (table 3).

As early as the 1970s, IR in the UK were 0.04 and 0.05 in females and males, respectively, and in the range of 0.0–0.15 in the pre-SEER databases (lowest in white females and highest in black males) [19, 20, 26, 27, 46]. More recent reports have shown a low incidence of malignant colon NETs, such as the one from Austria between 2004 and 2005 (0.06) and from Taiwan in 2008 (0.09) [15, 24], while in other parts of the world higher IR (up to 0.32) have been reported [21, 30, 31] (fig. 1). With time, IR of CNEN have increased only mildly (up to a 2.5-fold increase) in the UK, Norway and the USA [19–21, 49]. In Taiwan, absolute IR are low but increased 4-fold from 0.02 in 1996 to 0.09 in 2008 [24]. This increase in incidence of NEN of the colon around the world has been partly attributed to the increased use of screening colonoscopy and other imaging modalities.

Data on gender differences in IR of CNEN are conflicting [9, 14, 27, 31, 33–35, 49]. IR of CNEN in the US SEER database are higher in African Americans compared to whites [21, 26, 27, 29, 49]. The mean age at presentation with CNEN is 63–68 years in the USA, and even younger, between 54–61 years, in European series and in a series from Taiwan [24, 29, 31, 32, 49], with most patients (53–86%) presenting with either regional or distant spread [14, 26, 29, 46, 49].

The 5-year survival rates of CNEN in Europe have been reported over different time periods and range as low as 36% between 1976 and 1999 in Burgundy, France, 41% in Norway between 1993 and 2004, and as high as 65% in Spain between 2001 and 2008 [14, 21, 35, 50], and 60–67% in the pan SEER database (1973–2007) [19, 49]. Outside of Europe and the USA, 5-year survival rates were reported to be 64% in Australia (1980–2006) and only 48% in Taiwan (1996–2008) [24, 30].

Rectum

Rectal NEN (RNEN) are the most common GEP NEN in several parts of the world, and in some countries or ethnic groups these are the most common of all NEN, comprising 18–27% of all NEN (including the BP tree; table 4) [19, 21, 24, 29]. In the US SEER database RNEN have gradually become the second most common site for all NEN as of the years 2000–2007, and in black Americans they are the most common site [19, 21, 29]. In the Far East, reports from Taiwan, Korea and Japan show that RNEN are the most common of all NEN/GEP NEN [7, 13, 17, 24, 37]. In Europe, rectal NENs are much less common within all NEN/GEP NEN, in the range of 5.8–9% [14, 20, 21].

Early reports on the IR of RNEN were as low as 0.01 in the UK between 1970 and 1989, but higher in other European countries when reported from the mid-1980s on (0.1–0.22) [20, 21, 31, 34]. The IR of malignant rectal NENs in Austria between 2004 and 2005 was 0.08 [15]. In the USA, IR from the 1970s, as reported several times, were in the range of 0.09–0.4. With time, the IR of RNEN has been rising more than 10-fold in the UK and in the USA (1973–2007) [19, 20, 29, 49]. IR have also increased, albeit less dramatically, in other parts of the world [7, 21, 24, 30]. The dramatic increase in

IR of RNEN is partially attributed to higher rates of colonoscopy and sigmoidoscopy in more recent years (fig. 1).

Having said that, despite a similar fold increase in IR of RNEN in the US SEER database and in the UK, absolute IR over similar time periods are about 10 times as high in the US SEER database compared to the UK (US SEER 2003–2007: 1.05; UK 2000–2006: 0.12 in males and 0.1 in females), and are even higher in Japan where the incidence of all hindgut NEN was 2.12 as of 2010 [7, 19, 20]. These differences in the IR of RNEN between different countries and ethnic groups point to both genetic and environmental factors that influence the development of these tumors.

RNEN are diagnosed at a mean age of 52–57 years, and most patients present with local disease [9, 14, 26, 27, 29, 31, 37, 46]. In some countries and populations, the IR of RNEN is higher in males compared to females [14, 21, 24, 29]. In the USA, the IR of RNEN is much higher in the male and female black population compared to whites [21, 29]. Five-year survival rates of RNEN are very good, reaching over 90% in the US SEER database and 80–86% in Taiwan, with lower 5-year survival rates in Norway and Spain of 74 and 64%, respectively [14, 19, 21, 24, 27, 46, 49].

Appendix

Appendiceal NEN (ANEN) is most commonly an incidental finding on appendectomy performed for acute appendicitis. When trying to draw the picture of the epidemiology of ANEN one faces several issues. These include that the reporting of ANEN varied with time in different countries between only malignant or all ANEN, in some registries ANEN of the appendix were included as part of all 'large bowel' NEN, and goblet cell tumor of the appendix was inconsistently included as a NEN in different registries.

ANEN are considered one of the least common among several national cancer registries (table 3): 3.44–4.88% of all NEN in the SEER database (1973–2007), Norway (1993–2004), Taiwan and in other countries in the Far East [13, 17, 19, 21, 24, 27, 29, 37, 49]. In some European countries the relative frequency of ANEN is among the highest; in the UK it is as high as 38% of all gastrointestinal NEN (2000–2006) and about 38% of all GEP NEN in Girona, Spain (1994–2004) [20, 36] (table 4). Part of these differences in the frequency of ANEN around the world are explained again by differences in classification (benign vs. malignant) and registration policy.

IR of ANEN from Europe were as low as 0.03 in the UK in the early 1970s, with higher rates up to 0.4 occurring later on in Tuscany, Italy, Norway, Australia and Sweden [20, 21, 30, 31, 34]. IR of only malignant ANEN from Austria (2004–2005) were as low as 0.08. In the USA, between 1969 and 1971, TNCS IR were 0.79 in white females, while the early SEER database reported lower IR between 0.07 and 0.15. These differences are explained by the registration of only malignant ANEN by the SEER registry [19, 26, 27].

The IR of ANEN have increased in many parts of the world (fig. 1). The most dramatic increase has been observed in the UK, with a 10-fold increase in females and 11-fold increase in males. Such an increase is only partially explained by the inclusion of benign tumors in cancer registration in recent years, since there was also a 5-fold increase in the rates of malignant ANEN in the UK in this time period [20]. Milder increases in IR were also observed in Australia, Sweden and Norway [21, 30, 31]. In the USA, there was an early decrease and then a stabilization of IR, attributed to differences in the registration of all versus only malignant ANEN [19, 26, 27, 29, 49].

ANEN present at a younger age compared to other NEN, ranging between 31 and 49 years of age in different series, and with a very low rate of regional or distant metastasis [9, 16, 27, 29, 31, 32, 49]. The IR of ANEN is about twice as high in females compared to males in Europe and in the USA [14, 20, 27, 29, 32], an event partially explained by the higher rates of appendectomies and gynecological procedures in females. In the USA, no consistent racial differences between blacks and whites have been shown [29].

The 5-year survival rates of ANEN are better than most other NEN/GEP NEN. In Europe, Australia and Taiwan, 5-year survival rates in the range of 74–95% have been reported [14, 24, 30, 32]. In Norway, the inclusion of goblet cell tumors as ANEN lowered 5-year survival rates significantly [21]. The 5-year survival rates between 1973 and 2008 in the US SEER database were as high as 90% according to one report, but only 81% by another [19, 49]. Higher survival rates were reported in series from the 1970s when benign tumors comprised the majority of NEN at this site [26, 27]. The good prognosis of ANEN is mainly explained by the incidental discovery and early curative surgery performed for these tumors.

Bronchopulmonary Tree

For many years, NEN of the BP tree were classified into 4 subtypes: low-grade typical carcinoid tumor (TC), intermediate-grade atypical carcinoid tumor (AC), and 2 high-grade malignancies: large cell neuroendocrine carcinoma and small cell lung carcinoma [5]. Recently, a grading system based on the Ki-67 index for BP NEN, similar to GEP NEN, has been introduced, but has not yet been officially accepted [6]. BP NEN were not included in all NET registries; furthermore, some registries documented the occurrence of all 4 subtypes of BP NEN, while others included only low-grade TC and AC. In the last 2 decades, BP NEN have emerged as the most common type of NEN in many but not all parts of the world, as reflected both by national, regional and institutional registries (table 4), and comprise as high as 25–31% of all NEN [8, 21, 26, 27, 29, 30, 32–34, 36, 56].

IR of BP NEN vary around the world, with the lowest IR reported from Italy, Sweden and the UK (0.12–0.2) during the 1980s, and higher rates during the same time periods in Switzerland, Australia and the USA (0.37–0.48) [21, 30, 31, 33, 34, 57]. In registries reporting serial IR with time, there is a clear increase in IR of BP NEN [21, 24, 27, 29, 33, 58], which was most dramatic in the USA, rising from 0.32 in males in the years 1973–1991 to a rate of 1.3 (black and white) between the years 2000 and 2004. The highest rates of BP NEN were reported by the SEER database in females (1.49 between 2000 and 2004), making them the most common NEN (fig. 2) [29]. Whether this dramatic rise in IR is a true biologic phenomenon or reflects increased use of bronchoscopy and other anatomic imaging techniques of the chest is an unsolved question.

When reporting only the low-grade tumors (TC and AC), these tumors are revealed to be more common in females in some parts of the world, including the USA, Sweden and Australia [26, 29–31]. In the USA, IR in blacks are lower than in whites of both genders [21, 29]. The mean age at presentation according to most registries is in the 6th to 7th decade of life (1 decade earlier than non-NEN lung cancer) [5, 26, 31, 36, 56]. Five-year survival rates from BP NEN vary according to aggressiveness, being worst for large and small cell lung carcinoma, much better for AC and the highest for TC [36, 56, 58]. Relative 5-year survival for TC and AC vary around the world from 70 to 90% [26, 30, 32–34, 36, 56, 57]. As is true for other NEN, there is a clear trend for a worse prognosis when the disease is at a more advanced stage (i.e. distant spread compared to localized disease) [26, 27, 29, 32]. The 5-year survival rates decrease with age [24, 57], is worse in males compared to females [24, 33, 34, 57] and in blacks compared to whites [21]. In countries reporting 5-year survival rates for sequential time periods, there is a trend for better prognosis with time in some [30, 33], but not in others [27], an improvement that may be partially explained by the incidental diagnosis of small, low-grade tumors.

References

1 Modlin IM, Oberg K, Chung DC, Jensen RT, de Herder WW, Thakker RV, Caplin M, Delle Fave G, Kaltsas GA, Krenning EP, Moss SF, Nilsson O, Rindi G, Salazar R, Ruszniewski P, Sundin A: Gastroenteropancreatic neuroendocrine tumours. Lancet Oncol 2008;9:61–72.

2 Klöppel G, Perren A, Heitz PU: The gastroenteropancreatic neuroendocrine cell system and its tumors: the WHO classification. Ann NY Acad Sci 2004;1014:13–27.

3 Klimstra DS, Modlin IR, Adsay NV, Chetty R, Deshpande V, Gonen M, Jensen RT, Kidd M, Kulke MH, Lloyd RV, Moran C, Moss SF, Oberg K, O'Toole D, Rindi G, Robert ME, Suster S, Tang LH, Tzen CY, Washington MK, Wiedenmann B, Yao J: Pathology reporting of neuroendocrine tumors: application of the Delphic consensus process to the development of a minimum pathology data set. Am J Surg Pathol 2010;34:300–313.

4 Klimstra DS, Modlin IR, Coppola D, Lloyd RV, Suster S: The pathologic classification of neuroendocrine tumors: a review of nomenclature, grading, and staging systems. Pancreas 2010;39:707–712.

5 Gustafsson BI, Kidd M, Chan A, Malfertheiner MV, Modlin IM: Bronchopulmonary neuroendocrine tumors. Cancer 2008;113:5–21.

6 Rindi G, Klersy C, Inzani F, Fellegara G, Ampollini L, Ardizzoni A, Campanini N, Carbognani P, De Pas TM, Galetta D, Granone PL, Righi L, Rusca M, Spaggiari L, Tiseo M, Viale G, Volante M, Papotti M, Pelosi G: Grading the neuroendocrine tumors of the lung: an evidence-based proposal. Endocr Relat Cancer 2014;21:1–16.
7 Ito T, Igarashi H, Nakamura K, Sasano H, Okusaka T, Takano K, Komoto I, Tanaka M, Imamura M, Jensen RT, Takayanagi R, Shimatsu A: Epidemiological trends of pancreatic and gastrointestinal neuroendocrine tumors in Japan: a nationwide survey analysis. J Gastroenterol 2015;50:58–64.
8 Younes RN: Neuroendocrine tumors: a registry of 1,000 patients. Rev Assoc Med Bras 2008;54:305–307.
9 Ploeckinger U, Kloeppel G, Wiedenmann B, Lohmann R: The German NET-Registry: an audit on the diagnosis and therapy of neuroendocrine tumors. Neuroendocrinology 2009;90:349–363.
10 Lombard-Bohas C, Mitry E, O'Toole D, Louvet C, Pillon D, Cadiot G, Borson-Chazot F, Aparicio T, Ducreux M, Lecomte T, Etienne PL, Cacheux W, Legoux JL, Seitz JF, Ruszniewski P, Chayvialle JA, Rougier P: Thirteen-month registration of patients with gastroenteropancreatic endocrine tumours in France. Neuroendocrinology 2009;89:217–222.
11 Malik L, Chua YJ, Butt NS, Yip D: Single institutional series of neuroendocrine tumors managed in the Australian Capital Territory. Asia Pac J Clin Oncol 2013, Epub ahead of print.
12 Amarapurkar DN, Juneja MP, Patel ND, Amarapurkar AD, Amarapurkar PD: A retrospective clinicopathological analysis of neuroendocrine tumors of the gastrointestinal tract. Trop Gastroenterol 2010;31:101–104.
13 Cho MY, Kim JM, Sohn JH, Kim MJ, Kim KM, Kim WH, Kim H, Kook MC, Park do Y, Lee JH, Chang H, Jung ES, Kim HK, Jin SY, Choi JH, Gu MJ, Kim S, Kang MS, Cho CH, Park MI, Kang YK, Kim YW, Yoon SO, Bae HI, Joo M, Moon WS, Kang DY, Chang SJ: Current trends of the incidence and pathological diagnosis of gastroenteropancreatic neuroendocrine tumors (GEP-NETs) in Korea 2000–2009: multicenter study. Cancer Res Treat 2012;44:157–165.
14 Garcia-Carbonero R, Capdevila J, Crespo-Herrero G, Diaz-Perez JA, Martinez Del Prado MP, Alonso Orduna V, Sevilla-Garcia I, Villabona-Artero C, Beguiristain-Gomez A, Llanos-Munoz M, Marazuela M, Alvarez-Escola C, Castellano D, Vilar E, Jimenez-Fonseca P, Teule A, Sastre-Valera J, Benavent-Vinuelas M, Monleon A, Salazar R: Incidence, patterns of care and prognostic factors for outcome of gastroenteropancreatic neuroendocrine tumors (GEP-NETs): results from the National Cancer Registry of Spain (RGETNE). Ann Oncol 2010;21:1794–1803.
15 Niederle MB, Hackl M, Kaserer K, Niederle B: Gastroenteropancreatic neuroendocrine tumours: the current incidence and staging based on the WHO and European Neuroendocrine Tumour Society classification: an analysis based on prospectively collected parameters. Endocr Relat Cancer 2010;17:909–918.
16 Faggiano A, Ferolla P, Grimaldi F, Campana D, Manzoni M, Davi MV, Bianchi A, Valcavi R, Papini E, Giuffrida D, Ferone D, Fanciulli G, Arnaldi G, Franchi GM, Francia G, Fasola G, Crino L, Pontecorvi A, Tomassetti P, Colao A: Natural history of gastro-entero-pancreatic and thoracic neuroendocrine tumors: data from a large prospective and retrospective Italian epidemiological study: the NET Management Study. J Endocrinol Invest 2012;35:817–823.
17 Lim T, Lee J, Kim JJ, Lee JK, Lee KT, Kim YH, Kim KW, Kim S, Sohn TS, Choi DW, Choi SH, Chun HK, Lee WY, Kim KM, Jang KT, Park YS: Gastroenteropancreatic neuroendocrine tumors: incidence and treatment outcome in a single institution in Korea. Asia Pac J Clin Oncol 2011;7:293–299.
18 Wang YH, Lin Y, Xue L, Wang JH, Chen MH, Chen J: Relationship between clinical characteristics and survival of gastroenteropancreatic neuroendocrine neoplasms: a single-institution analysis (1995–2012) in South China. BMC Endocr Disord 2012;12:30.
19 Lawrence B, Gustafsson BI, Chan A, Svejda B, Kidd M, Modlin IM: The epidemiology of gastroenteropancreatic neuroendocrine tumors. Endocrinol Metab Clin North Am 2011;40:1–18.
20 Ellis L, Shale MJ, Coleman MP: Carcinoid tumors of the gastrointestinal tract: trends in incidence in England since 1971. Am J Gastroenterol 2010;105:2563–2569.
21 Hauso O, Gustafsson BI, Kidd M, Waldum HL, Drozdov I, Chan AK, Modlin IM: Neuroendocrine tumor epidemiology: contrasting Norway and North America. Cancer 2008;113:2655–2664.
22 Fraenkel M, Kim MK, Faggiano A, Valk GD: Epidemiology of gastroenteropancreatic neuroendocrine tumours. Best Pract Res Clin Gastroenterol 2012;26:691–703.
23 Fraenkel M, Kim M, Faggiano A, de Herder WW, Valk GD: Incidence of gastroenteropancreatic neuroendocrine tumours: a systematic review of the literature. Endocr Relat Cancer 2014;21:R153–R163.
24 Tsai H-J, Wu C-C, Tsai C-R, Lin S-F, Chen L-T, Chang JS: The epidemiology of neuroendocrine tumors in Taiwan: a nation-wide cancer registry-based study. PLoS One 2013;8:e62487.
25 Berge T, Linell F: Carcinoid tumours: frequency in a defined population during a 12-year period. Acta Pathol Microbiol Scand A 1976;84:322–330.
26 Godwin JD 2nd: Carcinoid tumors: an analysis of 2,837 cases. Cancer 1975;36:560–569.

27 Modlin IM, Lye KD, Kidd M: A 5-decade analysis of 13,715 carcinoid tumors. Cancer 2003;97:934–959.

28 Zarate X, Williams N, Herrera MF: Pancreatic incidentalomas. Best Pract Res Clin Endocrinol Metab 2012;26:97–103.

29 Yao JC, Hassan M, Phan A, Dagohoy C, Leary C, Mares JE, Abdalla EK, Fleming JB, Vauthey JN, Rashid A, Evans DB: One hundred years after 'carcinoid': epidemiology of and prognostic factors for neuroendocrine tumors in 35,825 cases in the United States. J Clin Oncol 2008;26:3063–3072.

30 Luke C, Price T, Townsend A, Karapetis C, Kotasek D, Singhal N, Tracey E, Roder D: Epidemiology of neuroendocrine cancers in an Australian population. Cancer Causes Control 2010;21:931–938.

31 Hemminki K, Li X: Incidence trends and risk factors of carcinoid tumors: a nationwide epidemiologic study from Sweden. Cancer 2001;92:2204–2210.

32 Quaedvlieg PF, Visser O, Lamers CB, Janssen-Heijen ML, Taal BG: Epidemiology and survival in patients with carcinoid disease in The Netherlands: an epidemiological study with 2,391 patients. Ann Oncol 2001;12:1295–1300.

33 Levi F, Te VC, Randimbison L, Rindi G, La Vecchia C: Epidemiology of carcinoid neoplasms in Vaud, Switzerland, 1974–97. Br J Cancer 2000;83:952–955.

34 Caldarella A, Crocetti E, Paci E: Distribution, incidence, and prognosis in neuroendocrine tumors: a population based study from a cancer registry. Pathol Oncol Res 2011;17:759–763.

35 Lepage C, Bouvier AM, Phelip JM, Hatem C, Vernet C, Faivre J: Incidence and management of malignant digestive endocrine tumours in a well defined French population. Gut 2004;53:549–553.

36 Alsina M, Marcos-Gragera R, Capdevila J, Buxo M, Ortiz RM, Barretina P, Vilardell L, Brunet J, Beltran M, Izquierdo A: Neuroendocrine tumors: a population-based study of incidence and survival in Girona province, 1994–2004. Cancer Epidemiol 2011;35: e49–e54.

37 Li AF, Hsu CY, Li A, Tai LC, Liang WY, Li WY, Tsay SH, Chen JY: A 35-year retrospective study of carcinoid tumors in Taiwan: differences in distribution with a high probability of associated second primary malignancies. Cancer 2008;112:274–283.

38 Habal N, Sims C, Bilchik AJ: Gastrointestinal carcinoid tumors and second primary malignancies. J Surg Oncol 2000;75:310–316.

39 Prommegger R, Ensinger C, Steiner P, Sauper T, Profanter C, Margreiter R: Neuroendocrine tumors and second primary malignancy – a relationship with clinical impact? Anticancer Res 2004;24:1049–1051.

40 Tsai HJ, Wu CC, Tsai CR, Lin SF, Chen LT, Chang JS: Second cancers in patients with neuroendocrine tumors. PLoS One 2013;8:e86414.

41 Amin S, Warner RR, Itzkowitz SH, Kim MK: The risk of metachronous cancers in patients with small-intestinal carcinoid tumors: a US population-based study. Endocr Relat Cancer 2012;19:381–387.

42 Zar N, Garmo H, Holmberg L, Hellman P: Risk of second primary malignancies and causes of death in patients with adenocarcinoma and carcinoid of the small intestine. Eur J Cancer 2008;44:718–725.

43 Kamp K, Damhuis RA, Feelders RA, de Herder WW: Occurrence of second primary malignancies in patients with neuroendocrine tumors of the digestive tract and pancreas. Endocr Relat Cancer 2012;19: 95–99.

44 Cote ML, Wenzlaff AS, Philip PA, Schwartz AG: Secondary cancers after a lung carcinoid primary: a population-based analysis. Lung Cancer 2006;52:273–279.

45 Scherubl H, Cadiot G, Jensen RT, Rosch T, Stolzel U, Klöppel G: Neuroendocrine tumors of the stomach (gastric carcinoids) are on the rise: small tumors, small problems? Endoscopy 2010;42:664–671.

46 Maggard MA, O'Connell JB, Ko CY: Updated population-based review of carcinoid tumors. Ann Surg 2004;240:117–122.

47 Modlin IM, Lye KD, Kidd M: A 50-year analysis of 562 gastric carcinoids: small tumor or larger problem? Am J Gastroenterol 2004;99:23–32.

48 Abraham NS: Proton pump inhibitors: potential adverse effects. Curr Opin Gastroenterol 2012;28:615–620.

49 Tsikitis VL, Wertheim BC, Guerrero MA: Trends of incidence and survival of gastrointestinal neuroendocrine tumors in the United States: a SEER analysis. J Cancer 2012;3:292–302.

50 Lepage C, Ciccolallo L, De Angelis R, Bouvier AM, Faivre J, Gatta G: European disparities in malignant digestive endocrine tumours survival. Int J Cancer 2010;126:2928–2934.

51 Lepage C, Bouvier AM, Manfredi S, Dancourt V, Faivre J: Incidence and management of primary malignant small bowel cancers: a well-defined French population study. Am J Gastroenterol 2006;101: 2826–2832.

52 Modlin IM, Champaneria MC, Chan AK, Kidd M: A three-decade analysis of 3,911 small intestinal neuroendocrine tumors: the rapid pace of no progress. Am J Gastroenterol 2007;102:1464–1473.

53 Halfdanarson TR, Rubin J, Farnell MB, Grant CS, Petersen GM: Pancreatic endocrine neoplasms: epidemiology and prognosis of pancreatic endocrine tumors. Endocr Relat Cancer 2008;15:409–427.

54 Halfdanarson TR, Rabe KG, Rubin J, Petersen GM: Pancreatic neuroendocrine tumors (PNETs): incidence, prognosis and recent trend toward improved survival. Ann Oncol 2008;19:1727–1733.

55 Thakker RV, Newey PJ, Walls GV, Bilezikian J, Dralle H, Ebeling PR, Melmed S, Sakurai A, Tonelli F, Brandi ML: Clinical practice guidelines for multiple endocrine neoplasia type 1 (MEN1). J Clin Endocrinol Metab 2012;97:2990–3011.
56 Skuladottir H, Hirsch FR, Hansen HH, Olsen JH: Pulmonary neuroendocrine tumors: incidence and prognosis of histological subtypes: a population-based study in Denmark. Lung Cancer 2002;37:127–135.
57 Gatta G, Ciccolallo L, Kunkler I, Capocaccia R, Berrino F, Coleman MP, De Angelis R, Faivre J, Lutz JM, Martinez C, Moller T, Sankila R: Survival from rare cancer in adults: a population-based study. Lancet Oncol 2006;7:132–140.
58 Naalsund A, Rostad H, Strom EH, Lund MB, Strand TE: Carcinoid lung tumors – incidence, treatment and outcomes: a population-based study. Eur J Cardiothorac Surg 2011;39:565–569.

Merav Fraenkel, MD
Endocrinology Unit, Soroka University Medical Center and the Faculty of Health Sciences
Ben-Gurion, University of the Negev
Beer Sheva (Israel)
E-Mail meravfr@bgu.ac.il

Papotti M, de Herder WW (eds): Neuroendocrine Tumors: A Multidisciplinary Approach.
Front Horm Res. Basel, Karger, 2015, vol 44, pp 24–39 (DOI: 10.1159/000381981)

Biochemical Testing in Patients with Neuroendocrine Tumors

Dan Granberg

Department of Medical Sciences, Uppsala University, Uppsala, Sweden

Abstract

Neuroendocrine tumors are usually slow-growing tumors. Many of these are capable of secreting peptide hormones or biogenic amines that may lead to endocrine syndromes. Nonfunctioning tumors can either secrete no hormones at all, or secrete hormones not giving rise to endocrine symptoms, such as chromogranin A, chromogranin B or pancreatic polypeptide. Chromogranin A is produced by the majority of endocrine tumors, both functioning and nonfunctioning, and is the best available marker for diagnosis, follow-up and treatment monitoring of patients with differentiated neuroendocrine tumors. Examples of endocrine syndromes are classical carcinoid syndrome caused by serotonin (measured in the urine as its metabolite 5-HIAA), insulinoma syndrome caused by insulin or proinsulin, Zollinger-Ellison syndrome resulting from gastrin secretion, glucagonoma syndrome caused by glucagon, WDHA syndrome caused by vasoactive intestinal peptide, or Cushing's syndrome resulting from ectopic production of adrenocorticotropic hormone or corticotropin-releasing hormone. In case there is uncertainty about the diagnosis, specific tests can be applied, such as the secretin test for diagnosis of gastrinomas and the 72-hour fast for diagnosis of an insulinoma. In patients with suspicion of an inherited syndrome, such as multiple endocrine neoplasia (MEN) 1 and MEN2 syndromes, genetic testing is indicated.

Neuroendocrine tumors may arise in the whole gastrointestinal tract, lungs, thymus, paraganglia, adrenal medulla or parafollicular cells (C cells) in the thyroid gland. They were previously divided into foregut (lungs, thymus, stomach, duodenum, endocrine pancreas), midgut (small bowel and proximal large bowel) and hindgut (distal large bowel and rectum) tumors according to their embryological origin. Nowadays, a new classification has been introduced, grading the tumors into

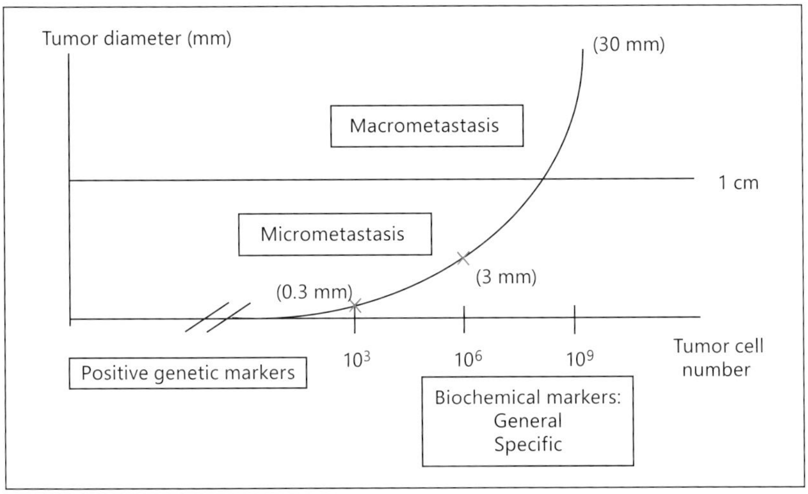

Fig. 1. The detection of tumors in relation to size and cellular number. Modified after Vinik et al. [4].

grade 1 through 3 neuroendocrine tumors (generally well differentiated) and neuroendocrine carcinomas (generally poorly differentiated), according to their mitotic count and proliferative rate (Ki-67) [1, 2]. In addition, the functional activity is included in the classification. Most neuroendocrine tumors are able to produce peptide hormones or biogenic amines leading to various endocrine syndromes. Examples are serotonin, causing classical carcinoid syndrome (diarrhea, flushing, bronchoconstriction and right-sided heart affection with valve fibrosis), tachykinins (neuropeptide K and substance P) also involved in carcinoid syndrome, histamine causing an atypical carcinoid syndrome (flushing, generalized swelling, edema, bronchoconstriction, lacrimation and diarrhea), glucagon leading to glucagonoma syndrome (necrolytic migratory erythema, diabetes mellitus or impaired glucose tolerance, muscle wasting, weight loss and elevated erythrocyte sedimentation rate), insulin or proinsulin causing insulinoma syndrome (hypoglycemia on fasting and exercise leading to adrenergic or neuroglycopenic symptoms), gastrin leading to Zollinger-Ellison syndrome (multiple gastric and duodenal ulcers, esophagitis and diarrhea), vasoactive intestinal peptide (VIP) causing Verner-Morrison or WDHA syndrome (watery diarrhea, hypokalemia and achlorhydria), adrenocorticotropic hormone (ACTH) leading to an ectopic Cushing's syndrome, calcitonin causing flushing or diarrhea, and the catecholamines epinephrine and norepinephrine leading to hypertension, tachycardia, headache, pallor, sweating and anxiety. In many patients, liver metastases are necessary before hormonal symptoms occur, but other patients may have small tumors and endocrine syndrome is the first symptom, leading to diagnosis of the tumor (fig. 1). Apart from hormones causing endocrine symptoms, neuroendocrine tumors may also secrete peptides not giving rise to hormonal symptoms, such as the chromogranins A and B, pancreatic polypeptide

(PP), neuron-specific enolase (NSE) and human chorionic gonadotropin (HCG) subunits alpha and beta. Tumors secreting only these latter hormones are called nonfunctioning tumors. Both functional and nonfunctional hormones may be used for diagnosis and treatment monitoring. In addition to plain measurement of the secreted hormones, various tests are available, such as the secretin test, 72-hour fast and the meal stimulation test.

General Markers

Chromogranin A

Human chromogranin A is a 439-amino acid, approximately 50-kDa acid glycoprotein, found throughout the neuroendocrine system and stored in the dense core vesicles containing peptide hormones or catecholamines. It belongs to the granin family of proteins, which also include chromogranin B and chromogranin C (sometimes called secretogranin II). Chromogranin A is cosecreted with the other peptides or amines stored in the same vesicles. The chromogranin A molecule contains 10 potential sites where it may be cleaved by proteases into biologically active fragments, such as pancreastatin, vasostatin and chromostatin. Chromogranin A may be used both as an immunohistochemical marker and for plasma measurements. Plasma chromogranin A is elevated in a variety of patients with neuroendocrine tumors, both functioning and nonfunctioning, including small and large bowel neuroendocrine tumors, gastric and duodenal carcinoids, pancreatic endocrine tumors, lung and thymic carcinoids, pheochromocytomas and paragangliomas, and medullary thyroid carcinomas (MTCs). The highest levels are found in patients with metastatic midgut carcinoids and endocrine pancreatic tumors. It is the best available marker for diagnosis, follow-up and treatment monitoring of patients with differentiated neuroendocrine tumors. There are several commercially available assays for measurement of chromogranin A, including radioimmunoassays and ELISA (enzyme-linked immunosorbent assays), using monoclonal or polyclonal antibodies [3, 4]. The most sensitive kits measure the whole chromogranin A molecule and not specified cleavage parts, such as pancreastatin [3–5]. Plasma measurements of chromogranins are more useful than measurements in urine [5]. The sensitivity of plasma chromogranin A varies between 60 and 100%, and the specificity between 70 and 100%, depending on the tumor type, amount of tumor, cut-off value and which assay is used [3, 4]. Chromogranin A has been found to be more sensitive than NSE [6, 7], and HCG alpha subunit [7]. The level correlates to tumor burden [6]. Chromogranin A may have a prognostic implication in patients with midgut tumors [8]. Plasma chromogranin A is also useful for the detection of early recurrences of small bowel carcinoids [9]. False positive elevation of chromogranin A can be found in patients with impaired renal function, chronic atrophic gastritis type A, chronic liver disease, inflammatory bowel disease, untreated hypertension, and in patients treated with proton pump inhibitors such as omeprazole [3]. Chromogranin A in plasma has a high spontaneous day-to-day variation, both in patients with neuroendocrine tumors and in healthy subjects [10]. Repeated measurements are thus necessary when used for treatment monitoring, and slight elevations should be interpreted with caution.

Chromogranin B

Chromogranin B is a 70-kDa acidic glycoprotein, containing 657 amino acids. Chromogranin B is present in the secretory granules of neuroendocrine cells, usually costored together with chromogranin A. The plasma level of chromogranin B is not affected by impaired renal function, chronic atrophic gastritis type A or treatment with proton pump inhibitors. Hence, chromogranin B in plasma may serve as a marker for neuroendocrine tumors, complementary to chromogranin A [11]. However, today there is no existing commercially available kit for the measurement of chromogranin B.

Pancreastatin

Pancreastatin is a cleavage product from chromogranin A, consisting of 49 amino acids. It has biological activity, inhibiting the release of parathyroid hormone and chromogranin A, as well as the glucose-induced secretion of insulin. Elevated plasma or serum levels of pancreastatin are found in many patients with neuroendocrine tumors, including gastrointestinal carcinoids, endocrine pancreatic tumors, gastrinomas and MTCs [5, 12]. In a study by Stridsberg et al. [5], measurement of plasma pancreastatin was inferior to chromogranin A and B in patients with carcinoids and endocrine pancreatic tumors. Others, however, have found pancreastatin to have prognostic value. In one study, a >20% decrease of pancreastatin after chemoembolization was associated with a good prognosis, while a <20% decrease correlated to a poor outcome [13]. In another study of patients with carcinoids treated with chemoembolization, significantly elevated pretreatment levels of pancreastatin were the only predictor of poor survival [14]. Elevated pretreatment levels of pancreastatin have also been demonstrated to predict poor outcome after somatostatin analog therapy [15].

Neuron-Specific Enolase

NSE is an enzyme occurring in the cytoplasm of neuroendocrine and neuronal cells. It is often elevated in patients with poorly differentiated neuroendocrine carcinomas such as small cell lung cancer, but also in 30–50% of patients with carcinoids, endocrine pancreatic tumors, MTCs and pheochromocytomas [4]. Raised levels of NSE are correlated to poor tumor differentiation [6]. The sensitivity of NSE may be improved by the simultaneous measurement of chromogranin A [16].

Neurokinin A

Neurokinin A, previously known as substance K, is a neuropeptide belonging to the tachykinins. It has strong prognostic value in patients with midgut carcinoids. In one study, it was the only independent predictor of survival in multivariate analysis.

Patients in whom neurokinin A continued to rise despite somatostatin analog treatment had significantly shorter survival compared to those in whom neurokinin A was reduced or stabilized [17].

Pancreatic Polypeptide

PP is a 36-amino acid linear peptide secreted by PP cells in the pancreatic islets and gut mucosa. PP is a member of the same family as neuropeptide Y and peptide tyrosine tyrosine. The secretion of PP is stimulated by the ingestion of meals (especially protein-containing foods), exercise and hypoglycemia, and is impaired by intravenous glucose. PP is often elevated in patients with neuroendocrine tumors and has a sensitivity of 50–80% [18], which is increased to 95% in nonfunctioning endocrine pancreatic tumors when combined with chromogranin A [4]. However, PP is also elevated in several nontumor conditions, including diarrhea, laxative abuse, inflammatory bowel disease, chronic renal disease and old age [18].

Human Chorionic Gonadotropin

HCG is a glycoprotein consisting of one alpha and one beta subunit. Usually, neuroendocrine tumor cells lack the ability to mount the two subunits together. Free alpha or beta subunits may be elevated in patients with endocrine pancreatic tumors, but are less sensitive and specific and hence less useful than chromogranin A. Elevation of beta subunits is a marker of shorter survival [19].

Specific Markers

5-Hydroxyindoleacetic Acid

Serotonin (5-hydroxytryptamine, 5-HT) is a biogenic amine derived from tryptophan by decarboxylation of 5-hydroxytryptophan, stored in granules in the enterochromaffin cells in the gastrointestinal tract and pancreas, in platelets and in neurons in the central nervous system. The synthesis and metabolism of serotonin is shown in figure 2. Serotonin causes smooth muscle contraction and vasoconstriction and is involved in blood pressure regulation and neurotransmission. Serotonin is an important factor causing classical carcinoid syndrome, in addition to tachykinins such as neuropeptide K and substance P. Serotonin is degraded to 5-hydroxyindoleacetic acid (5-HIAA), which is excreted in the urine. Urinary 5-HIAA is most frequently measured by high-performance liquid chromatography with detection by electrochemical, mass spectrometry or fluorometric methods [3]. Because of intermittent secretion of serotonin and hence intraindividual variation in 5-HIAA levels, two 24-hour urinary collections are recommended. The sensitivity varies between 52 and 68% and the specificity varies between 89 and 98% for the detection of a carcinoid tumor, depending on the cut-off value [20]. Since the following foods are rich in tryptophan and may affect the urinary 5-HIAA level, they should be avoided during and

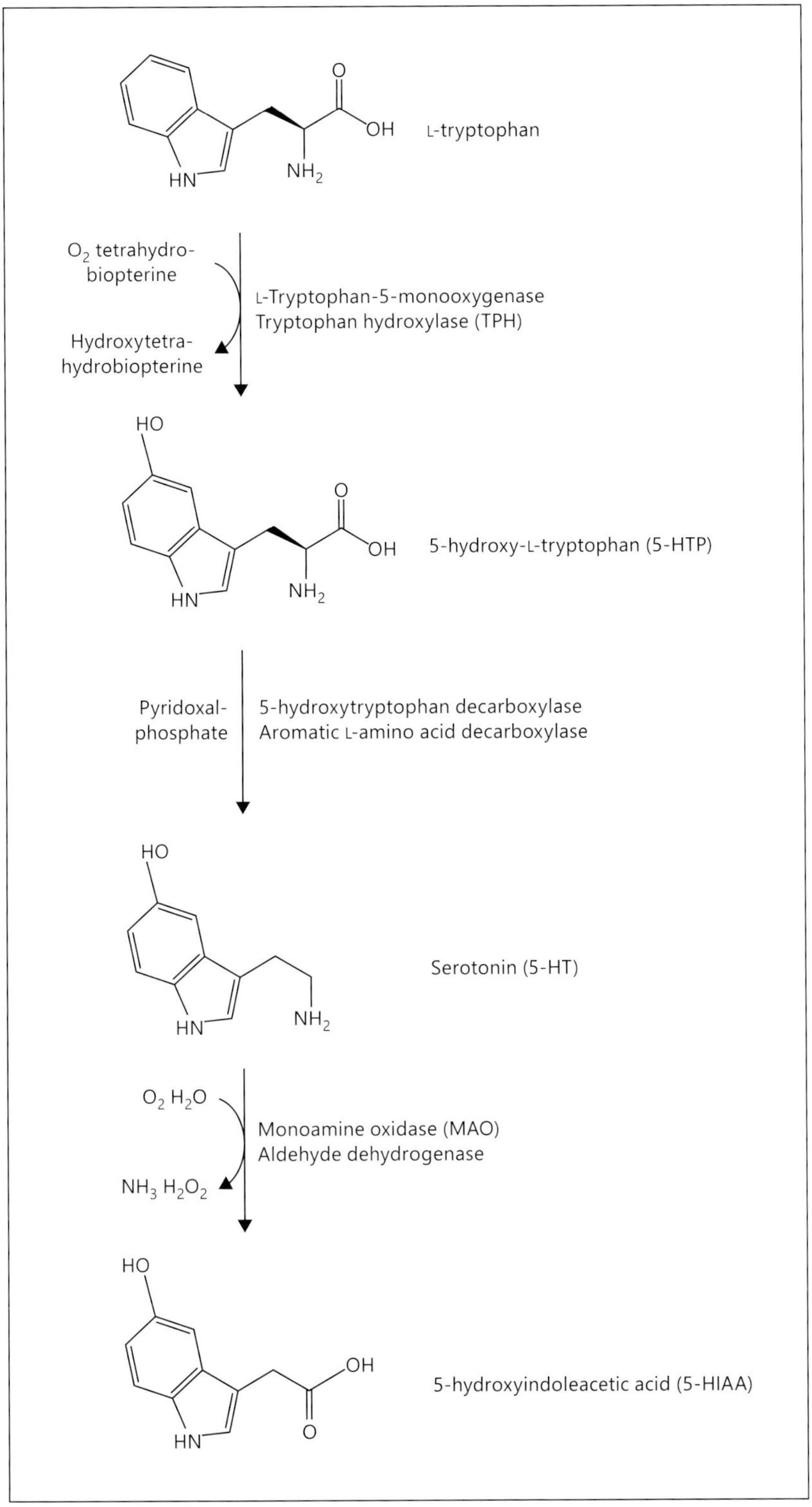

Fig. 2. The synthesis and metabolism of serotonin.

3 days prior to the collection: tomatoes, pineapples, bananas, avocados, plums, aubergines (eggplant), chocolate, kiwi, walnuts, coffee and tea. Patients with malabsorption due to coeliac disease (gluten-sensitive enteropathy), tropical sprue, Whipple's disease or cystic fibrosis may also have falsely high urinary 5-HIAA [3]. Drugs that may increase the 5-HIAA level include reserpine, fluorouracil, melphalan, cisplatin, acetanilide and phenacetin. Many patients with neuroendocrine tumors are treated with somatostatin analogs, which lower urinary 5-HIAA. Decreased 5-HIAA levels may also be caused by tricyclic antidepressants such as imipramine, SSRIs such as fluoxetine, phenothiazines including chlorpromazine, promethazine, heparin, monoamine oxidase inhibitors, isoniazid, chlorophenylalanine, methyldopa and corticotropin [3]. The highest levels of 5-HIAA in urine are found in patients with metastatic midgut tumors, especially those with massive liver metastases, while lower levels may be seen in patients with foregut tumors such as lung or gastric carcinoids or endocrine pancreatic tumors [20, 21]. Most patients with elevated 5-HIAA have carcinoid syndrome with diarrhea and/or flushing, yet the correlation between the 5-HIAA level and the severity of carcinoid syndrome seems to be inconsistent [3]. The role of 5-HIAA as a prognostic marker has not been definitely settled [3], but several studies indicate better survival in patients with lower 5-HIAA levels [8, 17, 22, 23].

Gastrin

Gastrin is a peptide hormone existing in three forms, containing 14, 17 and 34 amino acids, respectively. It is produced in the G cells in the antrum of the stomach. The release is stimulated by distension of the antrum, vagal stimulation, the presence of digested proteins, especially amino acids, and hypercalcemia, and is inhibited by low gastric pH, somatostatin, glucagon and calcitonin. Since gastrin secretion is stimulated by food intake, the test for serum gastrin should be taken after an overnight fast. Gastrin causes secretion of gastric juice including pepsinogen, stimulates pancreatic secretion and gall bladder emptying, influences the absorption and transportation of water and electrolytes through the intestinal mucosa, and has a trophic effect on the gastric mucosa. The main conditions leading to hypergastrinemia are gastrin-producing tumors (gastrinomas) in the duodenum or pancreas with Zollinger-Ellison syndrome (multiple gastric and duodenal ulcers, hypertrophic gastropathy, esophagitis and diarrhea), chronic atrophic gastritis type A with high gastric pH and often pernicious anemia, treatment with proton pump inhibitors such as omeprazole, antral G cell hyperplasia, *Helicobacter pylori* infection, pyloric obstruction and renal failure. Since proton pump inhibitors affect the serum gastrin level, they should be withdrawn, with H_2 blocker coverage, for at least 1 week prior to testing, if possible [24]. In order to differentiate between hypergastrinemia caused by a gastrinoma and chronic atrophic gastritis type A, it is important to check for gastric acid. A gastric pH <2 in combination with >10-fold elevated fasting serum gastrin is diagnostic for a gastrinoma [24], while the absence of gastric acid indicates chronic atrophic gastritis. In patients with <10-fold elevated serum gastrin and gastric pH ≤2, a secretin test and basal acid output should be performed to discriminate between a gastrinoma and more benign conditions causing hypergastrinemia [3, 24].

Secretin Test

Secretin is a 27-amino acid basic polypeptide, produced in the S cells in the small bowel with highest concentration in the distal duodenum and jejunum. Secretin is released by low duodenal pH and is inhibited by somatostatin. In normal subjects, secretin inhibits secretion of hydrochloric acid and gastrin from the stomach, but in patients with gastrinomas gastrin release is instead stimulated. The secretin test is performed as follows: after an overnight fast, secretin 2 U/kg is injected intravenously; serum gastrin is measured at 15 and 1 min before and 2, 5, 10, 15, 20 and 30 min after secretin injection. An increase of serum gastrin of ≥120 pg/ml over basal gastrin is diagnostic for Zollinger-Ellison's syndrome, with 94% sensitivity and 100% specificity [3, 24, 25].

Insulin

Insulin is a 6-kDa polypeptide hormone consisting of two peptide chains, an A-chain containing 21 amino acids and a B-chain containing 30 amino acids, linked together by 2 disulfide bonds. Insulin is synthesized in the pancreatic islet β-cells as a prohormone (proinsulin) which is cleaved into insulin and the inactive C-peptide. Insulin has a central role in the energy balance, causing increased glucose uptake in muscles and fat, increased synthesis of glycogen, protein and fat, decreased lipolysis and lowering of blood glucose. Elevated levels of insulin are seen in insulin-producing tumors (insulinomas), impaired glucose tolerance and diabetes mellitus type 2, factitious hypoglycemia from insulin and sulfonylurea-induced hypoglycemia. Insulinomas occur almost exclusively in the pancreas and are the most common functioning endocrine pancreatic tumor [3]. About 10% are malignant, and 5–10% are associated with multiple endocrine neoplasia (MEN) 1 syndrome [26]. Patients with insulinomas suffer from hypoglycemic symptoms, usually both adrenergic (hunger, sweating, tremor, palpitations, tachycardia, anxiety, feelings of warmth, nausea, weakness) and neuroglycopenic (diplopia, blurred vision, headache, dizziness, confusion, abnormal behavior, lethargy, amnesia, seizures, coma). Classically, symptoms are present in the morning before breakfast or induced by exercise, but may occur any time of the day. Differential diagnoses in patients with hypoglycemia include noninsulinoma pancreatogenous hypoglycemia syndrome, nesidioblastosis, factitious hypoglycemia from exogenously administered insulin, sulfonylurea-induced hypoglycemia, hypoglycemia mediated by insulin-like growth factor and Addison's disease. An insulinoma should be suspected in the presence of Whipple's triad, consisting of: (1) symptoms of hypoglycemia, (2) plasma glucose ≤2.2 mmol/l (≤40 mg/dl) and (3) relief of symptoms with the administration of glucose [3, 26]. By using the following six criteria, the insulinoma diagnosis can be determined [24, 26]:

(1) Blood glucose <3 mmol/l (<55 mg/dl);
(2) Concomitant insulin ≥3 mU/l (≥18 pmol/l);

(3) C-peptide ≥0.2 nmol/l (≥0.6 ng/ml);
(4) Proinsulin ≥5 pmol/l;
(5) β-Hydroxybutyrate ≤2.7 mmol/l;
(6) Absence of sulfonylurea (metabolites) in the plasma and/or urine.

If these criteria are not present, a 72-hour fast should be performed, which is the gold standard for the diagnosis of an insulinoma [26].

72-Hour Fast

A 72-hour supervised fast is performed as follows [3]. The patient is hospitalized during the test, is only allowed to drink water, black tea and coffee, to take essential medications and should be active during waking hours. Blood (venous) glucose and insulin are sampled every 6 h and whenever the patient has symptoms of hypoglycemia. When hypoglycemia is documented, blood is also drawn for C-peptide and proinsulin. At the end of the test, β-hydroxybutyrate or urinary ketones should be measured to confirm that the patient has been fasting. The fast is terminated when the plasma glucose level is 3 mmol/l (<55 mg/dl) and the patient has symptoms or signs of hypoglycemia, which will appear within 12 h in one third, within 24 h in 80%, within 48 h in 90% and within 72 h in almost 100% of cases [3]. If no definite results are obtained during the test, a supervised exercise test or a glucagon test may be performed immediately after the 72-hour fasting. When blood glucose drops to 2.5 mmol/l any measurable insulin is abnormal. An insulinoma is diagnosed when blood glucose is <3 mmol/l (<55 mg/dl) and the insulin level is ≥3 mU/l (≥18 pmol/l), and/or C-peptide is ≥0.2 nmol/l (≥0.6 ng/ml) and/or proinsulin is ≥5 pmol/l and β-hydroxybutyrate is ≤2.7 mmol/l and sulfonylurea is absent in the plasma [24, 26]. The ratio of insulin to glucose, as was previously used, is no longer recommended.

Glucagon

Glucagon is a 29-amino acid polypeptide, synthesized in the pancreatic α-cells as a prohormone (proglucagon) from which glucagon is enzymatically cleaved. Proglucagon is also produced in the intestinal L cells, where it is cleaved into glicentin and two glucagon-like peptides. Glucagon has important functions in glucose homeostasis, by stimulating glycogenolysis and gluconeogenesis. Elevated plasma glucagon is seen in glucagon-producing endocrine pancreatic tumors (glucagonomas), giving rise to glucagonoma syndrome with necrolytic migratory erythema, diabetes mellitus or impaired glucose tolerance, muscle wasting and weight loss. Elevated glucagon levels may also be found in untreated diabetes mellitus.

Vasoactive Intestinal Peptide

VIP is a 28-amino acid basic polypeptide present in gastrointestinal nerve fibers and nerve terminals, the pancreas, urogenital canal and in the central nervous system. Elevation of VIP is mainly seen in VIP-producing endocrine pancreatic tumors

(VIPomas), but may also occur in MTCs, pheochromocytomas, bronchial carcinoids and neuroblastomas. Patients with VIPomas present with the Verner-Morrison or WDHA syndrome with profuse watery diarrhea, hypokalemia and achlorhydria.

Ghrelin

Ghrelin is a 28-amino acid peptide produced mainly in the oxyntic mucosa of the stomach, but also in the pancreatic islets. Ghrelin stimulates secretion of growth hormone, ACTH, cortisol and prolactin, and increases appetite and food intake. Despite ghrelin-immunoreactive cells being frequent both in the gastric mucosa and in gastric and intestinal carcinoids, plasma ghrelin levels usually remain normal [27]. However, a patient affected by an endocrine tumor and with high circulating ghrelin was reported by Tsolakis et al. [28] in 2004.

Meal Stimulation Test

MEN1 is an autosomal dominantly inherited genetic disorder. The main lesions are primary hyperparathyroidism, endocrine pancreatic tumors and pituitary tumors. Other lesions are carcinoids in the stomach, duodenum, lungs and thymus, and adrenal hyperplasia. Endocrine pancreatic tumors occur in about 75% of the patients and are malignant in about half of these. Skogseid et al. [29] developed a standardized meal stimulation test aimed at early detection of the pancreatic tumors. The test is performed as follows: after an overnight fast a 563-calorie mixed meal composed of 66 g of carbohydrate, 18 g of protein and 22 g of fat is eaten during 20 min. Blood for analysis of gastrin and PP is collected 5 min before starting, just before starting, and at 10, 20, 30, 45 and 60 min after starting the meal. It was found that an elevated basal or exaggerated PP and/or gastrin response to the meal could detect pancreatic tumors earlier than a CT scan. The value of the meal stimulation test has since been questioned. In a more recent study, only raised basal PP and gastrin levels correlated to the presence of endocrine pancreatic tumors [30]. The laborious meal stimulation test is hence no longer recommended in the ENETS consensus guidelines for biochemical diagnosis of endocrine pancreatic tumors in patients with MEN1 [31].

Calcitonin

MTC is derived from the parafollicular C cells in the thyroid gland. The majority (75–80%) are sporadic, but 20–25% are hereditary. Lymph node metastases are present in 35–50% and distant metastases in 10–15% of the patients at diagnosis. The most important tumor marker for diagnosis and follow-up of patients with MTC is calcitonin, a 32-amino acid polypeptide produced in the C cells, and the calcitonin level is positively correlated to the tumor volume [32]. Calcitonin may, however, also be elevated in other neuroendocrine tumors, such as endocrine pancreatic tumors or carcinoids, although the levels are usually lower than in patients with metastatic MTC. The diagnostic sensitivity for MTC of basal calcitonin, which is about 75–90%, can be increased by stimulation with pentagastrin, which is, however, no longer available

[33]. Calcitonin may cause a carcinoid-like syndrome with flushing and diarrhea. Another useful marker for MTC is carcinoembryonic antigen (CEA), which is elevated in more than 50% of patients. CEA has prognostic implication, since high levels are associated with extensive lymph node and distant metastases, and rising CEA in the presence of stable calcitonin indicates dedifferentiation and worse prognosis [32].

Catecholamines
The catecholamines epinephrine and norepinephrine are biogenic amines. Norepinephrine is especially synthesized in the peripheral sympathetic nerve cells, functioning as a transmitter, while epinephrine is mainly produced in the adrenal medulla. Elevated levels of epinephrine are seen in patients with pheochromocytomas, while elevation of norepinephrine may be seen in both pheochromocytomas and functioning (sympathetic) paragangliomas. Other causes of elevated catecholamines include hypertension and various stress factors. Epinephrine and norepinephrine, as well as their metabolites (metoxiepinephrine = metanephrine, metoxinorepinephrine = normetanephrine, homovanillic acid, vanillyl mandelic acid) can be measured in the urine. Usually, two 24-hour collections are sampled. According to more recent research, free metanephrines in plasma measured by immunoassays is the best biochemical method for the diagnosis of pheochromocytomas and functioning paragangliomas [34]. Plasma chromogranin A is also, in the absence of renal insufficiency, highly efficient in diagnosing pheochromocytomas. By combining metanephrines with chromogranin A, the diagnostic yield is even higher, with 100% sensitivity and 95% accuracy [35].

Tumor Markers in Neuroendocrine Tumors

A summary of tumor markers in neuroendocrine tumors is given in table 1. Almost all neuroendocrine tumors may produce chromogranin A, which should be part of the routine biochemical diagnosis and follow-up in all these patients.

Foregut Carcinoids
Lung carcinoids may secrete various hormones, including serotonin, ACTH, corticotropin-releasing hormone (CRH) and growth hormone-releasing hormone. In the absence of clinical symptoms of Cushing's syndrome or carcinoid syndrome, analysis of ACTH, urinary cortisol or 5-HIAA is not necessary. About one third of patients with thymic carcinoids present with Cushing's syndrome, which may be silent, and these patients should be tested for ACTH and cortisol. Carcinoid syndrome has so far not been described in patients with thymic carcinoids. Gastric carcinoids may be gastrin dependent (type 1 and 2) and nongastrin dependent (type 3). Apart from serum gastrin, *H. pylori* antibodies, parietal cell antibodies, thyroid functional test and thyroperoxidase antibodies should be assessed at diagnosis, and

Table 1. Summary of general and specific biochemical analyses in relation to tumor type

Tumor	Markers
Lung carcinoid	Chromogranin A (5-HIAA, ACTH, U-cortisol; only if clinical symptoms)
Thymic carcinoid	Chromogranin A, ACTH, U-cortisol
Gastric carcinoid	Chromogranin A, gastrin, gastric pH (5-HIAA, ACTH, U-cortisol; only if clinical symptoms)
Duodenal carcinoid/gastrinoma	Chromogranin A, gastrin, gastric pH, secretin test (5-HIAA; only if clinical symptoms)
Midgut carcinoid	Chromogranin A, 5-HIAA
Hindgut carcinoid	Chromogranin A, PP
Endocrine pancreatic tumors	Chromogranin A, PP, gastrin, glucagon, calcitonin, insulin, proinsulin, VIP (72-hour fast, GT)
Medullary thyroid cancer	Chromogranin A, calcitonin, CEA, GT
Pheochromocytoma, paraganglioma	Chromogranin A, metanephrines, U-epinephrine, U-norepinephrine, GT
MEN1	Chromogranin A, PP, gastrin, glucagon, calcitonin, insulin, proinsulin, VIP, calcium, PTH, prolactin, IGF-1, GT
MEN2	Chromogranin A, metanephrines, U-epinephrine, U-norepinephrine, calcitonin, CEA, calcium, PTH, GT

GT = Genetic testing.

gastric pH may be of value. In patients with duodenal neuroendocrine tumors, serum gastrin, ACTH, cortisol and 5-HIAA may be indicated depending on the clinical symptoms. If there is doubt whether an elevated gastrin level is dependent on a gastrinoma or chronic atrophic gastritis type A, a secretin test may aid in the differential diagnosis.

Midgut Tumors
Most of these tumors produce serotonin, and classical carcinoid syndrome with flushing, diarrhea, asthma and right-sided heart affection is common in patients with metastatic tumors. Chromogranin A is of value for the early detection of recurrences [9] and together with 5-HIAA for monitoring of treatment. If the cardiac valves are affected, NT-proBNP can aid in the grading and monitoring of cardiac insufficiency.

Hindgut Tumors
These are usually nonfunctioning with normal 5-HIAA, but may produce chromogranin A, PP or β-HCG.

Endocrine Pancreatic Tumors

A large proportion (40–50%) of endocrine pancreatic tumors are nonfunctioning, i.e. without endocrine symptoms. These tumors may either have normal hormones or produce peptides with low biological activity such as chromogranin A and/or PP. Unless clinical symptoms are present, extensive hormonal screening is not indicated [31]. Endocrine symptoms may be caused by secretion of gastrin, insulin, proinsulin, glucagon, calcitonin, VIP, ACTH, CRH and parathormone (PTH)-related peptide. The most common functioning tumors are gastrinomas and insulinomas. The diagnosis of Zollinger-Ellison syndrome is based on the measurement of fasting serum gastrin, gastric pH and the secretin test. The gold standard for diagnosis of insulinomas is the 72-hour supervised fast [26]. It is not uncommon that multiple hormones are secreted at the same time, making the patient suffer from a mixture of endocrine symptoms, and that the hormone production is changed over time. Patients with a family history or multiple tumors should be suspected of having MEN1 syndrome and screened with ionized calcium, PTH and prolactin; additional laboratory testing include IGF-1 and pancreatic hormones depending on clinical symptoms. Genetic testing is only justified if there is a strong suspicion of MEN1 [24]. The meal stimulation test is not indicated for the detection of endocrine pancreatic tumors in patients with MEN1 syndrome [31].

Medullary Thyroid Carcinoma

Serum calcitonin is the most important tumor marker, and CEA is also of value, having prognostic implication [32]. Since 20–25% are inherited, either isolated or part of MEN2 syndrome, screening for germline mutations in the *RET* proto-oncogene is indicated.

Pheochromocytoma, Paraganglioma

The biochemical diagnosis and follow-up of pheochromocytomas and functioning (sympathetic) paragangliomas include measurement of plasma metanephrines, chromogranin A and urinary catecholamines (epinephrine and norepinephrine). About 25% of pheochromocytomas and paragangliomas are inherited and part of genetic syndromes, including MEN2, von Hippel-Lindau, neurofibromatosis and familial paraganglioma, and up to 60% of the tumors are caused by somatic or germline mutations in 1 of 11 known genes [36]. Genetic testing for *RET*, *VHL*, *NF1*, *SDHD*, *SDHB* and *SDHC* genes should be considered in all patients with pheochromocytomas and paragangliomas [4].

Conclusion

Neuroendocrine tumors are usually slow-growing neoplasms. The majority of the tumors are able to secrete peptides and other hormones that may or may not give rise to endocrine symptoms, such as carcinoid syndrome, Cushing's syndrome, hypoglycemia, glucagonoma syndrome or WDHA syndrome. Biochemical testing is an important part of the diagnostic work-up in these patients, both for the diagnosis of specific syndromes, early detection of small tumors and recurrences, as well as for treatment monitoring. Chromogranin A is the most useful general marker and is produced by the majority of endocrine tumors. In patients with normal renal function and not taking proton pump inhibitors, it is valuable both for treatment monitoring and early detection of recurrences. In addition, specific markers are used for the diagnosis and monitoring of patients presenting with various endocrine syndromes; these markers include gastrin, insulin, proinsulin, glucagon, VIP, ACTH, urinary cortisol and 5-HIAA, plasma metanephrines and urinary catecholamines. In the future, with the development of newer and simplified methods, such as next-generation sequencing and the detection of novel prognostic and predictive markers, biochemical testing and laboratory medicine will probably play an even more important role in the diagnostic work-up and follow-up of patients with neuroendocrine tumors.

References

1 Rindi G, Klöppel G, Alhman H, Caplin M, Couvelard A, de Herder WW, Erikssson B, Falchetti A, Falconi M, Komminoth P, Korner M, Lopes JM, McNicol AM, Nilsson O, Perren A, Scarpa A, Scoazec JY, Wiedenmann B: TNM staging of foregut (neuro)endocrine tumors: a consensus proposal including a grading system. Virchows Arch 2006;449:395–401.

2 Rindi G, Klöppel G, Couvelard A, Komminoth P, Korner M, Lopes JM, McNicol AM, Nilsson O, Perren A, Scarpa A, Scoazec JY, Wiedenmann B: TNM staging of midgut and hindgut (neuro) endocrine tumors: a consensus proposal including a grading system. Virchows Arch 2007;451:757–762.

3 O'Toole D, Grossman A, Gross D, Delle Fave G, Barkmanova J, O'Connor J, Pape UF, Plöckinger U: ENETS consensus guidelines for the standards of care in neuroendocrine tumors: biochemical markers. Neuroendocrinology 2009;90:194–202.

4 Vinik AI, Silva MP, Woltering EA, Go VL, Warner R, Caplin M: Biochemical testing for neuroendocrine tumors. Pancreas 2009;38:876–889.

5 Stridsberg M, Öberg K, Li Q, Engström U, Lundqvist G: Measurement of chromogranin A, chromogranin B (secretogranin I), chromogranin C (secretogranin II) and pancreastatin in plasma and urine from patients with carcinoid tumours and endocrine pancreatic tumours. J Endocrinol 1995;144:49–59.

6 Baudin E, Gigliotti A, Ducreux M, Ropers J, Comoy E, Sabourin JC, Bidart JM, Cailleux AF, Bonacci R, Ruffie P, Schlumberger M: Neuron-specific enolase and chromogranin A as markers of neuroendocrine tumours. Br J Cancer 1998;78:1102–1107.

7 Nobels FRE, Kwekkeboom DJ, Coopmans W, Schoenmakers CHH, Lindemans J, De Herder WW, Krenning EP, Bouillon R, Lamberts SWJ: Chromogranin A as a serum marker for neuroendocrine neoplasia: comparison with neuron-specific enolase and the α-subunit of glycoprotein hormones. J Clin Endocrinol Metab 1997;82:2622–2628.

8 Janson ET, Holmberg L, Stridsberg M, Eriksson B, Theodorsson E, Wilander E, Öberg K: Carcinoid tumors: analysis of prognostic factors and survival in 301 patients from a referral center. Ann Oncol 1997; 8:685–690.

9 Welin S, Stridsberg M, Cunningham J, Granberg D, Skogseid B, Öberg K, Eriksson B, Janson ET: Elevated plasma chromogranin A is the first indication of recurrence in radically operated midgut carcinoid tumors. Neuroendocrinology 2009;89:302–307.

10 Granberg D, Stridsberg M, Seensalu R, Eriksson B, Lundqvist G, Öberg K, Skogseid B: Plasma chromogranin A in patients with multiple endocrine neoplasia type 1. J Clin Endocrinol Metab 1999;84:2712–2717.

11 Stridsberg M, Eriksson B, Fellström B, Kristiansson G, Tiensuu Janson E: Measurements of chromogranin B can serve as a complement to chromogranin A. Regul Pept 2007;139:80–83.

12 Conlon JM: Granin-derived peptides as diagnostic and prognostic markers for endocrine tumors. Regul Pept 2010;165:5–11.

13 Desai DC, O'Dorisio TM, Schirmer WJ, Jung SS, Khabiri H, Villanueva V, Martin EW: Serum pancreastatin levels predict response to hepatic artery chemoembolization and somatostatin analogue therapy in metastatic neuroendocrine tumors. Regul Pept 2001;96:113–117.
14 Bloomston M, Al-Saif O, Klemanski D, Pinzone JJ, Martin EW, Palmer B, Guy G, Khabiri H, Ellison EC, Shah MH: Hepatic artery chemoembolization in 122 patients with metastatic carcinoid tumor: lessons learned. J Gastrointest Surg 2007;11:264–271.
15 Stronge RL, Turner GB, Johnston BT, McCance DR, McGinty A, Patterson CC, Ardill JE: A rapid rise in circulating pancreastatin in response to somatostatin analogue therapy is associated with poor survival in patients with neuroendocrine tumours. Ann Clin Biochem 2008;45:560–566.
16 Korse CM, Taal BG, Vincent A, van Velthuysen ML, Baas P, Buning-Kager JC, Linders TC, Bonfrer JM: Choice of tumour markers in patients with neuroendocrine tumours is dependent on the histological grade: a marker study of chromogranin A, neuron specific enolase, progastrin-releasing peptide and cytokeratin fragments. Eur J Cancer 2012;48:662–671.
17 Turner GB, Johnston BT, McCance DR, McGinty A, Watson RG, Patterson CC, Ardill JE: Circulating markers of prognosis and response to treatment in patients with midgut carcinoid tumours. Gut 2006; 55:1586–1591.
18 Metz DC, Jensen RT: Gastrointestinal neuroendocrine tumors: pancreatic endocrine tumors. Gastroenterology 2008;135:1469–1492.
19 Shah T, Srirajaskanthan R, Bhogal M, Toubanakis C, Meyer T, Noonan A, Witney-Smith C, Amin T, Bhogal P, Sivathasan N, Warner B, Hochhauser D, Caplin ME: α-Fetoprotein and human chorionic gonadotrophin-β as prognostic markers in neuroendocrine tumour patients. Br J Cancer 2008;99:72–77.
20 Meijer WG, Kema IP, Volmer M, Willemse PH, de Vries EG: Discriminating capacity of indole markers in the diagnosis of carcinoid tumors. Clin Chem 2000;46:1588–1596.
21 Baudin E, Bidart J-M, Rougier P, Lazar V, Ruffie P, Ropers J, Ducreux M, Troalen F, Sabourin J-C, Comoy E, Lasser P, DeBaere T, Schlumberger M: Screening for multiple endocrine neoplasia type 1 and hormonal production in apparently sporadic neuroendocrine tumors. J Clin Endocrinol Metab 1999;84:69–75.
22 Formica V, Wotherspoon A, Cunningham D, Norman AR, Sirohi B, Oates J, Chong G: The prognostic role of WHO classification, urinary 5-hydroxyindoleacetic acid and liver function tests in metastatic neuroendocrine carcinomas of the gastroenteropancreatic tract. Br J Cancer 2007;96:1178–1182.
23 van der Horst-Schrivers AN, Post WJ, Kema IP, Links TP, Willemse PH, Wymenga AN, de Vries EG: Persistent low urinary excretion of 5-HIAA is a marker for favourable survival during follow-up in patients with disseminated midgut carcinoid tumours. Eur J Cancer 2007;43:2651–2657.
24 Jensen RT, Cadiot G, Brandi ML, de Herder WW, Kaltsas G, Komminoth P, Scoazec JY, Salazar R, Sauvanet A, Kianmanesh R: ENETS consensus guidelines for the management of patients with digestive neuroendocrine neoplasms: functional pancreatic endocrine tumor syndromes. Neuroendocrinology 2012;95:98–119.
25 Berna MJ, Hoffmann KM, Long SH, Serrano J, Gibril F, Jensen RT: Serum gastrin in Zollinger-Ellison syndrome. II. Prospective study of gastrin provocative testing in 293 patients from the National Institutes of Health and comparison with 537 cases from the literature: evaluation of diagnostic criteria, proposal of new criteria, and correlations with clinical and tumoral features. Medicine 2006;85:331–364.
26 de Herder WW, Niederle B, Scoazec JY, Pauwels S, Klöppel G, Falconi M, Kwekkeboom DJ, Öberg K, Eriksson B, Wiedenmann B, Rindi G, O'Toole D, Ferone D: Well-differentiated pancreatic tumor/carcinoma: insulinoma. Neuroendocrinology 2006;84: 183–188.
27 Tsolakis AV, Stridsberg M, Grimelius L, Portela-Gomes GM, Falkmer SE, Waldum HL, Janson ET: Ghrelin immunoreactive cells in gastric endocrine tumors and their relation to plasma ghrelin concentration. J Clin Gastroenterol 2008;42:381–388.
28 Tsolakis AV, Portela-Gomes GM, Stridsberg M, Grimelius L, Sundin A, Eriksson BK, Öberg KE, Janson ET: Malignant gastric ghrelinoma with hyperghrelinemia. J Clin Endocrinol Metab 2004;89:3739–3744.
29 Skogseid B, Öberg K, Benson L, Lindgren PG, Lörelius LE, Lundqvist G, Wide L, Wilander E: A standardized meal stimulation test of the endocrine pancreas for early detection of pancreatic endocrine tumors in multiple endocrine neoplasia type I syndrome: five years experience. J Clin Endocrinol Metab 1987;64:1233–1240.
30 Langer P, Wild A, Celik I, Kopp I, Bergenfelz A, Bartsch DK: Prospective controlled trial of a standardized meal stimulation test in the detection of pancreaticoduodenal endocrine tumours in patients with multiple endocrine neoplasia type 1. Br J Surg 2001;88:1403–1407.
31 Falconi M, Bartsch DK, Eriksson B, Kloppel G, Lopes JM, O'Connor JM, Salazar R, Taal BG, Vullierme MP, O'Toole D: ENETS consensus guidelines for the management of patients with digestive neuroendocrine neoplasms of the digestive system: well-differentiated pancreatic non-functioning tumors. Neuroendocrinology 2012;95:120–134.

32 Sippel RS, Kunnimalaiyaan M, Chen H: Current management of medullary thyroid cancer. Oncologist 2008;13:539–547.

33 Öberg K, Metz DC: Diagnostic pathways; in Caplin M, Yao JC (eds): Handbook of Gastroenteropancreatic and Thoracic Neuroendocrine Tumours. Bristol, BioScientifica, 2011, pp 93–114.

34 Unger N, Deutschbein T, Walz MK, Mann K, Petersenn S: The value of immunoassays for metanephrines in the biochemical diagnosis of pheochromocytomas. H Horm Metab Res 2009;41:676–679.

35 d'Herbomez M, Forzy G, Bauters C, Tierny C, Pigny P, Carnaille B, Pattou F, Wemeau JL, Rouaix N: An analysis of the biochemical diagnosis of 66 pheochromocytomas. Eur J Endocrinol 2007;156:569–575.

36 Crona J, Verdugo AD, Granberg D, Welin S, Stålberg P, Hellman P, Björklund P: Next-generation sequencing in the clinical genetic screening of patients with pheochromocytoma and paraganglioma. Endocr Connect 2013;2:104–111.

Dan Granberg
Department of Endocrine Oncology
University Hospital
SE–751 85 Uppsala (Sweden)
E-Mail dan.granberg@medsci.uu.se

Papotti M, de Herder WW (eds): Neuroendocrine Tumors: A Multidisciplinary Approach.
Front Horm Res. Basel, Karger, 2015, vol 44, pp 40–57 (DOI: 10.1159/000382053)

Clinical Syndromes Related to Gastrointestinal Neuroendocrine Neoplasms

Georgios Boutzios · Gregory Kaltsas

Endocrine Unit, Department of Pathophysiology, National University of Athens, Athens, Greece

Abstract

Neuroendocrine neoplasms (NENs) comprise a heterogeneous group of tumors derived from multipotent neuroendocrine cells that have the inherent ability to synthesize and secrete a variety of substances (peptides and amines). When these substances are bioactive, NENs can present with a related clinical syndrome (functioning NENs) and/or symptoms of mass effects (functioning and nonfunctioning NENs). NENs differ in their pathogenesis, clinical syndromes produced, aspects of biological behavior and response to certain antitumor treatment. The carcinoid syndrome (CS) is the clinical constellation of secretory diarrhea, flushing, wheezing and dyspnea as a result of serotonin production mainly from small intestinal NENs. Complications of CS are frequent and include extensive mesenteric fibrosis, carcinoid heart disease and the life-threatening carcinoid crisis. A variety of substances (mainly hormones) are produced from NENs originating from the pancreas associated with specific symptoms that can lead to their precise diagnosis. NENs may also secrete substances characteristic of other sites of origin and produce a variety of paraneoplastic syndromes and/or change their secretory status with time. Surgery remains the best option for complete tumor resection and symptom relief. Surgery may also be used when medical treatment fails to obtain control of the symptoms along with cytoreductive techniques. Somatostatin analogs (octreotide and lanreotide) constitute the backbone of medical treatment for the majority of functioning NENs as they can alleviate symptoms, stabilize tumor growth and improve the quality of life. Telotristat etiprate is a novel oral agent that inhibits tryptophan hydroxylase, the key enzyme responsible for serotonin production, and can improve the symptoms of CS. Nonspecific and supportive therapies are also used for refractory cases. In this chapter the clinical features of functioning NENs will be analyzed as well as aspects of their diagnosis based on secretory substances and treatment of the hormonal excess.

Neuroendocrine neoplasms (NENs) comprise a heterogeneous group of malignancies derived from multipotent neuroendocrine cells that belong to the diffuse endocrine system. These are highly specialized cells that have the ability to produce, store and secrete peptides and biogenic amines that when bioactive can lead to distinct clinical syndromes [1]. The classification of NENs as functioning or nonfunctioning is based on the presence of symptoms related to these syndromes, although both can present with symptoms of mass effect due to local or distant metastases. Although named nonfunctioning, some of these tumors are either capable of producing low levels of peptides/amines that are insufficient to cause symptoms related to a syndrome or these compounds may be metabolically inactive or inappropriately processed [1]. Specific tumor markers facilitate the identification of functioning tumors and are characterized according to the presenting clinical syndrome and the site of the primary tumor location. However, all NENs irrespective of their tissue of origin secrete general markers of neuroendocrine differentiation such as chromogranins, neuron-specific enolase, pancreatic polypeptide and alpha subunits that can also facilitate their diagnosis. Serum chromogranin A is the most useful general tumor marker available for NEN patients that also bears prognostic significance [2]. Although the secretion of specific biogenic compounds leading to a clinical syndrome characterizes the tissue of origin (eutopic secretion), these substances can also be secreted from other nondesignated tissues (ectopic secretion). The clinical syndromes produced in this setting are named paraneoplastic humoral syndromes (PNS) and, although traditionally considered to be relatively rare, are now being increasingly recognized [3, 4]. In addition, the secretory component and functionality of NENs can change over time [1]. This may lead to a change in their phenotype as the secretion of one set of neurohormones may transform into another, with a consequent change in the clinical picture, or even a previously nonfunctioning tumor becoming a functioning one [5].

Since the great majority of NENs express somatostatin receptors on their surface, long-acting somatostatin analogs (SS-analogs; including octreotide and lanreotide) have extensively been used as therapeutic options. These compounds exert an inhibitory effect in the secretory component of these tumors and can alleviate related symptoms; in addition, through an inhibitory effect on tumor growth, they can stabilize NENs and improve the quality of life of these patients [6]. However, surgery remains the only potentially curative therapeutic option in patients with localized disease. Surgery can also be utilized, along with other cytoreductive techniques, when medical therapy with either SS-analogs and/or other systemic or supportive treatment fails to control the functional syndrome [6].

Following the introduction of successful treatments for the humoral symptoms, it became apparent that the great majority of patients with NENs succumb due to disease progression [1]. Currently, the most important prognostic determinants of disease progression are the tissue of origin of the primary tumor, extent of the disease based on TNM classification and tumor grading based on the Ki67 labeling index. It is therefore important to be able to diagnose patients with humoral syndromes at an early stage, not only to achieve symptomatic relief, but also to influence the overall prognosis. In this chapter, the clinical manifestations and symptomatic treatment of functioning gastroenteropancreatic NENs (GEP-NENs) along with those derived from the respiratory system (so called lung 'carcinoids') will be presented.

Clinical Syndromes Secondary to Gastrointestinal Neuroendocrine Neoplasms

Gastrointestinal NENs (GI-NENs; formerly named carcinoid tumors) are attributed to the neoplastic proliferation of neuroendocrine cells that are ubiquitous, but predominate in the gastrointestinal (GI) tract (55%), bronchial epithelium (30%) and urogenital tract; these tumors exhibit a wide range of biological behavior from relatively indolent local growth to highly aggressive rapidly metastasizing lesions [4, 6–9]. The most prominent secretory product of GI-NENs is serotonin (5-hydroxytryptamine; 5-HT), which is synthesized from tryptophan through its precursor 5-hydroxytryptophan (5-HTP) by the enzyme aromatic acid decarboxylase, and is further metabolized by monoamino-oxidase to 5-hydroxyindoloacetic acid (5-HIAA), which is excreted in the urine [4, 7]. In normal subjects, 99% of tryptophan is used for the synthesis of nicotinic acid and the remaining for 5-HT, but in NENs there is a shift towards 5-HT production [4, 6, 7]. When 5-HT is secreted in the portal circulation, it is efficiently metabolized; however, in the presence of hepatic metastases, or when the primary NENs are in the ovary/bronchus, the systemic features of the carcinoid syndrome (CS) may develop [4, 6, 7]. Serotonin is involved in the majority of the manifestations of CS as it stimulates intestinal motility and inhibits intestinal absorption [4, 6, 7]. The diversion of tryptophan to serotonin may also lead to nicotinic acid deficiency and the development of the clinical manifestations of pellagra [4, 6, 7]. Excess serotonin stimulates receptor fibroblast growth and fibrogenesis via the 5HT2B that may lead to peritoneal and valvular fibrosis [4, 6, 7]. In addition to serotonin, GI-NENs may secrete a number of other substances, such as the peptides substance P, neurotensin, prostaglandins, kallikrein and tachykinins [4, 6, 7]. Kallikrein is a potent vasodilator and may be involved in the development of the characteristic flushing of the CS which is not serotonin related [2, 7].

Carcinoid Syndrome

The CS results from the synergistic action of 5-HT, kinins and prostaglandins that enter the systemic circulation after by-passing their metabolism in either the portal or the pulmonary arterial circulation [2, 4, 6, 7]. The cardinal presenting features of the CS are diarrhea and flushing; CS is mainly produced by small intestinal NENs with hepatic metastases or when the primaries are in the lung and ovary even in the absence of hepatic involvement [8–10]. A typical patient with CS may present with flushing (60–85%), secretory diarrhea (60–80%), abdominal pain (40%), telangiectasia (25%), valvular heart disease (20%), intermittent bronchial wheezing (<10%) and pellagra (5%; table 1) [11, 12]. Consumption of food, alcohol intake and stress are well-known participants of CS, particularly of flushing [13]. The diarrhea may be initially intermittent accompanied by abdominal cramping, but may become continuous when complicated by lymphangiectasia and bacterial overgrowth [1, 7]. As CS diarrhea is a secretory one, it is not alleviated by food restriction and wakes up the patient during the night. The typical flush is of sudden onset, pink to red color, involving the face

Table 1. Clinical features of CS

Clinical features	Frequency %	Characteristics	Mediators
Flushing	60–85	Typical flush: sudden onset, pink to red color, involving the face and upper trunk, lasting for only a few minutes and can occur several times a day	5-HT, histamine, kallikrein, substance P, prostaglandins
Diarrhea	60–80	Secretory: initially intermittent accompanied by abdominal cramping but may become continuous when complicated by lymphangiectasia and bacterial overgrowth	5-HT, histamine, Vasoactive intestinal peptide, prostaglandins, gastrin
Abdominal pain	40	Long history	Tumor obstruction, hepatomegaly, intestinal ischemia
Telangiectasia	25	Face	Unknown
CHD	≤20	Dyspnea holosystolic murmur radiating to the right side of the chest, suggestive of tricuspid valve regurgitation	Substance P, 5-HT
Wheezing	<10		5-HTP, histamine
Pellagra	5	Dermatitis, diarrhea, dementia	Niacin deficiency

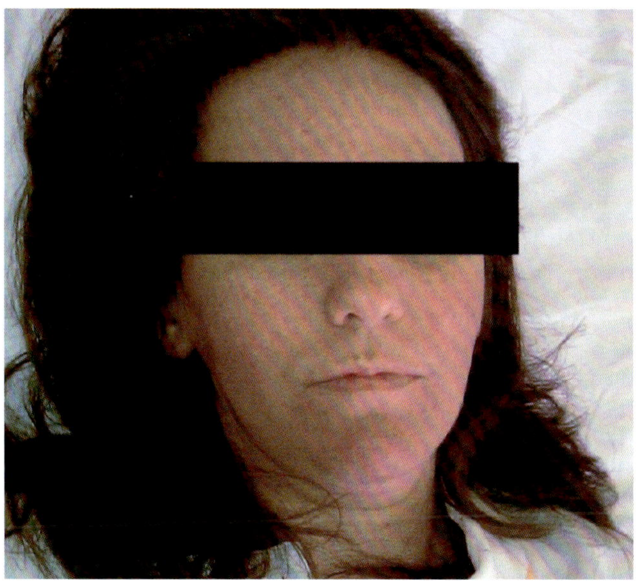

Fig. 1. A 41-year-old patient with ileal NEN and hepatic metastases, with CS demonstrating a typical flush.

and upper trunk, lasting for only a few minutes, which can occur several times a day, mainly caused by small intestinal NENs (fig. 1). An atypical CS that is thought to be 5-HTP and/or histamine induced can occur in approximately 5% of cases consisting of a purplish color flush that may be of prolonged duration (hours) associated with telangiectasia, hypertrophy of the skin and acrocyanosis [4, 6, 7]. An extremely rare, bright-red, patchy, histamine-induced flush may be seen in patients with chronic atrophic gastritis and enterochromaffin cell hyperplasia [14]. There is no evidence that the CS per se and independently from the presence of metastatic disease can influence overall prognosis except in the presence of carcinoid heart disease (CHD) [15]. In rare cases, nicotinic acid synthesis is impaired, which is associated with reduced protein synthesis and hypoalbuminemia and the development of pellagra (skin rashes, glossitis, stomatitis, confusion/dementia) [4, 6, 7].

The diagnosis is made on clinical suspicion and substantiated by elevated 5-HIAA levels in the urine that exert up to 100% sensitivity and 85–90% specificity [16]. As a variety of substances can interfere with the measurement of urinary 5-HIAA, collections should be made under strict dietary restrictions to avoid false positive results. Previous studies recommend at least two 24-hour urine collections for the evaluation of 5-HIAA but a single specimen may be sufficient for follow-up purposes [13]. As urinary 5-HIAA levels may depend on tumor volume they are frequently normal in patients with nonmetastatic GI-NENs, even in the presence of CS, particularly in patients without diarrhea [13]. Chromogranin A has a high sensitivity in identifying patients with NENs, and thus verifying the diagnosis of symptoms suggestive of CS, but has lower specificity as high chromogranin A levels can be found in patients taking proton pump inhibitors (PPIs), in atrophic gastritis and in the presence of renal and heart failure [17].

Carcinoid Crisis

This is a severe and potentially life-threatening exacerbation of hormonal symptoms of the CS, due to the release of large amounts of amines in the circulation. Hypotension, rarely hypertension, tachycardia, arrhythmias, bronchial wheezing, flushing and central nervous system dysfunction dominate the clinical presentation [14]. Carcinoid crisis can occur spontaneously after anesthesia or interventional procedures, or may be precipitated by catecholamine and histamine-releasing drugs used routinely in patients undergoing valve surgery [8, 18].

CHD (Hedinger's Syndrome)

A severe complication of CS is CHD, which may develop in 60–80% of patients with the CS as shown by echocardiography, although it is clinically significant in a much smaller percentage [1]. CHD is echocardiographically characterized by plaque-like, fibrous endocardial thickening that principally involves the right side of the heart, causing retraction and fixation of the tricuspid leaflets and pulmonary valves as well as diminished right ventricular function [19]. Tricuspid valves are affected in 90% of patients, while pulmonary valves are less frequently involved [20]. Concomitant mitral and aortic regurgitation has occasionally been demonstrated and is mainly seen in patients with patent foramen ovale or bronchial NENs [21]. Brain natriuretic peptide (BNP), especially N-terminal pro-brain BNP, has been shown to be a quite sensitive indicator of early CHD, exerts a high negative predictive value and is used for monitoring CHD [22, 23]. Patients with CHD have significantly higher levels of 5-HIAA, suggesting that serotonin per se may be implicated in its pathogenesis, a view supported by the finding of similar lesions in patients receiving anorectic drugs that interfere with serotonin metabolism [23]. When severe CHD develops, the median survival is only 1–4 years, although this has improved over recent years, probably due to successful valve replacement [24]. Reconstructive valve replacement surgery has been reported to be of value in patients with advanced heart disease and right ventricular failure, with low mortality in young patients but higher risk in patients older than 60 years of age [20]. Biosynthetic valve replacement should be considered in patients who have obtained control of hormonal symptoms and tumor growth [25].

Carcinoid Fibrosis
Small intestinal NENs that secrete serotonin can also be associated with mesenteric metastases characterized by extensive mesenteric fibrosis. This fibrosis results from the effects of serotonin and growth factors, such as connective tissue growth factor and other substances released from the carcinoid metastases [14]. The fibrosis causes shrinkage and fixation of the mesentery and mesenteric root to the retroperitoneum that may cause obstruction of the duodenum and parts of the colon. Retroperitoneal fibrosis can also obstruct the ureters and cause obstructive uropathy with impairment of renal function [26]. The mesenteric vessels may also become entrapped or occluded, leading to venous stasis and impairment of arterial circulation [7, 12].

Clinical Syndromes of Gastrointestinal Neuroendocrine Neoplasms According to the Tissue of Origin

The recent classification of NENs according to the tissue of origin has revealed the heterogeneity of these tumors that is also reflected by their ability to produce tissue-specific substances and cause relevant clinical syndromes [13]. Although the majority of the symptoms of CS are due to serotonin-producing cells of the small intestine, it can occasionally be produced from the same cells from other primary sites. Bronchial NENs account for approximately 1–2% of all lung carcinomas and are divided according to biologic aggressiveness and prognosis into low-grade typical carcinoids, intermediate-grade atypical carcinoids (well-differentiated lung carcinoids), and high-grade (poorly differentiated) large cell neuroendocrine carcinomas, and small cell carcinomas [26, 27]. These tumors have a low content of 5-HT and often secrete the serotonin precursor 5-HTP, histamine and various polypeptidic hormones [4, 6, 7]. The majority of well-differentiated lung NENs are nonfunctioning, but a subset may develop an atypical CS with prolonged flushing, headache, palpitations and bronchoconstriction or secrete various peptides leading to different pananeoplastic syndrome (PNS) (table 2) [28]. In atypical CS, histamine is one of the main mediators and the diagnosis is made by measuring the urinary metabolites of histamine along

Table 2. Ectopic humoral syndromes (paraneoplastic) secondary to NENs

Syndrome	Mediator	Tumor	Clinical biochemical features	Endocrine testing	Radiology imaging
Hypercalcemia	PTHrP, and growth factors/ cytokines	SCLC pNEN Carcinoid Pheochromocytoma	↑ Ca, ↓ P, ↑ cAMP urine	↓ PTH ↑ PTHrP ↑ TGFβ ↑ IL, PG	(–) Parathyroid imaging (+) Lesion elsewhere Conventional imaging (+) Octreoscan[1]
Acromegaly	GHRH GH	Carcinoid pNEN Pheochromocytoma	Acromegalic features	↑ GH, IGF1 failure to suppress GH on OGTT	Lesion elsewhere (+) Octreoscan
Cushing's syndrome	ACTH, CRH	SCLC pNEN Carcinoid Pheochromocytoma MTC	↓ K, cachexia, Cushing phenotype	↑ ACTH CRH/DDAVP test	Normal pituitary MRI (–) IPSS Lesion elsewhere (+) Octreoscan (+) MIBG scan
Hyponatremia (SIADH)	ADH and ANP	SCLC	↓ Na ↑ Plasma ↓ Urine osmolality	Water deprivation test	(+) Radiology (–) Octreoscan
Hypoglycemia	Insulin IGF1 IGF2 (pro-IGF2)	Carcinoid	Autonomic and neurological symptoms of hypoglycemia	↑ Insulin ↑ IGF1, N proIGF2 ↑ proIGF2 ↓ GH	Normal pancreas EUS Lesion elsewhere (+) Octreoscan
Other pituitary hormones	FSH/LH TSH PRL	pNEN	Hyperandrogenism Hyperthyroidism ± Gynecomastia	↑ LH, androgens ↑ fT4, T3, TSH ↑ PRL	Normal pituitary MRI Lesion elsewhere (+) Octreoscan
Vasoactive peptides	CGRP Ct	SCLC pNEN Pheochromocytoma	Vasodilation Flushing Hypotension	↑ CT Calcium/ pentagastrin stimulation	(–) Thyroid imaging Lesion elsewhere (+) Octreoscan
Gynecomastia menstrual irregularities	hCG HPL	SCLC pNEN Pheochromocytoma	Gynecomastia Menstrual irregularities Precocious puberty	↑ Androgens ↑ hCG	Normal adrenal Ovarian imaging Lesion elsewhere (+) Octreoscan
Hypertension	Renin	Carcinoid Pheochromocytoma	Malignant Hypertension Hypokalemic alkalosis	↑ Prorenin ↑ Aldosterone	(+) Radiology (+) Octreoscan
Gut hormones	Ghrelin Gastrin VIP GLP-1, 2	pNEN Carcinoid	ZES Diarrhea Hypoglycemia?	↑ Ghrelin ↑ Gastrin ↑ VIP	(+) Radiology (+) Octreoscan (+) Radiology (+) Octreoscan Endoscopy, EUS (+) Radiology (+) Octreoscan

PTH = Parathyroid hormone; PTHrP = parathyroid hormone-related peptide; SCLC = small cell lung carcinoma; TGF = tumor growth factor; IL = interleukin; PG = prostaglandin; DDAVP = desmopressin; MRI = magnetic resonance imaging; MTC = medullary thyroid carcinoma; MIBG = metaiodobenzylguanidine; ADH = vasopressin; ANP = atrial natriuretic peptide; hCG = chorionic gonadotropin; IGF = insulin growth factor; Ct = calcitonin; EUS = endoscopic ultrasound; fT4 = free thyroxine; ZES = Zollinger-Ellison syndrome; GH = growth hormone; FSH = follicle-stimulating hormone; LH = luteinizing hormone; TSH = thyroid-stimulating hormone; ACTH = adrenocorticotropic hormone; CRH = corticotropin-releasing hormone; T3 = triiodothyronine; HPL = human placenta lactogen; CGRP = calcitonin gene-related peptide; GLP = glucagon-like peptide; PRL = prolactin; IPSS = inferior petrosal sinus sampling; N = normal.

[1] Usually negative in poorly differentiated tumors.

with nonspecific markers of NENs [28]. Poorly differentiated lung NENs may also cause PNS, such as Cushing's syndrome, due to ectopic adrenocorticotrophin production or acromegaly due to ectopic growth hormone-releasing hormone secretion; these PNS may also be caused from typical/atypical carcinoids [13, 27]. Thymic NENs are exceedingly rare, accounting for only 2% of all NENs; CS has rarely been described in approximately 2% of cases [29]. Gastric NENs represent up to 23% of all GI-NENs and are classified further into types 1 and 2 that are related to hypergastrinemia in the context of chronic gastritis (type 1) or a gastrin-secreting neoplasm (duodenal or pancreatic, type 2 gastric NENs) in patients with multiple endocrine neoplasia type 1 (MEN1) and Zollinger-Ellison syndrome (ZES), respectively [30]. Although the majority of type 1 gastric NENs are not associated with a functional syndrome, they may occasionally develop an atypical CS due to histamine production. Type 3 gastric NENs are not gastrin related and only rarely develop features of the typical CS; however, 5–10% may develop an atypical CS [31]. Duodenal NENs (d-NENs) are usually small (<1 cm) and are classified further into gastrin- and somatostatin-producing tumors, and nonfunctional d-NENs [31, 32]. Although originally thought to be uncommon, recent findings suggest that they make up 50–88% of sporadic gastrinomas and 70–100% of gastrinoma in MEN1 cases, and rarely (4%) can produce a typical CS [31–33]. Periampullary d-NENs are distinct from other d-NENs, are associated with von Recklinghausen's disease and show somatostatin immunoreactivity, but almost never produce the clinical features of somatostatinoma syndrome [34]. Gastrin-secreting d-NENs along with pancreatic (p)NENs cause the ZES (see below). Appendiceal NENs are mostly localized and the CS has only very rarely been described (<1%), mainly in the rare patients with metastatic disease [7, 35–37]. Colonic and rectal NENs cannot convert tryptophan to serotonin and other metabolites and rarely cause CS (<5%) even in the presence of hepatic metastases [1, 6, 7]. However, these tumors can secrete pancreatic peptide, somatostatin and peptide YY, but rarely cause related syndromes (table 3) [38].

Treatment of the Carcinoid Syndrome and Related Syndromes

As flushing and diarrhea may be associated with particular habits, lifestyle adjustments may be required and patients should be advised to avoid alcohol, spicy foods and strenuous exercise [1]. Surgery constitutes the best therapeutic option for localized tumors or as a debulking procedure along with other cytoreductive techniques for more advanced disease [31]. However, this is not always feasible, although debulking procedures can be used along with medical treatment. SS-analogs effectively reduce hypersecretion-related symptoms in patients with CS, achieving symptomatic improvement in 40–80% of patients and reduction in biochemical markers in 40–60% [31]. As the duration and effects can be limited due to tachyphylaxis or desensitization, these can be managed, at least temporarily, by an increase in dose and/or by

Table 3. Clinical syndromes related to pNENs

Functioning GEP-NENs				
Tumor	Tumor-specific markers/ active peptides	Incidence (new cases/10^6 population/year)	Tumor location	Signs and symptoms
Insulinoma	Fasting insulin Fasting proinsulin C-peptide	1–3	Pancreas (>99%): head, body tail (evenly distributed)	Hypoglycemia, dizziness sweating, tachycardia confusion, seizures
Gastrinoma (ZES)	Fasting and stimulating gastrin	0.5–2	Gastrinoma triangle Duodenum (70%) Pancreas (25%) Other sites (5%)	Gastric acid hypersecretion peptic ulcer, diarrhea esophagitis, epigastric pain
VIPoma	Fasting VIP	0.1	Pancreas: distal pancreas, body and tail mainly (90%); neural, adrenal paraganglionic (10%)	Watery diarrhea, hypokalemia achlorhydria (or acidosis) dehydration
Glucagonoma	Fasting glucagon	0.01–0.1	Pancreas: body and tail, often large and spread outside pancreas	Diabetes mellitus, necrolytic, migratory, erythema, stomatitis, glossitis, angular cheilitis, weight loss
Somatostatinoma	Fasting somatostatin	Rare	Pancreaticoduodenal groove ampullary, periampullary Pancreas (50–60%) Duodenal/jejunal (40–50%)	Gallstones, diabetes mellitus, weight loss, steatorrhea
GHRoma	GHRH	Very rare	Lung mainly (54%) Pancreas (30%) Small intestine (jejunum 7%) Other sites (13%)	Acromegaly (excessive sweating, enlarged facial features, glucose intolerance)
ACTHoma	ACTH or POMC or high-molecular-weight precursor form of ACTH	Rare	Pancreas (4–16% all ectopic Cushing's syndrome)	Cushing's syndrome (weight gain and fatty tissue deposits, striae, easily bruising)
pNEN causing hypercalcemia	PTH-related peptide	Rare	Pancreas	Hypercalcemia, abdominal pain due to hepatic metastases

PTH = Parathyroid hormone; ACTH = adrenocorticotropic hormone; VIP = vasoactive intestinal peptide; GHRH = growth hormone releasing hormone; POMC = pro-opiomelanocortin products.

alternating between the different SS-analogs [31]. Tolerance and efficacy should be tested by initiating therapy with the short-acting SS-analog octreotide before starting long-acting analogs. This treatment is associated with only minor side effects, the most important being steatorrhea, which can be easily managed with pancreatic enzyme replacement. Interferon-α (IFN-α) is given for the same indications as SS-analogs, mainly as a second-line treatment, except for carcinoid crisis; however, this treatment is associated with more severe side effects. Whether the combination of both SS-analogs and IFN-α is more efficacious in ameliorating the symptoms of CS than SS-analogs alone remains to be proven. To prevent a carcinoid crisis, SS-analogs should be administered intravenously during anesthesia or interventional procedures. Acute administration of intravenous octreotide (500 μg in 500 ml saline starting from a 50- to 200-μg/h infusion) has been reported to provide rapid reversal of symptoms of carcinoid crisis, although the current focus is to prevent its development with octreotide prophylaxis. Adrenergic drugs should be avoided as these may cause further release of serotonin and tachykinins [1]. CS-induced diarrhea is not exclusively related to excessive hormonal production, as it may occasionally deteriorate or start following surgical resection mainly in the terminal ileum. In such cases, the diarrhea may be related to bile acid loss and/or increased bacterial contamination of the small intestine with subsequent deconjugation of bile acids, needing treatment with cholestyramine and antibiotics, respectively [1]. Patients with atypical CS due to histamine production should avoid histamine-liberating drugs and when needed be pretreated with SS-analogs, histamine receptor blockage and glucocorticoids. In addition, traditionally used medication such as loperamide and morphine for diarrhea and vitamin B replacement for pellagra are still of value. Telotristat etiprate is an investigational oral agent (currently on a phase III clinical trial) that inhibits tryptophan hydroxylase, the key enzyme responsible for serotonin production. Telotristat administration leads to reduced serotonin production and symptoms of the CS [39]. The multitarget SSA pasireotide has also been used in refractory cases but larger studies are needed to define its precise role. Recent data have shown that subcutaneous pasireotide was effective and generally well tolerated in controlling the symptoms of CS in 27% of patients with advanced NENs refractory or resistant to octreotide LAR therapy [40].

Clinical Syndromes Related to Pancreatic Neuroendocrine Neoplasms

pNENs are relatively rare with an estimated incidence of 0.5–1/100,000; these tumors carry a better prognosis than exocrine tumors but are often metastatic at diagnosis [41]. It was previously thought that the majority of these tumors are functioning but recently there has been a sharp rise of nonfunctioning pNENs, which account for more than 50% of currently diagnosed pNENs [42]. Functioning pNENs are often diagnosed earlier due to hormonal production and this may account for a relatively better prognosis in a subset, such as in insulinomas. A number of distinct clinical syndromes have been attributed to pNENs creating concern regarding the multitude of presenting symptoms (table 3).

Table 4. Currently used biochemical criteria for the diagnosis of endogenous hyperinsulinemia

(1)	Documented blood glucose levels <3.0 mmol/l (<55 mg/dl)
(2)	Concomitant insulin levels ≥3 μU/ml (≥18 pmol/l)
(3)	C-peptide levels ≥0.6 ng/ml (≥0.2 nmol/l)
(4)	Proinsulin levels ≥5 pmol/l
(5)	β-Hydroxybutyrate levels ≤2.7 mmol/l
(6)	Absence of sulfonylurea (metabolites) in the plasma and/or urine

The normal range for fasting serum insulin levels is 14.3–122 pmol/l (2–17 mIU/l). The normal range for fasting C-peptide levels is 0.26– 0.63 nmol/l (0.78–1.89 ng/ml). Normal fasting serum proinsulin levels are 7.9 ± 1.5 pmol/l. β-Hydroxybutyrate levels are measured by an automated kinetic method in samples collected in Vacutainer tubes containing sodium fluoride and potassium oxalate.

Insulinoma

Insulinomas characteristically present between 40 and 50 years of age with an estimated incidence of 1–3/1,000,000/year. These tumors are the most common functioning pNENs and the most common cause of endogenous hyperinsulinemia [43, 44]. Insulinomas are typically small with 30% measuring <1 cm; their relative small size at diagnosis probably reflects their functional status and relatively benign behavior [7, 45]. Insulinomas are characterized by symptoms of neuroglycopenia (headache, lethargy, blurred vision, diplopia and, rarely, seizures) and adrenergic symptoms (tremor, anxiety, palpitations and sweating) [1, 7, 45, 46]. Symptoms of catecholamine excess are not always present and neuroglycopenic symptoms may be the only manifestation of an underlying insulinoma [1, 7, 45, 46]. Hypoglycemic episodes typically occur early in the morning, although postprandial episodes are increasingly being recognized [7, 30, 47]. The mean duration of symptoms at diagnosis is 3 years and a recent increase in body weight is present in the majority of patients [43, 44]. The presence of symptoms/signs of hypoglycemia along with low glucose levels that are relieved with glucose administration constitute the main diagnostic criteria (Whipple's triad) [1, 7]. The diagnosis is substantiated by the finding of unsuppressed insulin levels in the presence of hypoglycemia and in equivocal cases by provoking hypoglycemia with prolonged fasting (up to 72 h; table 4). Almost all insulinomas are located within the pancreas, though aberrant cases have been described in the duodenum, ileum, lung and cervix [1, 7]. In some cases, islet cell hypertrophy and nesidioblastosis, rather than a distinct tumor, may be responsible for the symptoms; in such cases, neuroglycopenic symptoms usually develop within 4 h following meal ingestion [1, 7, 46].

Gastrinoma

Gastrinomas are gastrin-secreting tumors derived from the duodenum or the pancreas causing ZES with an incidence of 0.5–2/1,000,000/year [7, 26, 32]. The majority of gastrinomas arise in the gastrinoma triangle (defined by the duodenum, pancreatic head and hepatoduodenal ligament) and are either sporadic or in association with MEN1 syndrome in up to 25% of cases; MEN1-related gastrinomas are usually small, located in the duodenum and often multifocal [7, 26, 31, 32]. The diagnosis is considered in patients with complicated peptic ulcer disease refractory to treatment with PPIs and *Helicobacter pylori* eradication. Ulceration of the upper GI mucosa develops in 90% of patients and may also involve the distal duodenum and/or jejunum [7, 26, 32]. Ulcers can be single or multiple and are less than 1 cm in diameter; esophageal involvement occurs in 10–60% of patients and is associated with heartburn and dysphagia due to gastroesophageal reflux [7, 26, 32]. Diarrhea develops in up to 70% of cases and can proceed, accompany or follow the ulcer disease while being the only initial symptom in 7–35% of patients [7, 26]. Diarrhea develops as a result of the large amount of gastric acid produced that enters the small bowel inactivating pancreatic enzymes and fat bile acid emulsification and directly damaging the villi of intestinal epithelial cells, causing malabsorption; a secretory component is also present due to diminished water and sodium absorption caused by hypergastrinemia [1, 7, 32]. Other symptoms, such as abdominal pain, nausea/vomiting, weight loss and bleeding, may also be present [7, 26]. In up to 6% of gastrinomas, Cushing's syndrome may develop secondary to ectopic adrenocorticotrophin secretion and carries a worse prognosis [7, 31]. When the gastrinoma is found in the context of MEN1, the trophic effect of prolonged hypergastrinemia on enterochromaffin cells leads to the formation of gastric NEN type 2 in the body and fundus of the stomach. The diagnosis is established in the presence of relevant symptoms after finding high gastrin levels in the absence of PPI administration or documentation of low gastric pH; in equivocal cases, a secretin or calcium stimulation test is used, demonstrating a >200 pg/ml rise in gastrin levels [1].

Glucagonoma

Glucagonomas are rare, slowly growing tumors arising from the alpha cells of the pancreas with an incidence of 0.01–0.1/1,000,000/year [48]. The majority are sporadic but between 5 and 17% may be associated with MEN1 or familial adenomatous polyps [7, 33]. The most common presenting symptoms are weight loss (70–80%), rash (50–80%), diabetes mellitus (75%), cheilosis, stomatitis and diarrhea [1, 7, 32, 49]. The almost universal characteristic rash, necrolytic migratory erythema (NME), is a dermatitis-looking lesion that evolves over 7–14 days, starting as small erythematous papules in the groin extending to the perineum, lower extremities and perioral regions (fig. 2) [1, 7, 31, 32]. Other dermatological manifestations are dystrophic nails, angular cheilitis, atrophic glossitis and buccal mucosal inflammation. Fatty acid, zinc and amino acid deficiency, along with hepatic impairment, may be responsible for the NME as glucagon levels do not correlate with the presence or severity of the rash [7, 33]. Gastrointestinal symptoms (abdominal pains, cramps, anorexia, diarrhea or constipation) may also develop and may be the result of cosecretion of other substances, such as serotonin and VIP. Other common manifestations include psychiatric disorders and a predilection for thromboembolism (up to 30%) [1, 7, 33].

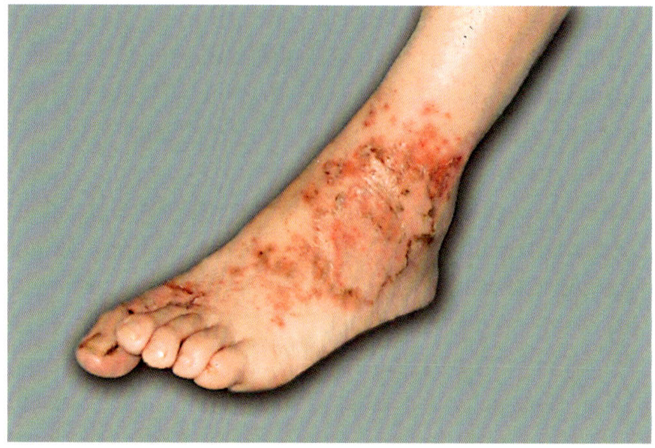

Fig. 2. Dermatosis affecting the lower legs that was shown to be NME in a patient with glucagonoma.

VIPoma (Verner-Morrison Syndrome, Pancreatic Cholera)

VIPoma is a rare pNEN with an estimated incidence about 1/10,000,000/year [32]; approximately 80% of the tumors arise from the pancreas, but they can also be of neural origin, particularly in children, as ganglioneuromas or neuroblastomas [1, 7, 33]. Severe secretory watery diarrhea as a result of excessive VIP secretion that binds to epithelial intestinal cells activating cellular adenyl cyclase occurs in almost all patients; diarrhea can be intermittent in 53% and continuous in 47% of cases [1, 7, 50]. Patients may produce more than 3 liters of stool per day that may be increased to 30 liters/day leading to severe fluid and electrolyte loss with subsequent asthenia, cramps, tetany and cardiac rhythm abnormalities [7, 50]. Severe hypokalemia (<2.5 mmol/l) with hyperchloremic acidosis develops and may be associated with carbohydrate intolerance; facial flushing in up to 20% of patients may be the direct vasodilatory effect of VIP.

Somatostatinoma

Somatostatinomas are rare tumors (1/40,000,000/year) of either the pancreas or small intestine and duodenum [7, 34, 51]. In contrast to other functioning tumors, somatostatinomas exert a relatively low incidence as a hypersecretory syndrome and may be associated with the MEN1 syndrome, von Hippel–Lindau syndromes, neurofibromatosis type 1, gangliocytic paragangliomas and pheochromocytomas [1, 7, 51]. Somatostatin exerts a general inhibitory role on the exo- and endocrine secretions and bowel motility leading to suppression of hormonal secretion and bowel functions and, in approximately 11% of cases, causes hyperglycemia, cholelithiasis and diarrhea due to steatorrhea [7, 51]. These typically occur in pancreatic tumors, whereas duodenal tumors most often present with obstructive symptoms.

Paraneoplastic Syndromes Secondary to Neuroendocrine Tumors

The term paraneoplastic syndrome is used to denote an array of symptom complexes that are manifested systemically as the result of the production of hormones, growth factors, cytokines and/or other substances by tumor cells from tissues not designated to secrete these particular substances [52, 53]. A significant number of these syndromes are caused by the secretory products, mainly peptide hormones, of neurendocrine cells that are widely dispersed throughout the lung, gastrointestinal tract, pancreas, thyroid gland, adrenal medulla, skin, prostate and breast [6, 53]. The pathophysiological mechanisms of PNS caused by NENs are related to the production and secretion of biologically active substances (amines/peptides), cytokines and antibodies against specific autoantigens causing mainly neurological syndromes [54]. Relevant clinical syndromes include the majority of those GEP-NENs that were previously considered as causing rare functional syndromes (table 2). Successful tumor treatment leads to clinical remission of the syndrome, whereas tumor recurrence leads to its reappearance; in parallel, these changes are accompanied by changes in hormonal levels [55, 56].

Treatment of Clinical Syndromes Related to Pancreatic Neuroendocrine Neoplasms

Surgery is the only potentially curative therapeutic strategy in localized disease. Reduction of tumor burden often leads to a reduction in hormone secretion and an improvement in symptom control. Surgical cytoreductive techniques for palliative purposes can be considered in patients with extensive liver metastasis and hormonal syndromes refractory to medical therapy. When surgery is not an option, regional control of liver metastases can be achieved by other cytoreductive techniques and adjuvant systemic therapy [31]. Medical treatment mainly based on SS-analogs has extensively been used to relieve the symptoms attributed to the majority of pNEN-related syndromes.

Insulinoma

These tumors are the least sensitive to SS-analogs, as approximately 50% lack SSTR2 receptors. It is therefore important to look for the presence of these receptors before initiating therapy as in their absence intractable hypoglycemia may develop due to SS-analog-induced suppression of counteractive to hypoglycemia hormones. Diazoxide at doses of 50–300 mg/day (up to 600 mg/day) usually diminishes insulin secretion but may be associated with edema, renal impairment and hirsutism [57]. Verapamil, glucocorticoids and phenytoin have been used, albeit with less efficacy, although the combination of high-dose glucocorticoids and growth hormone has been used in the past for refractory cases [1]. Recently, the mTOR inhibitor everolimus has been shown to substantially reduce hypoglycemic episodes in patients with malignant insulinomas [8]. In addition, the multipotent SS-analog pasireotide that is associated with hyperglycemia could also be a further therapeutic option.

Gastrinoma

The introduction of proton pump inhibitors has markedly improved the symptomatic control of such patients as they can achieve both short- and long-acting gastric acid suppression using doses of omeprazole of 40–80 mg or an equivalent drug. SS-analogs are also efficacious, but PPIs constitute the drugs of choice for symptomatic relief [1]. Recently, gastrin (CCK-B) antagonists have been shown to reduce gastrin-mediated effects; netazepide, an orally administered peripheral CCK-B inhibitor, has been shown to have rapid onset and prolonged duration, leading to gastric acid output suppression [12, 58].

Glucagonoma

SS-analogs improve the clinical manifestations of diabetes and NME, which responds irrespective of alterations in glucagon levels. In such patients, it is also important to correct hypoaminoacidemia and mineral deficiency and administer low-dose heparin to minimize the risk of thrombosis. SS-analogs can also be administered preoperatively [1].

VIPoma

Glucocorticoids have traditionally been used, but they have now been surpassed by SS-analogs which are also effective in the extremely rare somatostatinomas.

Conclusion

NENs of the gastrointestinal system are a heterogeneous group of tumors that have the ability to synthesize and secrete a variety of compounds (peptides and amines) that, when bioactive, can cause distinct clinical syndromes (functioning tumors). Although the presence of such a syndrome may occasionally be life threatening, it can also facilitate the diagnosis and help to identify tumors at an early stage. Small intestinal NENs are the most common causes of CS, which in the majority of cases develops when metastases to the liver have occurred. In contrast, the most common functioning pNENs, insulinomas, may be detected at an early stage, exhibiting a better prognosis. Other common functioning tumors are duodenal and pancreatic gastrinomas causing ZES, and pancreatic glucagonomas, VIPomas and, rarely, somatostatinomas causing relevant syndromes; ectopic secretion of bioactive substances leading to paraneoplastic syndromes are increasingly being recognized. Although curative surgery constitutes the main therapeutic procedure as it can remove the abnormal hormone-secreting tissue, it is rarely feasible and thus medical treatment with SS-analogs is used to alleviate symptoms and improve the quality of life. Evolving targeted therapies are required for a more specific drug effect directed against the relevant compound causing the clinical syndrome.

References

1 Kaltsas GA, Besser GM, Grossman AB: The diagnosis and medical management of advanced neuroendocrine tumors. Endocr Rev 2004;25:458–511.

2 Kanakis G, Kaltsas G: Biochemical markers for gastroenteropancreatic neuroendocrine tumours (GEP-NETs). Best Pract Res Clin Gastroenterol 2012;26: 791–802.

3 Engelbach M, Heerdt S, Görges R, Kunt T, Pfützner A, Forst T, Diefenbach K, Walgenbach S, Beyer J: Is there an ectopic secretion of monomeric calcitonin in the human being? Langenbecks Arch Surg 1998; 383:456–459.

4 Schneider R, Heverhagen AE, Moll R, Bartsch DK, Schlosser K: Differentiation between thyroidal and ectopic calcitonin secretion in patients with coincidental thyroid nodules and pancreatic tumors – a report of two cases. Exp Clin Endocrinol Diabetes 2010;118:520–523.

5 Furrer J, Hättenschwiler A, Komminoth P, Pfammatter T, Wiesli P: Carcinoid syndrome, acromegaly, and hypoglycemia due to an insulin-secreting neuroendocrine tumor of the liver. J Clin Endocrinol Metab 2001;86:2227–2230.

6 Modlin IM, Oberg K, Chung DC, de Herder WW, Thakker RV, Caplin M, Delle Fave G, Kaltsas GA, Krenning EP, Moss SF, Nilsson O, Rindi G, Salazar R, Ruszniewski P, Sundin A: Gastroenteropancreatic neuroendocrine tumours. Lancet Oncol 2008;9:61–72.

7 Caplin ME, Buscombe JR, Hilson AJ, Jones AL, Watkinson AF, Burroughs AK: Carcinoid tumour. Lancet 1998;352:799–805.

8 Kulke MH, Mayer RJ: Carcinoid tumors. N Engl J Med 1999;340:858–868.

9 Maggard MA, O'Connell JB, Ko CY: Updated population-based review of carcinoid tumors. Ann Surg 2004;240:117–122.

10 Quaedvlieg PF, Visser O, Lamers CB, Janssen-Heijen ML, Taal BG: Epidemiology and survival in patients with carcinoid disease in the Netherlands: an epidemiological study with 2391 patients. Ann Oncol 2001;12:1295–1300.

11 Pape UF, Berndt U, Müller-Nordhorn J, Böhmig M, Roll S, Koch M, Willich SN, Wiedenmann B: Prognostic factors of long-term outcome in gastroenteropancreatic neuroendocrine tumours. Endocr Relat Cancer 2008;15:1083–1097.

12 Ahmed A, Turner G, King B, Jones L, Culliford D, McCance D, Ardill J, Johnston BT, Poston G, Rees M, Buxton-Thomas M, Caplin M, Ramage JK: Midgut neuroendocrine tumours with liver metastases: results of the UKINETS study. Endocr Relat Cancer 2009;16:885–894.

13 O'Toole D, Grossman A, Gross D, Delle Fave G, Barkmanova J, O'Connor J, Pape UF, Plöckinger U, Mallorca Consensus Conference Participants, European Neuroendocrine Tumor Society: ENETS consensus guidelines for the standards of care in neuroendocrine tumors: biochemical markers. Neuroendocrinology 2009;90:194–202.

14 Oberg K: Neuroendocrine gastrointestinal tumors – a condensed overview of diagnosis and treatment. Ann Oncol 1999;10(suppl 2):S3–S8.

15 Jann H, Roll S, Couvelard A, Hentic O, Pavel M, Müller-Nordhorn J, Koch M, Röcken C, Rindi G, Ruszniewski P, Wiedenmann B, Pape UF: Neuroendocrine tumors of midgut and hindgut origin: tumor-node-metastasis classification determines clinical outcome. Cancer 2011;117:3332–3341.

16 Ardill JE, Erikkson B: The importance of the measurement of circulating markers in patients with neuroendocrine tumours of the pancreas and gut. Endocr Relat Cancer 2003;10:459–462.

17 Arnold R, Wilke A, Rinke A, Mayer C, Kann PH, Klose KJ, Scherag A, Hahmann M, Müller HH, Barth P: Plasma chromogranin A as marker for survival in patients with metastatic endocrine gastroenteropancreatic tumors. Clin Gastroenterol Hepatol 2008;6: 820–827.

18 Papadogias D, Makras P, Kossivakis K, Kontogeorgos G, Piaditis G, Kaltsas G: Carcinoid syndrome and carcinoid crisis secondary to a metastatic carcinoid tumour of the lung: a therapeutic challenge. Eur J Gastroenterol Hepatol 2007;19:1154–1159.

19 Bhattacharyya S, Toumpanakis C, Chilkunda D, Caplin ME, Davar J: Risk factors for the development and progression of carcinoid heart disease. Am J Cardiol 2011;107:1221–1226.

20 Akerström G, Falconi M, Kianmanesh R, Ruszniewski P, Plöckinger U, Mallorca Consensus Conference participants, European Neuroendocrine Tumor Society: ENETS consensus guidelines for the standards of care in neuroendocrine tumors: pre- and perioperative therapy in patients with neuroendocrine tumors. Neuroendocrinology 2009;90:203–208.

21 Bhattacharyya S, Toumpanakis C, Burke M, Taylor AM, Caplin ME, Davar J: Features of carcinoid heart disease identified by 2- and 3-dimensional echocardiography and cardiac MRI. Circ Cardiovasc Imaging 2010;3:103–111.

22 Zuetenhorst JM, Korse CM, Bonfrer JM, Bakker RH, Taal BG: Role of natriuretic peptides in the diagnosis and treatment of patients with carcinoid heart disease. Br J Cancer 2004;90:2073–2079.

23 Plöckinger U, Gustafsson B, Ivan D, Szpak W, Davar J, Mallorca Consensus Conference participants, European Neuroendocrine Tumor Society: ENETS consensus guidelines for the standards of care in neuroendocrine tumors: echocardiography. Neuroendocrinology 2009;90:190–193.
24 Castillo JG, Filsoufi F, Rahmanian PB, Anyanwu A, Zacks JS, Warner RR, Adams DH: Early and late results of valvular surgery for carcinoid heart disease. J Am Coll Cardiol 2008;51:1507–1509.
25 Mokhles P, van Herwerden LA, de Jong PL, de Herder WW, Siregar S, Constantinescu AA, van Domburg RT, Roos-Hesselink JW: Carcinoid heart disease: outcomes after surgical valve replacement. Eur J Cardiothorac Surg 2012;41:1278–1283.
26 Modlin IM, Kidd M, Latich I, Zikusoka MN, Shapiro MD: Current status of gastrointestinal carcinoids. Gastroenterology 2005;128:1717–1751.
27 Vinik AI, Silva MP, Woltering EA, Go VL, Warner R, Caplin M: Biochemical testing for neuroendocrine tumors. Pancreas 2009;38:876–889.
28 Oberg K, Hellman P, Kwekkeboom D, Jelic S, ESMO Guidelines Working Group: Neuroendocrine bronchial and thymic tumours: ESMO Clinical Practice Guidelines for diagnosis, treatment and follow-up. Ann Oncol 2010;21(suppl 5):v220–v222.
29 Hage R, de la Riviere AB, Seldenrijk CA, van den Bosch JM: Update in pulmonary carcinoid tumors: a review article. Ann Surg Oncol 2003;10:697–704.
30 Norton JA, Melcher ML, Gibril F, Jensen RT: Gastric carcinoid tumors in multiple endocrine neoplasia-1 patients with Zollinger-Ellison syndrome can be symptomatic, demonstrate aggressive growth, and require surgical treatment. Surgery 2004;136:1267–1274.
31 Delle Fave G, Kwekkeboom DJ, van Cutsem E, Rindi G, Kos-Kudla B, Knigge U, Sasano H, Tomassetti P, Salazar R, Ruszniewski P, Barcelona Consensus Conference participants: ENETS consensus guidelines for the management of patients with gastroduodenal neoplasms. Neuroendocrinology 2012;95:74–87.
32 Klöppel G, Perren A, Heitz PU: The gastroenteropancreatic neuroendocrine cell system and its tumors: the WHO classification. Ann NY Acad Sci 2004;1014:13–27.
33 Jensen RT, Niederle B, Mitry E, Ramage JK, Steinmuller T, Lewington V, Scarpa A, Sundin A, Perren A, Gross D, O'Connor JM, Pauwels S, Kloppel G, Frascati Consensus Conference, European Neuroendocrine Tumor Society: Gastrinoma (duodenal and pancreatic). Neuroendocrinology 2006;84:173–182.
34 Green BT, Rockey DC: Duodenal somatostatinoma presenting with complete somatostatinoma syndrome. J Clin Gastroenterol 2001;33:415–417.
35 Yesner R: Small cell tumors of the lung. Am J Surg Pathol 1983;7:775–785.
36 Groth SS, Virnig BA, Al-Refaie WB, Jarosek SL, Jensen EH, Tuttle TM: Appendiceal carcinoid tumors: predictors of lymph node metastasis and the impact of right hemicolectomy on survival. J Surg Oncol 2011;103:39–45.
37 Stinner B, Rothmund M: Neuroendocrine tumours (carcinoids) of the appendix. Best Pract Res Clin Gastroenterol 2005;19:729–738.
38 Oberg K: Circulating biomarkers in gastroenteropancreatic neuroendocrine tumours. Endocr Relat Cancer 2011;18(suppl 1):S17–S25.
39 Margolis KG, Stevanovic K, Li Z, Yang QM, Oravecz T, Zambrowicz B, Jhaver KG, Diacou A, Gershon MD: Pharmacological reduction of mucosal but not neuronal serotonin opposes inflammation in mouse intestine. Gut 2014;63:928–937.
40 Kvols LK, Oberg KE, O'Dorisio TM, Mohideen P, de Herder WW, Arnold R, Hu K, Zhang Y, Hughes G, Anthony L, Wiedenmann B: Pasireotide (SOM230) shows efficacy and tolerability in the treatment of patients with advanced neuroendocrine tumors refractory or resistant to octreotide LAR: results from a phase II study. Endocr Relat Cancer 2012;19:657–666.
41 Ekeblad S, Skogseid B, Dunder K, Oberg K, Eriksson B: Prognostic factors and survival in 324 patients with pancreatic endocrine tumor treated at a single institution. Clin Cancer Res 2008;14:7798–7803.
42 Bettini R, Boninsegna L, Mantovani W, Capelli P, Bassi C, Pederzoli P, Delle Fave GF, Panzuto F, Scarpa A, Falconi M: Prognostic factors at diagnosis and value of WHO classification in a mono-institutional series of 180 non-functioning pancreatic endocrine tumours. Ann Oncol 2008;19:903–908.
43 Kulke MH, Anthony LB, Bushnell DL, de Herder WW, Goldsmith SJ, Klimstra DS, Marx SJ, Pasieka JL, Pommier RF, Yao JC, Jensen RT, North American Neuroendocrine Tumor Society (NANETS): Treatment guidelines: well-differentiated neuroendocrine tumors of the stomach and pancreas. Pancreas 2010; 39:735–752.
44 Ekeblad S: Islet cell tumours. Adv Exp Med Biol 2010;654:771–789.
45 Niederle MB, Hackl M, Kaserer K, Niederle B: Gastroenteropancreatic neuroendocrine tumours: the current incidence and staging based on the WHO and European Neuroendocrine Tumour Society classification: an analysis based on prospectively collected parameters. Endocr Relat Cancer 2010;17: 909–918.
46 Corbetta S, Peracchi M, Cappiello V, Lania A, Lauri E, Vago L, Beck-Peccoz P, Spada A: Circulating ghrelin levels in patients with pancreatic and gastrointestinal neuroendocrine tumors: identification of one pancreatic ghrelinoma. J Clin Endocrinol Metab 2003;88:3117–3120.

47 Tsolakis AV, Portela-Gomes GM, Stridsberg M, Grimelius L, Sundin A, Eriksson BK, Oberg KE, Janson ET: Malignant gastric ghrelinoma with hyperghrelinemia. J Clin Endocrinol Metab 2004;89:3739–3744.
48 Chastain MA: The glucagonoma syndrome: a review of its features and discussion of new perspectives. Am J Med Sci 2001;321:306–320.
49 Metz DC, Jensen RT: Gastrointestinal neuroendocrine tumors: pancreatic endocrine tumors. Gastroenterology 2008;135:1469–1492.
50 Levy-Bohbot N, Merle C, Goudet P, Delemer B, Calender A, Jolly D, Thiefin G, Cadiot G, Groupe des Tumeurs Endocrines: Prevalence, characteristics and prognosis of MEN 1-associated glucagonomas, VIPomas, and somatostatinomas: study from the GTE (Groupe des Tumeurs Endocrines) registry. Gastroenterol Clin Biol 2004;28:1075–1081.
51 Garbrecht N, Anlauf M, Schmitt A, Henopp T, Sipos B, Raffel A, Eisenberger CF, Knoefel WT, Pavel M, Fottner C, Musholt TJ, Rinke A, Arnold R, Berndt U, Plöckinger U, Wiedenmann B, Moch H, Heitz PU, Komminoth P, Perren A, Klöppel G: Somatostatin-producing neuroendocrine tumors of the duodenum and pancreas: incidence, types, biological behavior, association with inherited syndromes, and functional activity. Endocr Relat Cancer 2008;15:229–241.
52 Baylin SB, Mendelsohn G: Ectopic (inappropriate) hormone production by tumors: mechanisms involved and the biological and clinical implications. Endocr Rev 1980;1:45–77.
53 Agarwala SS: Paraneoplastic syndromes. Med Clin North Am 1996;80:173–184.
54 Kaltsas G, Androulakis II, de Herder WW, Grossman AB: Paraneoplastic syndromes secondary to neuroendocrine tumours. Endocr Relat Cancer 2010;17:R173–R193.
55 Bollanti L, Riondino G, Strollo F: Endocrine paraneoplastic syndromes with special reference to the elderly. Endocrine 2001;14:151–157.
56 Keffer JH: Endocrinopathy and ectopic hormones in malignancy. Hematol Oncol Clin North Am 1996;10:811–823.
57 Jensen RT, Cadiot G, Brandi ML, de Herder WW, Kaltsas G, Komminoth P, Scoazec JY, Salazar R, Sauvanet A, Kianmanesh R: Barcelona Consensus Conference participants ENETS consensus guidelines for the management of patients with digestive neuroendocrine neoplasms: functional pancreatic endocrine tumor syndromes. Neuroendocrinology 2012;95:98–119.
58 Gustafsson BI, Kidd M, Modlin IM: Neuroendocrine tumors of the diffuse neuroendocrine system. Curr Opin Oncol 2008;20:1–12.

Georgios Boutzios
Endocrine Unit, Department of Pathophysiology
National University of Athens, Mikras Asias 75
GR–11527 Athens (Greece)
E-Mail gboutzios@gmail.com

Papotti M, de Herder WW (eds): Neuroendocrine Tumors: A Multidisciplinary Approach.
Front Horm Res. Basel, Karger, 2015, vol 44, pp 58–72 (DOI: 10.1159/000382056)

Radiological Imaging: Computed Tomography, Magnetic Resonance Imaging and Ultrasonography

Anders Sundin[a] · Mark Wills[b] · Andrea Rockall[c]

[a]Department of Radiology, Section for Molecular Imaging, Uppsala University Hospital, Uppsala, Sweden; [b]Salisbury NHS Foundation Trust, Salisbury, Wiltshire; [c]Department of Radiology, Imperial College Healthcare NHS Trust, London, UK

Abstract

Neuroendocrine tumor (NET) imaging is generally performed by a combination of radiological and functional methods. Conventional radiological imaging of morphology (anatomy) is usually performed by computed tomography (CT), magnetic resonance imaging (MRI) and ultrasound, whereas functional imaging of somatostatin receptor expression generally utilizes scintigraphy, but recently also positron emission tomography (PET). Because of the large variations in tumor characteristics (for example primary location, presence or absence of hormonal production, proliferation and metastatic spread) and disease presentation, the imaging requirements in different patients are very diverse. Imaging also needs to be adapted according to the imaging application in the individual patient (tumor localization, staging, detection of recurrent disease, monitoring of therapy). Familiarity with the contrast-enhancement technique for CT and MRI is important in the interpretation and understanding of the radiological findings. The choice of the optimal imaging techniques also needs to be considered in the light of the department's local availability and expertise. In this review, methodological aspects of radiological imaging are described, imaging requirements for various types of NETs are discussed, and typical image findings are illustrated.

Neuroendocrine tumors (NETs) as a group show large variations in several aspects. Some give rise to hormonal symptoms ('functioning') and others do not ('nonfunctioning'), although increased hormonal activity may be detected biochemically. Most NETs have low proliferation with a low ki-67 and grow slowly (G1 NETs; ki-67 up to 2%) whereas others are more clinically aggressive high-grade tumors (G3 neuroendocrine carcinomas; ki-67 >20%) and some show an intermediate proliferation (G2 NETs; ki-67 3–20%). Depending on the primary location, the NET may also show site-specific symptoms. Because of these variations, NET patients present at very different tumor stages, although more than 50% show metastatic disease at diagnosis. Patients with functioning NETs, however, tend to present earlier than those with nonfunctioning NETs. Consequently, the imaging requirements are very diverse, depending on the presentation of the disease, and need to be adapted for the individual patient. For those with clinically disseminated disease, computed tomography (CT) of the chest and abdomen in combination with somatostatin receptor imaging, usually by scintigraphy using OctreoScan™, is usually sufficient [1]. Localization of a functioning tumor producing severe hormonal symptoms may, by contrast, require the use of several imaging techniques, as the lesion may be very small in size. For some NETs, local radiological staging is of importance before surgery, for example to visualize the relation between a pancreatic NET (pNET) and the adjacent vessels, pancreatic duct and the external bile ducts. A combination of radiological and nuclear medicine imaging is used for surveillance of NET patients who have undergone surgical resection with curative intent in order to diagnose recurrent disease, and to monitor systemic therapy and locoregional ablative procedures.

Imaging Techniques

Computed Tomography

CT has developed to constitute one of the main radiological imaging techniques besides conventional radiography of bone and chest. With current spiral CT (helical CT) systems, applying multidetector technology (MDCT), usually 64 or more parallel detector rows are used to produce hundreds of 0.5- to 1-mm transversal sections per second. The fast scanning technique minimizes the risk of breathing artefacts and the chest and abdomen may be examined during one breath hold. The transverse images are routinely reformatted in the coronal and sagittal planes to facilitate the image reading. Three-dimensional maximum intensity projection images and volume rendering technique reformatted images may also be produced to assist in establishing vascular anatomy and the relation between tumors and adjacent structures and tissues [1].

The fast MDCT scanners also allow for better use of intravenous iodine-based contrast media, which is of utmost importance to visualize various types of NET lesions. The contrast-enhancement technique to visualize liver metastases is based on the fact that the tumor blood supply exclusively relies on the hepatic artery, whereas the blood to the normal liver parenchyma is mainly delivered by the portal vein (some 75%) and only partly (approximately 25%) by the hepatic artery. A precontrast examination of the liver and pancreas is usually performed because calcifications are more easily detected and occasionally liver metastases may be best visualized in the native examination. NETs and NET metastases are more commonly hypervascular compared to cancers in general oncology. Therefore, it is important to examine the liver and pancreas in the late arterial phase (portal-venous inflow phase). In this phase, the contrast-mixed blood has been ejected from the left ventricle into the aorta and has reached the small arterial branches to enhance hypervascular lesions in the liver. At this time point, very little of the contrast medium has reached the normal liver parenchyma through the hepatic artery and hypervascular contrast-enhancing metastases appear bright against the virtually unenhanced dark normal liver. Later, approximately 60–90 s from the start of the injection, the contrast-mixed blood is delivered to the normal liver parenchyma through the portal vein. In this phase, the venous (portal-venous) contrast-enhancement phase, hypovascular metastases are best depicted and appear hypoattenuating (dark) against the contrast-enhanced (bright) normal liver parenchyma [1]. Rarely, a dedicated CT angiography (early arterial contrast-enhancement phase) is needed because the arterial anatomy is usually sufficiently displayed in the late arterial phase. For the few patients in whom CT angiography is of essence, this is usually performed preoperatively as a separate examination. Hypervascular pNETs are generally also well displayed in the late arterial phase.

Magnetic Resonance Imaging

Magnetic resonance imaging (MRI) has the advantage of not using any ionizing radiation, which makes it an investigation of choice in patients who require longer-term follow-up or screening. However, the most widely used indication for MRI is in performing a focused examination for problem solving. Dedicated high-spatial resolution sequences are used for the detection of pNETs or liver metastases. More recently, whole-body MRI techniques have allowed the possibility of monitoring the full extent of disease, as well as being used in screening at-risk families.

For the detection of pNETs, high-resolution images through the pancreas are required to ensure optimal sensitivity. Patients are fasted for 4–6 h prior to the examination. Sequences should include axial T1 with and without fat saturation, T2 (with optional T2 with fat saturation), diffusion-weighted imaging (DWI) and axial three-dimensional volumetric dynamic contrast-enhanced T1 fat-saturated gradient echo sequence. The addition of DWI to the T2 image, with or without fusion of images, has been shown to improve the detection rate of small lesions [2].

MRI of a small bowel primary NET involves adequate distension of the bowel, either by ingestion of oral fluid (enterography) or by infusion of fluid through a naso-jejunal tube (enteroclysis), together with the use of an antispasmolytic agent. MR enteroclysis is the preferred technique for the identification of a small bowel mass lesion [3]. Overall, the best sequence for demonstrating the primary bowel NET has been reported to be postgadolinium T1 with fat saturation [4].

Recent studies have reported that MRI has 87–99% sensitivity for the detection of hepatic NET metastases [5, 6]. The MRI technique for the detection of metastases from NETs should include conventional T1- and T2-weighted sequences followed by contrast-enhanced sequences ideally using a dynamic acquisition to allow for evaluation of arterial and portal venous phase images. T1-weighted imaging with both in-phase and opposed-phase imaging is recommended in order to allow for differentiation between areas of focal fatty change and metastatic deposits. T2-weighted imaging with fat suppression typically provides greater lesion conspicuity than a T2-weighted sequence without fat suppression. DWI provides a high sensitivity for detection of focal liver lesions and the presence of restricted water diffusion, with high signal intensity on high b value images and corresponding low signal intensity on the apparent diffusion coefficient (ADC) map, may help to characterize liver lesions, as well as to evaluate the response to treatment, but further research is ongoing [7]. This group used three b values: 0, 50 and 800.

MRI for bone imaging is performed in selected patients and may include the spine or a specific bone region for problem solving, or may be performed as a whole-body scan to evaluate the full extent of disease. Suggested sequences include T1 and STIR images and DWI (b values of 0 and 600 are suggested) [8].

Ultrasonography

Ultrasonography (US) is generally performed by using a hand-held transducer that emits high-frequency (MHz) sound waves. Thus, there is no radiation exposure of the patient. These sound echoes are reflected by the tissues and picked up by the transducer, and are computed to form images. Air and bone cause 'total reflection' of the sound waves and, therefore, US cannot be used for examination of the lungs or tissues shielded by bone (e.g. the brain). Low-frequency transducers (approximately 3 MHz) are well suited for examination of the abdomen because of good penetration, but suffer from lower spatial resolution. Conversely, high frequency transducers (8–10 MHz) are best suited for high-spatial resolution examination of superficial structures (e.g. the thyroid) but the penetration is poor. The abdomen of thin adults and children can be examined with high-frequency transducers, but large patients are less well suited for examination of the abdomen by US, and CT is preferred instead.

US can also be performed during intravenous contrast-enhancement (CEUS) using micro bubbles and allows for the detection of very small (<0.5 cm) liver metastases. Equivocal liver lesions at CT and MRI may be characterized by dynamic CEUS based on the tumors' in- and outflow pattern of the contrast medium [9].

When the patient presents with NET disease, the initial diagnosis of liver metastases is often performed by US and the method is well suited to guide the biopsy needle to acquire a Tru-Cut biopsy specimen for histopathological examination. This is usually performed quicker and more easily than by CT which is, however, the method of choice for intrathoracic biopsies because of the inherent methodological restrictions of US in the thorax, as described above.

In order to decrease the radiation dose in young patients who undergo repeated CT examinations for surveillance, contrast-enhanced US every second follow-up can be considered when MRI is not available. Contrast-enhanced US as a part of the imaging surveillance may also be advantageous because new liver metastases may, in some patients, be earlier and better depicted by US than by CT. In occasional patients, the liver lesions may actually be clearly visible by US, but not at all seen by CT. Some drawbacks of US for surveillance and therapy monitoring are that examination of the whole abdomen is usually time consuming and in metastatic disease with a bulky liver it may be difficult to achieve an appropriate overview to accurately assess the liver tumor load. Consequently, US is not the standard method for therapy monitoring.

Endoscopic US, Intraoperative US

Endoscopic US (EUS) is used to evaluate gastric and duodenal NETs in relation to the stomach/bowel wall and is the best method to diagnose pNETs [10, 11]. The regional lymph nodes in the close vicinity of the tumor may also be assessed. Despite these advantages, the imaging work-up to diagnose a small pNET is usually initiated by using other methods, such as CT and MRI, due to the somewhat limited availability of EUS. EUS of the pancreas is, however, recommended preoperatively and is especially important in patients with MEN1 syndrome in whom several pNETs are generally present. In addition to tumor depiction, the relation between the pNET/pNETs and the pancreatic duct and the main bile duct needs to be evaluated. At preoperative or intraoperative US, the transducer is placed directly on the surface of the organ (liver, pancreas) to increase the image resolution, and it is mandatory to facilitate surgical resection of a pNET and of liver metastases.

For rectal NETs, local tumor staging and evaluation of regional lymph nodes is generally performed by EUS or MRI, depending on the local expertise. Biopsies may be guided by EUS, performing either fine-needle aspiration for cytology or Tru-Cut biopsy for histopathological examination.

Imaging Findings

Gastric and Duodenal NETs

Endoscopy and EUS is usually sufficient for the diagnosis and monitoring of gastric NETs type I and II and for duodenal NETs. Gastric NETs type III are usually large at diagnosis and CT/MRI is needed to assess the extension of the tumor outside the stomach and for staging of regional and distant metastases (fig. 1).

Pancreatic NETs

Generally, functioning pNETs are diagnosed at an earlier stage because the hormonal symptoms bring the patient to the doctor and the tumors are therefore usually smaller at presentation, for example insulinomas. Nonfunctioning pNETs, by contrast,

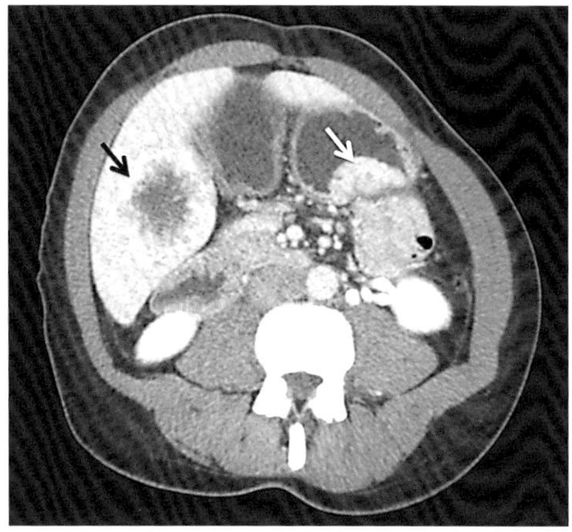

Fig. 1. Contrast-enhanced transverse CT image (late arterial phase) showing a gastric NET type III (white arrow) and a hypervascular liver metastasis (black arrow) with a hypovascular necrotic center.

typically give rise to local symptoms with abdominal discomfort and pain when the tumors become larger.

Diagnosis of a functioning pNET can be challenging because the tumor is usually small despite pronounced hormonal symptoms. The superiority of EUS for the diagnosis of pNETs is well documented in the literature, but CT and MRI are usually more widely available. EUS is therefore usually performed later in the imaging sequence than CT and/or MRI, which are frequently applied as the first step in the diagnostic work-up. It is important to describe the relation of the pNET relative to the pancreatic duct and the common bile duct in the radiological report since this has an impact on surgical planning – tumor enucleation versus pancreatic resection – and magnetic resonance cholangiopancreatography or EUS are preferred for this evaluation.

Calcifications are not uncommon in small pNETs and are usually seen more frequently in the larger tumors. They are best visualized by CT [12] (fig. 2). Pancreatic NETs are typically hypervascular and at CT appear as contrast-enhancing lesions, although there are exceptions to this rule (fig. 2). Consequently, most pNETs are usually best visualized in the late arterial contrast-enhancement phase. Gastrinomas are interesting among pNETs because they are frequently located outside the pancreas and may be found in the duodenum, stomach and hepatoduodenal ligament. Glucagonomas and the VIPomas are less frequent and patients usually present with larger tumors and disseminated disease. Regional lymph node metastases are typically hypervascular and are most frequent in the peripancreatic area and adjacent to the descending aorta and inferior vena cava (fig. 3).

On MRI, a pNET typically appears hypointense on T1 and T1 fat-saturated images and either iso- or hyperintense on T2-weighted images in relation to the adjacent pancreas. Following contrast administration, there is some variability in enhancement patterns, which may be homogeneously hyperintense (the most common pattern;

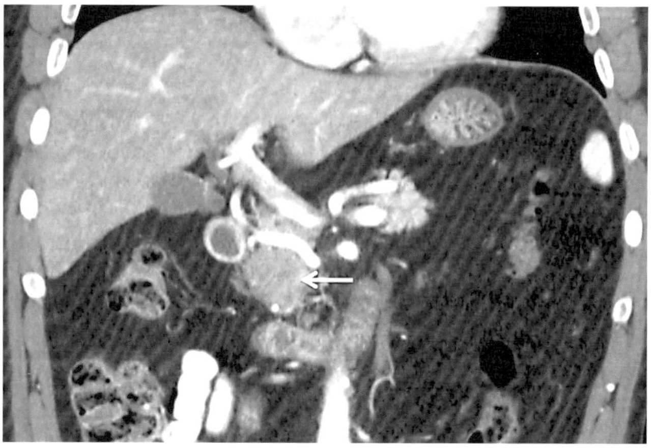

Fig. 2. Contrast-enhanced coronally reformatted CT image (late arterial phase) showing a hypovascular pNET (arrow) with calcification in its caudal part. Although most pNETs are hypervascular, the finding of a hypovascular pNET is fairly common.

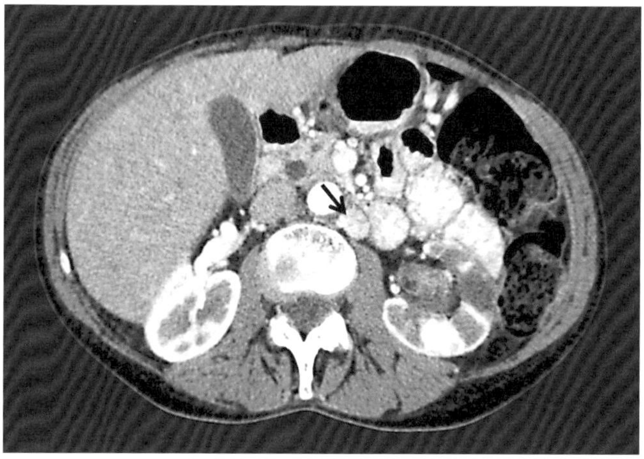

Fig. 3. Contrast-enhanced transversal CT image (late arterial phase) showing a paraaortic lymph node metastasis (arrow) from a pNET.

fig. 4) or may be peripherally hyperintense by centrally isointense [13, 14]. Tumors that contain a high collagen or fibrous tissue content may return a low signal intensity on T2-weighted images, but this is rare. In one study, benign pNETs were found to be more typically round or ovoid in shape, less hypovascular on arterial phase and have a significantly higher ADC than nonbenign lesions [15]. In addition, no benign lesion was found to cause pancreatic duct dilatation. Morphological features of malignant change in nonfunctioning pNETs include an irregular margin, absence of a cleavage plane with the main pancreatic duct, vascular encasement and metastatic sites [13]. Recent studies have reported high diagnostic performances of MRI, with sensitivities of 74–94% and specificities of 78–100% [16]. Sensitivity decreases for extrapancreatic lesions, small lesions and multiple tumors, as in patients with MEN. All of these features make detection more difficult.

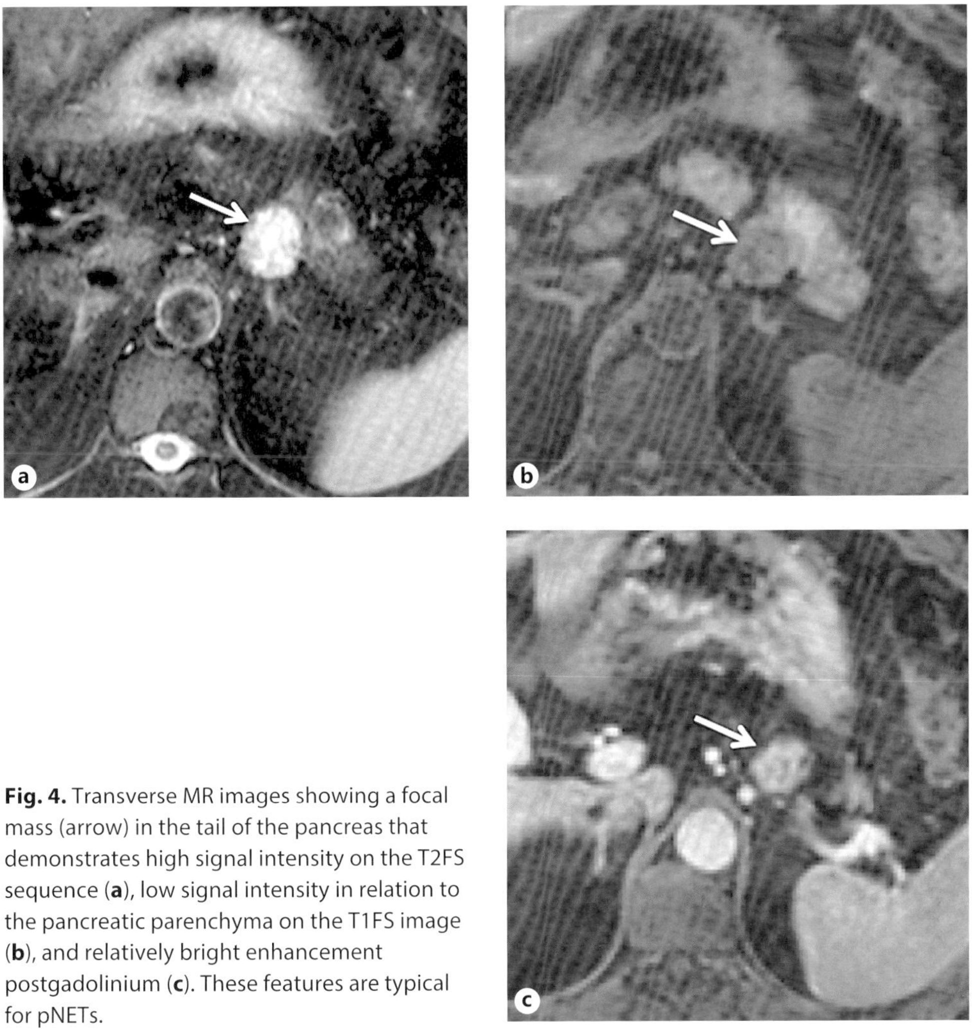

Fig. 4. Transverse MR images showing a focal mass (arrow) in the tail of the pancreas that demonstrates high signal intensity on the T2FS sequence (**a**), low signal intensity in relation to the pancreatic parenchyma on the T1FS image (**b**), and relatively bright enhancement postgadolinium (**c**). These features are typical for pNETs.

Small Bowel NETs

Primary small bowel NETs may not be seen on CT/MRI due to their small size. The lesions may be inconspicuous against the small bowel or the ascending/transverse colon from which it arises. There may be multiple primary sites. On MRI, small bowel lesions are usually hypointense on T1 and hyperintense on T2, and the best sequence for demonstrating the primary tumor has been reported to be the postgadolinium T1-weighted fat-suppressed image. MR enteroclysis has been reported to have a sensitivity of 67–94% [4, 17]. The tumor may appear as a smooth submucosal nodular mass arising from the bowel wall or as regional uniform bowel wall thickening. The primary tumor enhances moderately to intensely following gadolinium administration.

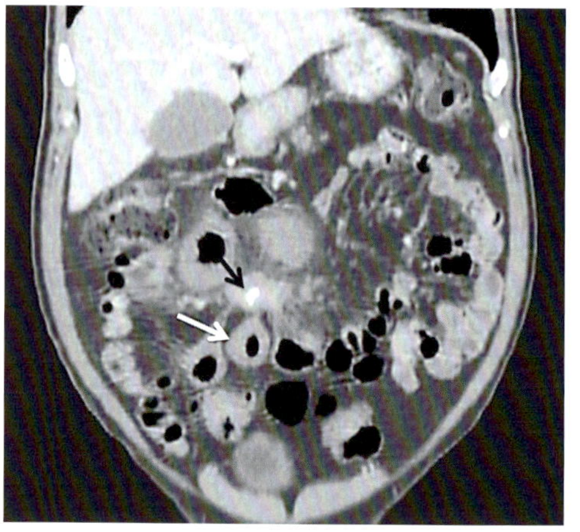

Fig. 5. Contrast-enhanced coronally reformatted CT image (venous phase) showing a mesenteric metastasis (black arrow) from a small bowel NET with typical calcifications and surrounding desmoplastic reaction creating the 'spoke wheel' pattern. This fibrosis has compromised the mesenteric vessels, leading to venous bowel ischemia with thickening of the bowel wall (white arrow).

A mesenteric metastasis from a small bowel NET is common (40–70%) and it is logical to describe its appearance in this paragraph in connection with that of the primary lesion(s). In most cases, a mesenteric small bowel NET metastasis shows typical image characteristics: mainly located to the right of the midline in the lower abdomen since the tumor is more frequently located in the distal ileum, often with course calcifications and a 'spoke-wheel' appearance, with radiating strands of soft-tissue density (fig. 5) because of mesenteric fibrosis that occurs secondary to the production of hormonally active substances (such as serotonin) [4, 18]. This so-called desmoplastic reaction may cause kinking of the small bowel and the mesenteric veins and lead to bowel obstruction and/or venous bowel ischemia that is fairly frequently the reason for the patient to present with his/her disease at the emergency department. A radiological sign of intestinal ischemia is a thickening of the small bowel wall (fig. 5).

A similar appearance is found on MRI (fig. 6). Mesenteric masses are typically isointense to muscle on T1 and T2 images and may show limited to marked gadolinium enhancement [17]. Because the risk of future bowel complications, patients with disseminated disease are considered for surgery with bowel resection of the primary tumor/tumors and of the mesenteric metastases, where feasible. Before surgery, CT is helpful to evaluate the extent of encasement and kinking of the mesenteric vessels by the mesenteric metastases and the radiological report needs to define the vascular anatomy and the number of arterial branches from the superior artery and number of tributaries to the superior mesenteric vein, proximal to the mesenteric metastasis/metastases.

Appendiceal NETs

Appendiceal NETs are usually incidental findings at surgery and are very rarely a radiological diagnosis. They may for instance be found at appendectomy because of appendicitis, or at elective abdominal surgery. An appendiceal NET may sometimes be an unexpected finding at histopathological examination of the resected appendix.

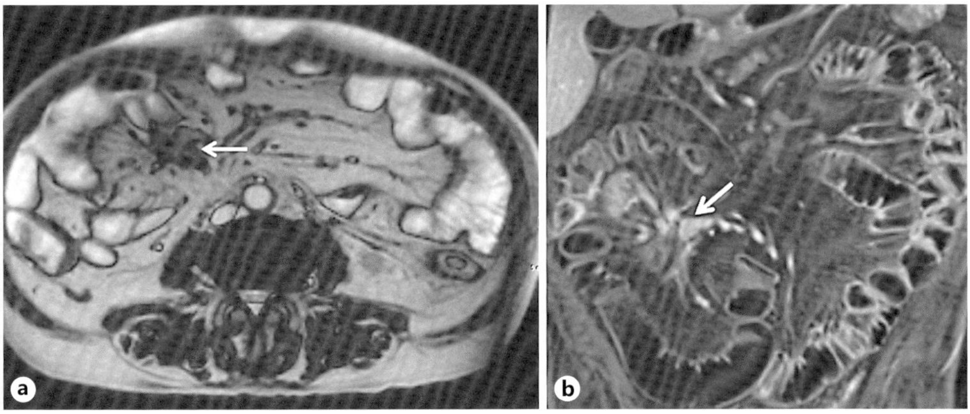

Fig. 6. A mesenteric mass (arrow) secondary to a small bowel NET demonstrates relatively low signal intensity on a T2-weighted transverse MR image (**a**) and some enhancement postgadolinium in the coronal MR image (**b**). Note the 'spoke wheel' configuration on the coronal image due to fibrotic indrawing of the mesentery. The patient drank water prior to the MRI in order to distend the small bowel loops to provide the best technical image for detecting the primary tumor.

Colonic NETs

Colonic NETs produce symptoms similar to colonic cancer. The patient often presents with a significant symptomatic mass, but sometimes a small colonic NET may be an endoscopic finding. Small rectal polyps are usually diagnosed at endoscopy whereas larger rectal NETs present similarly to rectal cancer and local staging and detection of regional lymph node metastases is performed by MRI or EUS, depending on the local routine and expertise. With colorectal NETs the whole colon needs to be examined for synchronous tumors.

Liver Metastases

At histology, the most common site of metastatic disease is nodal [19]. However, on imaging, the most frequent site of metastatic disease is the liver, followed by bone and lung [6].

On CT, the late arterial contrast-enhancement phase is best suited to visualize hypervascular liver metastases, which appear as typically rounded contrast-enhancing (bright) lesions in the nonenhanced (dark) normal liver parenchyma [20] (fig. 7a). Hypovascular metastases are also fairly common and appear in the venous (portal-venous) contrast-enhancement phase as a low-attenuating (dark) lesion in the contrast-enhanced (bright) normal liver parenchyma (fig. 7b). Notably, the same patient may harbor both types of liver metastases.

On MR imaging, the majority of NET liver metastases are of low signal intensity on T1-weighted imaging, and of high signal intensity on T2-weighted imaging. Following contrast administration, over 90% of lesions are hypervascular, typically demonstrating avid contrast enhancement in the arterial phase, and a proportion of these

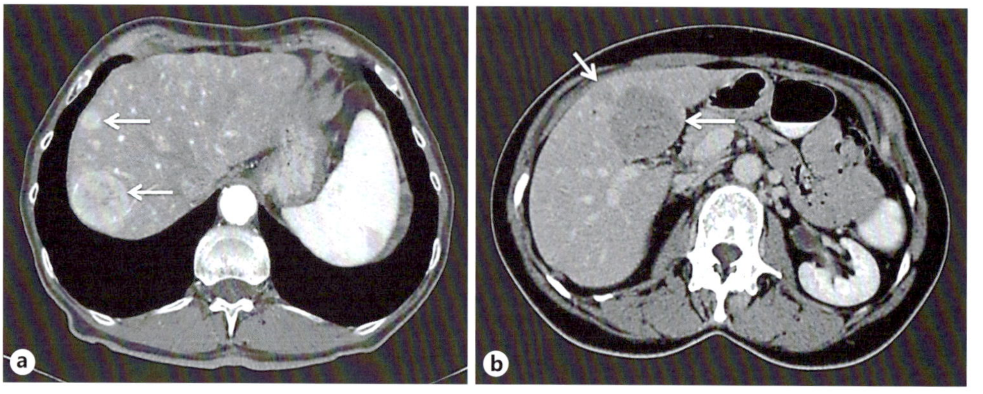

Fig. 7. Contrast-enhanced transverse CT images of the liver in the late arterial phase (**a**) showing hypervascular (bright) liver metastases (arrows) from a small bowel NET, and in the venous phase (**b**) showing hypovascular (dark) liver metastases (arrows) from a small bowel NET. Note the typical appearance of the spleen in the late arterial phase showing heterogeneous contrast enhancement.

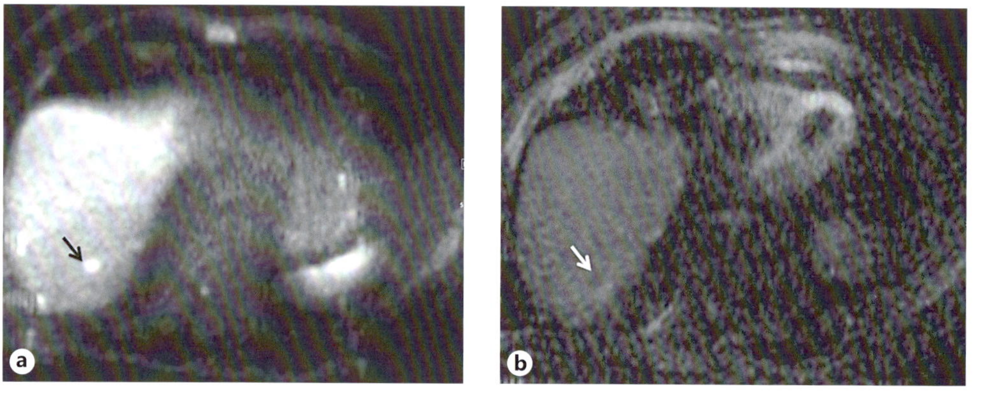

Fig. 8. Transverse MR images showing a small liver metastasis demonstrated on DWI. The lesion is highly conspicuous and of high signal intensity on the b800 image (**a**). The lesion is low in signal intensity on the ADC map (**b**), confirming restricted water diffusion. The primary lesion in this case was a small bowel NET.

lesions will be solely identifiable in this phase [4]. On DWI, NET liver metastases appear hyperintense at high b values and hypointense on the corresponding ADC map (fig. 8). DWI has been demonstrated as more sensitive than T2-weighted imaging for the detection of NET liver metastases, although will not reliably differentiate between metastases of different origins (e.g. NET from adenocarcinoma) [21].

Nodal Metastases

Retroperitoneal and precardiac lymph node metastases, especially in the right thorax, are other typical anatomical sites of lymphatic metastases. Retrocrural lymph node metastases are sometimes found, as are mediastinal and less frequently

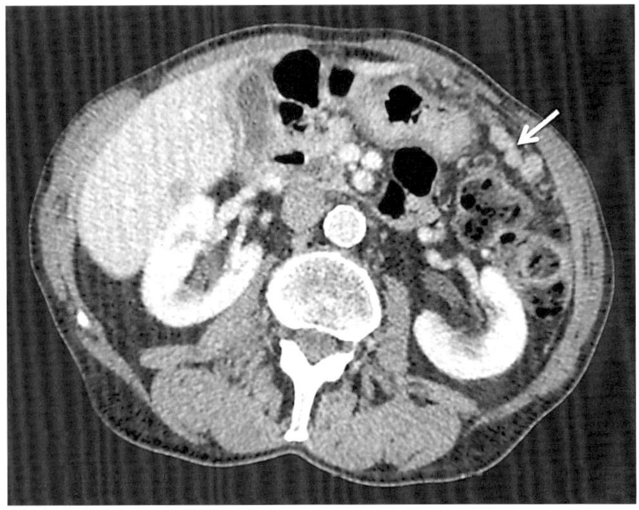

Fig. 9. A contrast-enhanced transverse CT image (venous phase) of a patient with a small bowel NET showing peritoneal metastases located in the ventral left lateral aspect of the abdomen (arrow). A hypovascular liver metastasis is also seen in the medial-dorsal aspect of the liver.

supraclavicular and cervical nodes. Similarly to pNETs, liver metastases from a small bowel NET may be hypervascular, hypovascular or mixed.

Diffuse peritoneal metastatic disease occurs in a smaller percentage (20–30%) of patients with gastrointestinal small bowel NETs. These often very small lesions are easily overlooked at the CT/MRI image reading. Gadolinium-enhanced T1 fat-saturated images and, more recently, DWI have been reported to increase the sensitivity for detecting small peritoneal tumor nodules [22]. They appear as foci of irregular nodularity throughout the mesentery and on the peritoneal surfaces, typically in the presence of ascites (fig. 9). Small nodular, usually elongated or flat deposits on the surface of the liver should not be mistaken as hepatic metastases. Paracolic tumor nodules and small pelvic deposits are not uncommon. In diffuse peritoneal carcinomatosis, the abdominal fat is infiltrated by irregular elongated strands with a reticular or sponge-like appearance, typically located in the ventral aspect of the abdomen near the ventral peritoneum and omentum. Occasionally ovarian metastases are found.

Bone Metastases

In patients with small bowel NETs and pNETs, bone metastases are predominantly sclerotic and are usually appearing in late-stage disease, as are lung and brain metastases. Bone scintigraphy is rarely needed because bone metastases that are not detected by CT are usually visualized by somatostatin receptor imaging by scintigraphy (OctreoScan™) or PET with ^{68}Ga-labelled somatostatin analogs. In patients with spine symptoms, MRI is best applied to detect bone metastases and to visualize any soft tissue components.

On MRI, bone metastases typically appear as lesions of reduced signal on T1-weighted imaging, with variable signal intensity on T2-weighted imaging dependent upon the extent of associated edema. Bone metastases from NETs may enhance following gadolinium administration [23]. Whole-body MR imaging has been found to have a sensitivity of 86–96% for the detection of bone metastases in patients with gastroenteropancreatic endocrine neoplasms, performing better for the detection of bone metastases, when compared directly to gallium ^{68}Ga-DOTATOC PET/CT [6].

Image Surveillance and Monitoring of Neuroendocrine Tumor Therapy

Surveillance of the patient is generally very long (sometimes life-long) because recurrences may be seen after many years. For low-grade tumors, monitoring of NET therapy by CT/MRI may initially be performed every 3–6 months and, in patients with stable disease, after the first year be extended to examination every 6 months. Somatostatin receptor scintigraphy (OctreoScan™) or PET/CT (^{68}Ga-labelled somatostatin analogs) is valuable after 1–2 years and, additionally, in patients for whom the results of radiology, biochemistry and the patient's clinical status are contradictory.

In some patients, liver metastases may be difficult to visualize by CT and occasionally the lesions may not be seen at all. Additionally, during therapy, the attenuation of the normal liver parenchyma may change and as a consequence metastases can become more difficult to delineate. US and CEUS are therefore helpful to include in the image monitoring, from time to time, as is MRI in centers where the technique is readily available. However, for patients included in clinical trials, US is generally not accepted for therapy monitoring. Likewise, it is generally not accepted to switch between CT and MRI for therapy monitoring during a clinical trial.

Several problems in the image monitoring of NET therapies are related to the inherent characteristic features of these tumors [24]. One of these features is that NET lesions are frequently hypervascular. The size of hypervascular liver metastases may vary as a reflection of different intravenous contrast-enhancement techniques at CT. When the CT acquisition is initiated too early after the start of contrast injection, the contrast medium will not have reached the small arterial branches in the liver and consequently not the tumor vessels, and the size of the liver metastases may be underestimated. Better timing of the CT acquisition in relation to contrast medium administration, at the time point of maximal enhancement of the tumor, will make the same lesions appear larger. Similarly, the injection rate, contrast medium concentration and the total amount of administered iodine may affect the lesion depiction. Consequently, an increase in lesion size and even appearance of new liver metastases, or the reverse, a decrease in size and disappearance of lesions, may sometimes be solely attributed to differences in examination technique. Therefore, the CT examination protocols need to be kept constant between examinations.

A second characteristic is that most NETs are low grade and slow growing. The response evaluation criteria in solid tumors (RECIST) that are applied in general oncology are therefore not optimal for the monitoring of NET therapy. The result of systemic NET therapies is usually stabilization of the disease, rather than a decrease of the tumor load. There is therefore a need for modified imaging evaluation criteria of NET therapy. PET using ^{68}Ga-labelled somatostatin analogs has been tried for monitoring of peptide receptor-targeted radiotherapy and the prediction of outcome [25, 26], but so far no convincing results have been reported.

References

1 Sundin A, Vullierme MP, Kaltsas G, Plöckinger U: ENETS consensus guidelines for the standards of care in neuroendocrine tumors: radiological examinations. Neuroendocrinology 2009;90:167–183.

2 Schmid-Tannwald C, Schmid-Tannwald CM, Morelli JN, Neumann R, Haug AR, Jansen N, Nikolaou K, Schramm N, Reiser MF, Rist C: Comparison of abdominal MRI with diffusion-weighted imaging to ^{68}Ga-DOTATATE PET/CT in detection of neuroendocrine tumors of the pancreas. Eur J Nucl Med Mol Imaging 2013;40:897–907.

3 Masselli G, Gualdi G: Evaluation of small bowel tumors: MR enteroclysis. Abdom Imaging 2010;35: 23–30.

4 Bader TR, Semelka RC, Chiu VC, Armao DM, Woosley JT: MRI of carcinoid tumors: spectrum of appearances in the gastrointestinal tract and liver. J Magn Reson Imaging 2001;14:261–269.

5 Schreiter NF, Nogami M, Steffen I, Pape UF, Hamm B, Brenner W, Röttgen R: Evaluation of the potential of PET-MRI fusion for detection of liver metastases in patients with neuroendocrine tumours. Eur Radiol 2012;22:458–467.

6 Schraml C, Schwenzer NF, Sperling O, Aschoff P, Lichy MP, Müller M, Brendle C, Werner MK, Claussen CD, Pfannenberg C: Staging of neuroendocrine tumours: comparison of [^{68}Ga]DOTATOC multiphase PET/CT and whole-body MRI. Cancer Imaging 2013;13:63–72.

7 Kukuk GM, Mürtz P, Träber F, Meyer C, Ullrich J, Gieseke J, Ahmadzadehfar H, Ezziddin S, Schild HH, Willinek WA: Diffusion-weighted imaging with acquisition of three b-values for response evaluation of neuroendocrine liver metastases undergoing selective internal radiotherapy. Eur Radiol 2014;24:267–276.

8 Cossetti RJ, Bezerra RO, Gumz B, Telles A, Costa FP: Whole body diffusion for metastatic disease assessment in neuroendocrine carcinomas: comparison with OctreoScan® in two cases. World J Surg Oncol 2012;10:82.

9 Massironi S, Conte D, Sciola V, Pirola L, Paggi S, Fraquelli M, Ciafardini C, Spampatti MP, Peracchi M: Contrast-enhanced ultrasonography in evaluating hepatic metastases from neuroendocrine tumours. Dig Liver Dis 2010;42:635–641.

10 Pais SA, Al-Haddad M, Mohamadnejad M, Leblanc JK, Sherman S, McHenry L, DeWitt JM: EUS for pancreatic neuroendocrine tumors: a single-center, 11-year experience. Gastrointest Endosc 2010;71: 1185–1193.

11 Ishikawa T, Itoh A, Kawashima H, Ohno E, Matsubara H, Itoh Y, Nakamura Y, Nakamura M, Miyahara R, Hayashi K, Ishigami M, Katano Y, Ohmiya N, Goto H, Hirooka Y: Usefulness of EUS combined with contrast-enhancement in the differential diagnosis of malignant versus benign and preoperative localization of pancreatic endocrine tumors. Gastrointest Endosc 2010;71:951–959.

12 Gallotti A, Johnston RP, Bonaffini PA, Ingkakul T, Deshpande V, Fernández-del Castillo C, Sahani DV: Incidental neuroendocrine tumors of the pancreas: MDCT findings and features of malignancy. AJR Am J Roentgenol 2013;200:355–362.

13 Manfredi R, Bonatti M, Mantovani W, Graziani R, Segala D, Capelli P, Butturini G, Mucelli RP: Nonhyperfunctioning neuroendocrine tumours of the pancreas: MR imaging appearance and correlation with their biological behaviour. Eur Radiol 2013;23: 3029–3039.

14 Daneshvar K, Grenacher L, Mehrabi A, Kauczor HU, Hallscheidt P: Preoperative tumor studies using MRI or CT in patients with clinically suspected insulinoma. Pancreatology 2011;11:487–494.

15 Jang KM, Kim SH, Lee SJ, Choi D: The value of gadoxetic acid-enhanced and diffusion-weighted MRI for prediction of grading of pancreatic neuroendocrine tumors. Acta Radiol 2014;55:140–148.

16 Sahani DV, Bonaffini PA, Fernández-Del Castillo C, Blake MA: Gastroenteropancreatic neuroendocrine tumors: role of imaging in diagnosis and management. Radiology 2013;266:38–61.

17 Masselli G, Polettini E, Casciani E, Bertini L, Vecchioli A, Gualdi G: Small-bowel neoplasms: prospective evaluation of MR enteroclysis. Radiology 2009; 251:743–750.

18 Druce MR, Bharwani N, Akker SA, Drake WM, Rockall A, Grossman AB: Intra-abdominal fibrosis in a recent cohort of patients with neuroendocrine ('carcinoid') tumours of the small bowel. QJM 2010; 103:177–185.

19 Berge T, Linell F: Carcinoid tumours: frequency in a defined population during a 12-year period. Acta Pathol Microbiol Scand A 1976;84:322–330.

20 Sundin A: Radiological and nuclear medicine imaging of gastroenteropancreatic neuroendocrine tumours. Best Pract Res Clin Gastroenterol 2012;26: 803–818.

21 d'Assignies G, Fina P, Bruno O, Vullierme MP, Tubach F, Paradis V, Sauvanet A, Ruszniewski P, Vilgrain V: High sensitivity of diffusion-weighted MR imaging for the detection of liver metastases from neuroendocrine tumors: comparison with T2-weighted and dynamic gadolinium-enhanced MR imaging. Radiology 2013;268:390–399.

22 Low RN, Sebrechts CP, Barone RM, Muller W: Diffusion-weighted MRI of peritoneal tumors: comparison with conventional MRI and surgical and histopathologic findings – a feasibility study. AJR Am J Roentgenol 2009;193:461–470.

23 Debray MP, Geoffroy O, Laissy JP, Lebtahi R, Silbermann-Hoffman O, Henry-Feugeas MC, Cadiot G, Mignon M, Schouman-Claeys E: Imaging appearances of metastases from neuroendocrine tumours of the pancreas. Br J Radiol 2001;74:1065–1070.

24 Sundin A, Rockall A: Therapeutic monitoring of gastroenteropancreatic neuroendocrine tumors: the challenges ahead. Neuroendocrinology 2012;96: 261–271.

25 Gabriel M, Oberauer A, Dobrozemsky G, Decristoforo C, Putzer D, Kendler D, Uprimny C, Kovacs P, Bale R, Virgolini IJ: ^{68}Ga-DOTA-Tyr^{3}-octreotide PET for assessing response to somatostatin-receptor-mediated radionuclide therapy. J Nucl Med 2009;50:1427–1434.

26 Haug AR, Auernhammer CJ, Wängler B, Schmidt GP, Uebleis C, Göke B, Cumming P, Bartenstein P, Tiling R, Hacker M: ^{68}Ga-DOTATATE PET/CT for the early prediction of response to somatostatin receptor-mediated radionuclide therapy in patients with well-differentiated neuroendocrine tumors. J Nucl Med 2010;51:1349–1356.

Anders Sundin
Department of Radiology, Section for Molecular Imaging
Uppsala University Hospital
SE–751 85 Uppsala (Sweden)
E-Mail anders.sundin@radiol.uu.se

Papotti M, de Herder WW (eds): Neuroendocrine Tumors: A Multidisciplinary Approach.
Front Horm Res. Basel, Karger, 2015, vol 44, pp 73–87 (DOI: 10.1159/000382059)

Nuclear Medicine Imaging of Neuroendocrine Tumors

Tessa Brabander[a] · Dik J. Kwekkeboom[a] · Richard A. Feelders[b] · Adrienne H. Brouwers[c] · Jaap J.M. Teunissen[a]

Departments of [a]Nuclear Medicine and [b]Internal Medicine, Division of Endocrinology, Erasmus Medical Centre, Rotterdam, and [c]Department of Nuclear Medicine and Molecular Imaging, University of Groningen, University Medical Centre Groningen, Groningen, The Netherlands

Abstract

An important role is reserved for nuclear imaging techniques in the imaging of neuroendocrine tumors (NETs). Somatostatin receptor scintigraphy (SRS) with ^{111}In-DTPA-octreotide is currently the most important tracer in the diagnosis, staging and selection for peptide receptor radionuclide therapy (PRRT). In the past decade, different positron-emitting tomography (PET) tracers have been developed. The largest group is the ^{68}Gallium-labeled somatostatin analogs (^{68}Ga-SSA). Several studies have demonstrated their superiority compared to SRS in sensitivity and specificity. Furthermore, patient comfort and effective dose are favorable for ^{68}Ga-SSA. Other PET targets like β-[^{11}C]-5-hydroxy-L-tryptophan (^{11}C-5-HTP) and 6-^{18}F-L-3,4-dihydroxyphenylalanine (^{18}F-DOPA) were developed recently. For insulinomas, glucagon-like peptide-1 receptor imaging is a promising new technique. The evaluation of response after PRRT and other therapies is a challenge. Currently, the official follow-up is performed with radiological imaging techniques. The role of nuclear medicine may increase with the newest tracers for PET. In this review, the different nuclear imaging techniques and tracers for the imaging of NETs will be discussed.

Nuclear imaging techniques play a pivotal role in the diagnosis and staging of neuroendocrine tumors (NETs). Furthermore, selection of patients for peptide receptor radionuclide therapy (PRRT) can only be done by scintigraphy with radiolabeled somatostatin analogs. Besides the above-mentioned indications, nuclear imaging can play an important role in follow-up after therapy and in the evaluation of therapy response.

In general, two different imaging modalities in nuclear medicine are used to image NETs. With the gamma camera, both planar (two-dimensional) and single-photon emission computed tomography (SPECT; three-dimensional) images can be made. A relative new image modality, the positron emission tomography (PET) camera can be used after the injection of a positron-emitting radionuclide-based tracer. The emitted positrons annihilate with a surrounding electron in the tumor or normal tissue, forming two gamma rays with an energy of 511 KeV in opposite directions. In this way, imaging with a PET camera ensures a better sensitivity and higher spatial resolution compared to the gamma camera. Currently, most PET cameras are combined with computed tomography (CT), allowing hybrid imaging in a single imaging procedure. The CT is used for attenuation correction, which improves the image quality. Furthermore, the CT can be used for anatomical correlation. This will improve the accuracy and makes it possible to distinguish between physiological and pathological activity, resulting in less false-positive findings [1, 2].

This review will focus on the different imaging modalities which nuclear medicine has to offer for the diagnosis and staging of NETs. Furthermore, selection for PRRT and the imaging options for the evaluation of therapy response will be discussed.

Imaging of Neuroendocrine Tumors

NETs are a heterogeneous group of tumors that can differ in location, function and growth. Variations in these characteristics make the presentation of a NET diverse and, therefore, the optimal diagnostic path for patients may be different. In order to perform the right type of diagnostic imaging, knowledge of the most recent World Health Organization (WHO) classification of gastroenteropancreatic NETs, as published in 2010 [3], is essential. This classification defines three tumor categories or grades, irrespective of their site of origin, based on the mitotic count (MC) and the number of cells positively staining with the proliferation marker Ki-67: low-grade (grade 1; G1) NETs with <2 mitoses/10 HPF (high-power field) and Ki-67 <3%; intermediate (grade 2; G2) NETs with 2–20 mitoses/10 HPF or Ki-67 3–20%, and high-grade (grade 3; G3) neuroendocrine carcinomas with >20 mitoses/10 HPF or Ki-67 >20%. This grading is important since there is an inverse association between grade and prognosis [4]. Besides the prognosis, the classification plays a role in the choice of imaging and/or subsequent therapy.

Somatostatin Receptor-Based Imaging

One of the characteristics of NETs is that they may express somatostatin receptors (SSTRs) on the cell surface. This receptor can be used to image tumors by using radiolabeled somatostatin analogs. In vivo visualization of somatostatin-positive tumors with radioiodine-labeled somatostatin analogs was first described in 1989 [5]. In the following years, somatostatin analogs labeled with different radionuclides were developed. These compounds have different affinities for the five subtypes of the SSTR (table 1) [6].

Table 1. Affinity profiles (IC50) for human SSTR (hsst1–5) of a series of somatostatin analogs

	hsst1	hsst2	hsst3	hsst4	hsst5
SS-28	5.2±0.3	2.7±0.3	7.7±0.9	5.6±0.4	4.0±0.3
Octreotide	>10,000	2.0±0.7	187±55	>1,000	22±6
DTPA-octreotide	>10,000	12±2	376±84	>1,000	299±50
In-DTPA-octreotide	>10,000	22±3.6	182±13	>1,000	237±52
DOTA-TOC	>10,000	14±2.6	880±324	>1,000	393±84
Ga-DOTA-TOC	>10,000	2.5±0.5	613±140	>1,000	73±21
In-DTPA-octreotate	>10,000	1.3±0.2	>10,000	433±16	>1,000
Ga-DOTATATE	>10,000	0.2±0.04	>1,000	300±140	377±18

All values are IC50 ± SEM in nM. Modified from Reubi et al. [6].

Most radiolabeled somatostatin analogs, which are currently available for imaging, have good affinity for the subtype 2 receptor, which is most frequently expressed by NETs.

In SSTR-positive NETs, unlabeled somatostatin analogs (e.g. octreotide or lanreotide) can be used for therapy. In case patients have NETs that produce hormones, which lead to specific symptoms or syndromes (e.g. carcinoid syndrome), treatment with somatostatin analogs results in a reduction of hormonal overproduction and, therefore, relief of these symptoms. Furthermore, it can lengthen the time to tumor progression compared to placebo in patients with midgut NETs [7]. Currently, many patients with NETs are treated with somatostatin analogs. This cold octreotide can compete for binding to the SSTR with the radiolabeled somatostatin analogs. This may influence the sensitivity of the imaging and effect of PRRT. To obtain the best quality of imaging, it is therefore advised to discontinue somatostatin analogs before SSTR-based imaging and PRRT. With the proper patient preparation and imaging acquisition SSTR imaging is very helpful in the optimal staging of the patient.

[^{111}In-DTPA^{0}]octreotide

Currently, the only registered radiopharmaceutical for SSTR scintigraphy (SRS) is [^{111}In-DTPA^{0}]octreotide (OctreoScan; Covidien, Petten, The Netherlands). The SNM guideline [8] recommends an administered activity of 222 MBq and 10 μg of pentetreotide. Furthermore, SPECT(-CT) of at least the upper abdomen is mandatory for optimal imaging and staging. Due to a relative long half-life of 2.8 days, it is possible to image at 24 h and an optional 48 h after injection.

Normal tissues, such as thyroid, spleen and the pituitary gland, express SSTR. Furthermore, the liver and kidneys excrete the tracer, so accumulation of radioactivity is seen in these organs as well [9]. More specifically, approximately 2% of the administered dose leaves the body by hepatobiliary excretion. Therefore, laxatives should be considered when visualizing tumors in the abdomen. In the last decade many studies have evaluated the sensitivity and specificity of ^{111}In-DTPA-octreotide for the detection of NETs, and the results vary considerably due to variations in the size and location of the tumor and different acquisition protocols. A large review of 1,200 patients with gastrointestinal NETs showed a median detection rate of 89% (range 67–100%) and sensitivity of 84% (range 57–93%) [10]. Besides the presence of unlabeled somatostatin or therapeutic use of somatostatin analogs blocking the SSTR, SRS can have a negative result due to high glucocorticoid levels, which has a downregulatory effect on tumoral SSTR expression. De Bruin et al. [11] described 2 patients with a negative SRS caused by hypercortisolism due to ectopic ACTH secretion. After treatment with the glucocorticoid receptor antagonist mifepristone, the SRS pointed towards the diagnosis of an ACTH-producing bronchial carcinoid in both patients.

Furthermore, imaging of NETs with ^{111}In-DTPA-octreotide is used to select patients for PRRT. PRRT is performed with somatostatin analogs labeled with a β-emitting radionuclide such as Yttrium-90 or Lutetium-177 (e.g. [^{90}Y-DOTA^{0},Tyr^{3}] octreotide and [^{177}Lu-DOTA^{0},Tyr^{3}]octreotate). The level of accumulation in the tumor on the pretherapeutic SRS is an important prognostic factor for the prediction of tumor regression. The uptake is expressed using a semiquantitative score, comparing the accumulation in the tumor to physiological accumulation in the liver and kidneys/spleen. In general, a high accumulation in the tumor will result in a good response to therapy [12].

^{99m}Tc-Labeled Somatostatin Analogs

As an alternative to ^{111}In-DTPA-octreotide, somatostatin analogs can be labeled with ^{99m}Technetium (^{99m}Tc). Currently, the most commonly used ^{99m}Tc-labeled somatostatin analogs are ^{99m}Tc-depreotide and ^{99m}Tc-EDDA/HYNIC-Tyr^{3}-octreotide (^{99m}Tc-EDDA/HYNIC-TOC). The latter is available under the commercial name ^{99m}Tc-Tektrotyd and most frequently used in (Eastern) Europe. The main advantage of ^{99m}Tc-labeled somatostatin analogs is the wide availability of ^{99m}Tc, which can be produced by the majority of nuclear medicine departments with the use of a ^{99m}Tc generator. This makes the production of this radionuclide relatively inexpensive. Another advantage is that the radiation burden is lower [13]. However, a disadvantage of ^{99m}Tc is the short half-life of 6 h. Because of this short half-life it is not possible to image at 24 h after injection. On the other hand, imaging can be performed on the day of the administration of the tracer and therefore disturbing bowel uptake is less of an issue. Still, it is recommended that an imaging protocol with ^{99m}Tc-EDDA/HYNIC-TOC should include acquisitions 2 and 4 h after injection, complemented with SPECT(-CT) of the upper abdomen. Using this protocol, a sensitivity of 80% and specificity of 94% could be achieved in 88 patients with NETs of the gastroenteropancreatic tract [14]. In a direct comparison between ^{111}In-DTPA-octreotide and ^{99m}Tc-EDDA/HYNIC-TOC SRS, both modalities performed similarly, with a slightly higher sensitivity for ^{99m}Tc-EDDA/HYNIC-TOC. However, the latter showed more false-positive results due to nonspecific abdominal tracer accumulation [15]. In summary, although ^{99m}Tc-EDDA/HYNIC-TOC is not widely used and only few studies have been performed with this tracer, somatostatin scintigraphy with ^{99m}Tc-EDDA/HYNIC-TOC seems a reasonable alternative for ^{111}In-DTPA-octreotide.

Somatostatin Receptor PET/CT

Imaging with a positron-emitting radionuclide-labeled compound allows imaging with a PET camera, which results in a better image quality compared to imaging with a gamma camera including SPECT. To image NETs with PET, most somatostatin analogs are labeled with the positron emitter Gallium-68 (^{68}Ga). The most commonly used somatostatin analogs labeled with ^{68}Ga are [^{68}Ga-DOTA^{0},Tyr^{3}]octreotide (^{68}Ga-DOTATOC), [^{68}Ga-DOTA,1-nal^{3}]octreotide (^{68}Ga-DOTANOC) and [^{68}Ga-DOTA^{0},Tyr^{3}]octreotate (^{68}Ga-DOTATATE). These ^{68}Ga-labeled somatostatin analogs (^{68}Ga-SSA) all have a different affinity profile for the different subtypes of the SSTR, but have in common that each analog can bind to SSTR2. ^{68}Ga-DOTATATE has the highest affinity for SSTR2. Despite the differences in the affinity profile, the different ^{68}Ga-SSAs perform similarly with regard to sensitivity and specificity [16].

Recently, the European Association of Nuclear Medicine (EANM) published the first guideline for imaging with ^{68}Ga-labeled somatostatin analogs. In order to obtain the best imaging quality, an administered activity of at least 100 MBq and less than 50 μg of ^{68}Ga-DOTA-conjugated peptide is recommended. Image acquisition should be done at 60 min after injection [17]. A recent meta-analysis in which studies were included using various somatostatin analogs labeled mainly with ^{68}Ga with a total of 2,105 patients with NETs in the thorax and abdomen showed a pooled sensitivity of 93% and specificity of 91% [16]. It is to be expected that the ^{68}Ga-labeled somatostatin analogs will become more widely available in the near future.

Comparison between ^{68}Ga-SSA and Non-PET SRS

Several studies have compared ^{68}Ga-SSA to SRS, including ^{111}In-DTPA-octreotide, ^{111}In-DOTATOC and ^{99m}Tc-EDDA/HYNIC-TOC [18–20]. Overall, ^{68}Ga-SSA have many advantages over non-PET SRS. Firstly, as mentioned before, ^{68}Ga is a positron-emitting radionuclide, which ensures a higher spatial resolution with PET imaging. Therefore, it is not surprising that, in a direct comparison, ^{68}Ga-SSA imaging shows a significantly higher detection rate compared to non-PET SRS [18]. Especially for the detection of metastatic lesions in the bones and lungs, ^{68}Ga-SSA is superior to ^{111}In-DTPA-octreotide [19]. Due to the higher detection rate, the clinical management can change. Secondly, imaging with a ^{68}Ga-SSA is performed 60 min after injection in contrast to imaging with ^{111}In-DTPA-octreotide after 24 h. Due to the short time between injection and image acquisition it is not necessary to use laxatives when performing PET with ^{68}Ga-SSA, which is an advantage as patients often experience the use of these laxatives as burdensome. Other advantages are that ^{68}Ga-SSA is performed in 1 day, and the radiation burden for a whole-body scan is lower compared to ^{111}In-DTPA-octreotide [21]. For these reasons, the ^{68}Ga-SSA are better tolerated by the patients than ^{111}In-DTPA-octreotide [20]. Furthermore, one cost-effectiveness study comparing ^{68}Ga-DOTATOC and ^{111}In-DTPA-octreotide demonstrated that

^{68}Ga-DOTATOC was less expensive with respect to materials and personnel costs [22]. Due to the higher sensitivity and specificity fewer additional examinations were needed.

A disadvantage of ^{68}Ga-SSA is the increase in false-positive results especially due to findings of high uptake in the pancreatic head [18, 23], which can be explained by the higher density of SSTRs in this area of the pancreas [24]. These false positive findings did not occur with ^{111}In-DTPA-octreotide, probably because of the lower sensitivity and resolution of the gamma camera. Another disadvantage remains the limited availability of ^{68}Ga-SSA. Currently, the most frequently used radiopharmaceutical for imaging of NETs is ^{111}In-DTPA-octreotide. This tracer is available in almost every nuclear medicine department and there is considerable shared experience with the interpretation of the images. Moreover, most literature is based on SRS with ^{111}In-DTPA-octreotide. Currently, the uptake on SRS can be used to assess whether a patient is eligible for PRRT. If the tumor shows less uptake than the physiological liver uptake on the SRS (grade 1 uptake), PRRT is not a suitable therapy. Such a scale is not available for ^{68}Ga-SSA and further studies are needed to translate the semiquantitative 'Krenning' score on SRS to quantitative uptake on a PET scan with ^{68}Ga-SSA.

In summary, PET imaging with ^{68}Ga-SSA performs better with regard to sensitivity and detection rate than ^{111}In-DTPA-octreotide. The discomfort for patients is lower, due to a 1-day protocol and there being no need to use laxatives. However, SRS has the advantage of better availability and larger clinical experience. It is expected that ^{68}Ga-SSA PET imaging will replace SRS in the daily practice of imaging NETs.

Other Imaging Modalities

^{123}I-Metaiodobenzylguanidine

Metaiodobenzylguanidine (MIBG) labeled with radioactive iodine (^{123}I) can be used to image NETs with planar and/or with SPECT(-CT) imaging. MIBG is structurally similar to norepinephrine and therefore utilizes the vesicular monoamine transporters and is incorporated into vesicles or neurosecretory granules in the cytoplasm of neuroendocrine cells [25]. For imaging of pheochromocytoma and paraganglioma, ^{123}I-MIBG scintigraphy has been the investigation of first choice with a high sensitivity and specificity of 87 and 99%, respectively [26]. However, new PET tracers (e.g. ^{18}F-DOPA), which will be discussed in the next paragraphs, may perform better in sensitivity and specificity, but their availability is limited. For the detection of NETs, the sensitivity of MIBG scintigraphy is lower than SRS with ^{111}In-DTPA-octreotide. In a large review, the median detection rate was 50% and the sensitivity 76% [27]. Therefore, MIBG has a limited role in the diagnosis of NETs. However, ^{123}I-MIBG scintigraphy can be used when other imaging modalities fail to detect the tumor and for the selection of therapy with ^{131}I-MIBG.

^{18}F-Fluorodeoxyglucose

^{18}F-fluorodeoxyglucose (^{18}F-FDG) is the most frequently used PET tracer in oncology. FDG is a glucose analog that accumulates in tumor cells with a high expression of glucose transporters. The FDG undergoes phosphorylation by hexokinase and is trapped intracellularly. However, in contrast to the wide use of ^{18}F-FDG in numerous types of tumors, it has a limited role in the imaging of NETs. Poorly differentiated tumors (G3) with a high proliferative activity have an increased glucose metabolism [28]. The majority of the more differentiated tumors (G1/G2) have a normal or slightly increased glucose metabolism. For these tumors, imaging with ^{18}F-FDG should not be the first choice of imaging technique for staging. However, some G2 tumors do have an increased glucose metabolism. For these tumors, the uptake on ^{18}F-FDG PET can predict the prognosis. Overall, a high FDG uptake predicts a poorer prognosis [29, 30].

Only a few studies have compared ^{18}F-FDG to ^{68}Ga-SSA [31, 32]. Kayani et al. [31] found a significant correlation between uptake of ^{68}Ga-DOTATATE and ^{18}F-FDG and tumor grade on histology. Low-grade tumors had a higher accumulation of ^{68}Ga-DOTATATE than ^{18}F-FDG. The reverse was true in high-grade tumors. The overall sensitivity in this study for ^{68}Ga-DOTATATE was 82%, and for ^{18}F-FDG was 66%. The highest sensitivity of 92% was achieved when combining these two different PET tracers [31]. SSTR imaging and glucose metabolism imaging seem to have a complementary role [32]. Although ^{18}F-FDG-PET seems to have no additional value for the staging of patients with low-grade tumors (G1/G2), positive findings on an ^{18}F-FDG PET might define specific NET subgroups. However, it is currently not common practice to perform both imaging modalities for staging or to use this functional or metabolic information as a guidance before starting the therapy. Additional clinical studies have to be performed to gain more insight.

^{18}F- L-3,4-Dihydroxyphenylalanine

The radiopharmaceutical 6-^{18}F-L-3,4-dihydroxyphenylalanine (^{18}F-DOPA) is one of the PET tracers for imaging NETs which makes use of the capability of neuroendocrine (tumor) cells to synthesize various hormones via amine precursor uptake and decarboxylation. In the catecholamine pathway, active in many NETs, phenylalanine and intermediate products such as L-DOPA are taken up via system L large amino acid transporters. Once inside the cell, decarboxylation to dopamine takes place via the enzyme AADC (aromatic amino acid decarboxylase). Dopamine is then transported into intracellular storage vesicles through the vesicular monoamine transporter. From these vesicles, the resulting end products can be released in the extracellular environment.

Nowadays, more and more PET centers are capable of producing ^{18}F-DOPA, and it is commercially available in several European countries. Usually, images are made 60–90 min after injection, although earlier images are advocated for some indications [33, 34]. Physiological variants and pitfalls have been described [34, 35]. Practices differ regarding premedicating patients with carbidopa for NET imaging. Carbidopa is

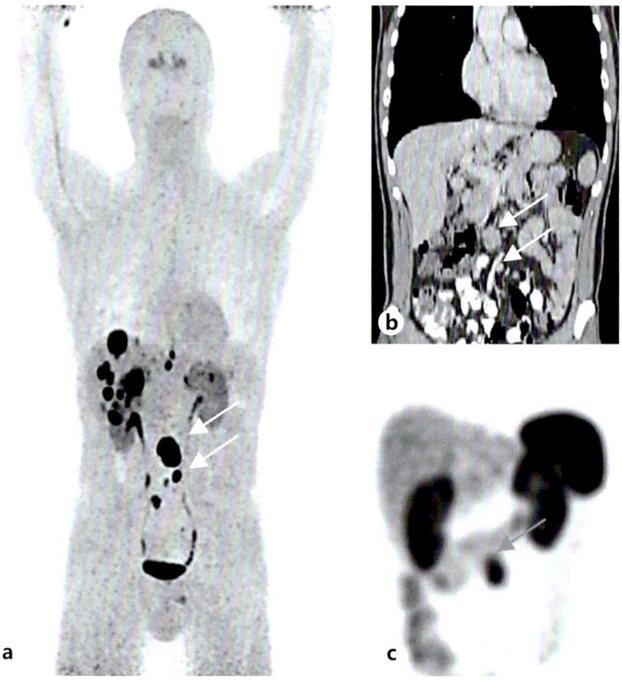

Fig. 1. A patient with liver and mesenteric lymph node metastases from a small bowel G1 NET. **a** Maximum intensity projection of whole-body ^{18}F-DOPA PET showing multiple liver lesions and metastases in the mesenterium. Physiologic uptake is seen in the striata. Physiological excretion is via the kidneys and ureters to the bladder. **b** Abdominal CT showing large and smaller (white arrows) malignant mesenteric lymph nodes. **c** On the ^{111}In-DTPA-octreotide SPECT scan 24 h after injection only the large mesenteric lymph node could be visualized (gray arrow).

an inhibitor of AADC, and it prevents early decarboxylation of ^{18}F-DOPA to ^{18}F-dopamine outside the brain. This results in decreased renal excretion and increased ^{18}F-DOPA uptake in NET cells, thus increasing image quality and sensitivity [36, 37]. However, carbidopa pretreatment is not recommended for the evaluation of pancreatic pathology, such as congenital hyperinsulinism/nesidioblastosis or insulinomas [38, 39].

Most studies with ^{18}F-DOPA PET have been performed for diagnosing and the (re-)staging of NET patients. Its superior role has been established in the following, more common subtypes of NETs: well-differentiated NETs of midgut origin, pheochromocytoma/paraganglioma and medullary thyroid carcinoma. In these NET types, ^{18}F-DOPA PET/CT can serve as the initial imaging technique, provided that it is available [40]. In well-differentiated NETs of midgut origin, overall (n = 76 patients) patient- and lesion-based sensitivity for ^{18}F-DOPA is 89 and 97%. This is significantly higher when compared to SRS with ^{111}In-DTPA-octreotide (80 and 49%, respectively; fig. 1), and is equal compared to CT/MRI (89% patient based) or higher (65% lesion based) [40]. Furthermore, in these patients, the extension of ^{18}F-DOPA uptake on the whole body PET scan reflects the total tumor load, and was correlated with various urinary and plasma hormonal products, but not with serum chromogranin A [41]. Thus far, patient series directly comparing ^{18}F-DOPA and ^{68}Ga-SSA in NET patients are small. Preliminary results suggest that they perform equally well [40]. An example is given in figure 2.

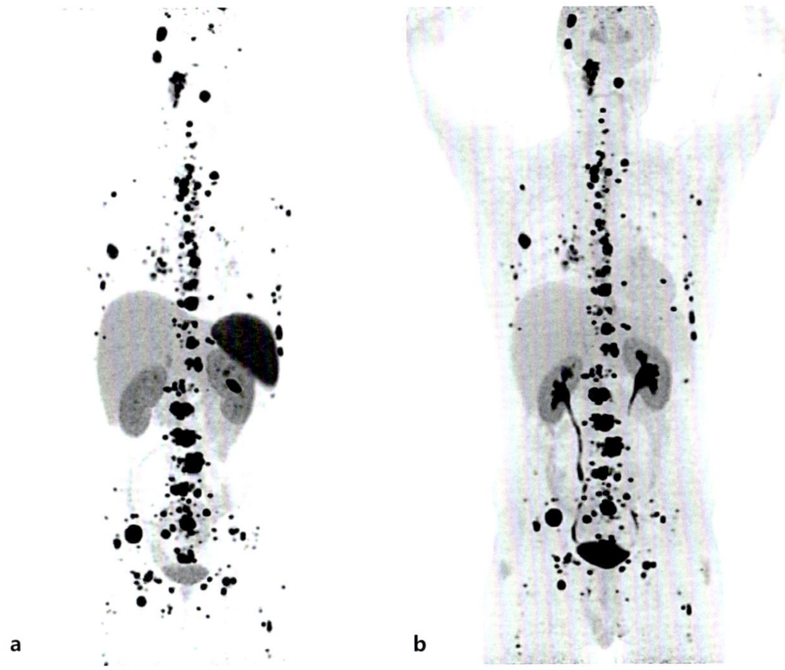

Fig. 2. A patient with paraganglioma with widespread (bone) metastases. **a** Maximum intensity projection (MIP) of whole-body ^{68}Ga-DOTATATE PET. **b** MIP of whole-body ^{18}F-DOPA PET. Note the similarity of uptake of ^{68}Ga-DOTATATE and ^{18}F-DOPA in the lesions. Only some lesions take up ^{68}Ga-DOTATATE (e.g. axillary regions), but this might be due to PD (the acquisition was 6 months after the ^{18}F-DOPA PET).

There are differences of opinion as to whether or not ^{18}F-DOPA should be advised as a first-choice functional imaging technique in patients with pancreatic NETs. Other functional imaging techniques such as ^{111}In-DTPA-ocetreotide SRS, ^{68}Ga-SSA PET or ^{11}C-5-HTP PET may be considered as well [35, 39, 40, 42].

β-[^{11}C]-5-Hydroxy-L-Tryptophan

PET imaging with β-[^{11}C]-5-hydroxy-L-tryptophan (^{11}C-5-HTP) PET can visualize the serotonin pathway, which is active in many NETs. The precursors tryptophan and 5-HTP are taken up via the L-amino acid transporter, and subsequently decarboxylated by aromatic L-amino acid decarboxylase (DOPA decarboxylase, tryptophan decarboxylase) ADCC. This results in serotonin, which is then also stored in vesicles through the vesicular monoamine transporter. When released into the extracellular environment, serotonin is thereafter degraded and eventually excreted as urinary 5-hydroxyindole acetic acid (5-HIAA).

^{11}C-5-HTP is produced in only a few centers worldwide, since the tracer synthesis is very complex. It is advised for the pretreatment of patients with carbidopa [43]. Whole-body imaging usually starts 10–20 min after injection of the tracer. Based on the limited studies that have been published, it can be concluded that ^{11}C-5-HTP is a

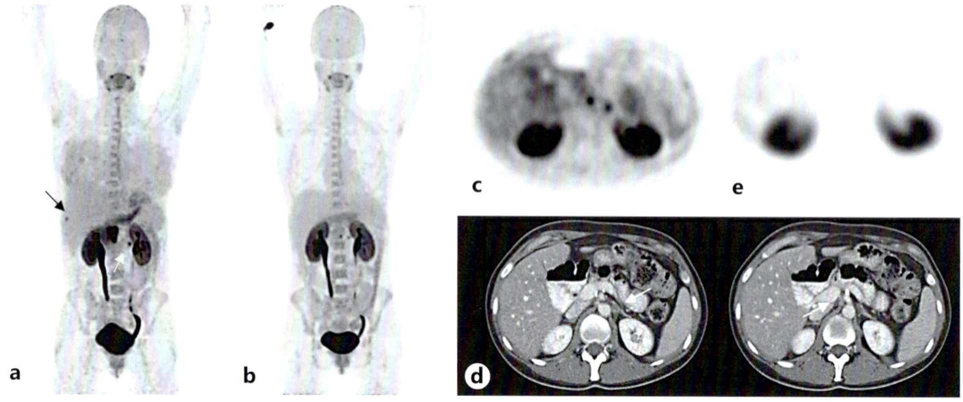

Fig. 3. A patient with insulinoma G2 of the pancreas, pT3N1M1. **a** Maximum intensity projection of whole-body ^{11}C-5-HTP PET before surgery. The primary tumor is seen in the head of the pancreas. Also, a liver metastasis (black arrow) and a locoregional lymph node metastasis were detected. All were surgically removed. Physiological uptake is seen in salivary and mammary glands, mucosa of the esophagus and bone marrow. Physiological excretion is via the kidneys and ureters to the bladder. **b** Six months later, during follow-up with ^{11}C-5-HTP PET and a diagnostic CT of the abdomen, two small new locoregional metastatic lymph nodes were detected. **c** Transverse slices of ^{11}C-5-HTP PET/CT showing the two new lesions, para-aortic right and left sided. **d** Transverse slices of the diagnostic CT of the abdomen (venous phase), also showing the two new lymph node metastases. **e** A follow-up ^{111}In-DTPA-octreotide SPECT scan (transverse slice) failed to detect these small metastases.

universal NET tracer for all tumors arising from the fore- to hindgut [44, 45]. It has been suggested that ^{11}C-5-HTP performs better compared to ^{18}F-DOPA, especially in foregut (e.g. bronchial) NETs, but this needs further confirmation [33]. In a recent study, Orlefors et al. [46] reported for ^{11}C-5-HTP PET a sensitivity of 83% and specificity of 100% in 38 patients with abdominal NETs, confirmed by surgery and histopathology results. An example of a ^{11}C-5-HTP PET is given in figure 3.

Based on a study by Koopmans et al. [47], it was concluded that ^{11}C-5-HTP PET outperforms ^{18}F-DOPA PET both in a patient- and a tumor lesion-based analysis in patients with predominantly advanced pancreatic islet cell tumors. However, as stated earlier, there are different opinions regarding the choice for a functional imaging PET tracer in this patient group. Not only for pancreatic NETs, but also for other (subsets) of NETs, further research is needed to define more precisely the role of both metabolic pathway tracers, ^{18}F-DOPA and ^{11}C-5-HTP, also in relation to other new functional PET tracers that are currently being developed or are already in use.

Glucagon-Like Peptide-1 Receptor

A rare type of NET is the insulinoma. The great majority (more than 90%) of insulinomas are benign, but they can be life threatening due to increased excretion of insulin and induction of episodes of hypoglycemia. Approximately 10% of the insulinomas are multiple, mainly in genetic polyendocrine syndromes. Insulinomas are the most common cause of endogenous hyperinsulinemic hypoglycemia in adults. Virtually all insulinomas are located in the pancreas, but 10–27% remain undetected even after surgery [48]. Preoperative localization is therefore essential to facilitate and optimize surgery. The sensitivity of ^{111}In-DTPA-octreotide for detection of insulinomas is only 50–60% [49]. Because of this relatively poor sensitivity, other imaging targets such as the glucagon-like peptide-1 receptor (GLP-1R) have been recently developed. GLP-1R is expressed at very high density in almost all benign insulinomas [50]. The first studies with GLP-1R agonists demonstrated very promising results [51, 52] with a high detection rate compared to conventional imaging. However, these agonists are not commercially available. Unlike benign insulinoma, malignant insulinomas often lack GLP1-R. In contrast, the malignant insulinomas often express SSTR type 2, which can be visualized by SRS [53].

Imaging Response after Therapy

Adequate assessment of response after therapy is important in NET patients. Not only will it predict the prognosis of the patient, but it will also influence the decision to continue the current therapy or to switch to other alternative therapies. The most frequently used assessment method during follow-up is the response evaluation criteria in solid tumors (RECIST). This assessment is based on the number and size of the lesions measured on CT and, in certain situations, MRI or chest X-ray. The latest guideline version was published in 2009 [54]. A partial response (PR) is defined as a decrease of at least 30% in the sum of the diameters of target lesions. Progressive disease (PD) is defined as a 20% increase in the sum of the diameters of target lesions. Stable disease is every change that is not sufficient for PD or PR. Another response evaluation assessment method is the Southwest Oncology Group (SWOG) solid tumor response criteria. The SWOG criteria use a slightly different method for tumor measuring and different definitions for PD and PR. In a direct comparison between the RECIST and SWOG criteria in patients treated with [^{177}Lu-DOTA^0,Tyr^3]octreotate, there were no significant differences in the evaluation of responses [55]. In general, NETs are slow-growing tumors and most therapies do not lead to shrinkage of tumors, but stable disease instead. Therefore, the RECIST criteria using morphological volume characteristics may not be the ideal response criteria for relatively slow-growing NETs (i.e. G1/G2 tumors). Different groups have tried to develop new criteria for response evaluation based on nuclear imaging techniques. A small study with 4 patients found a more appropriate evaluation with the tumor-to-nontumor ratio (T/nT) on SRS with ^{99m}Tc-EDDA/HYNIC-TOC in combination with volume and attenuation changes on CT [56]. With the newest ^{68}Ga-SSA, it is easier to measure the change in standardized uptake value (SUV). Haug et al. [57] measured the tumor-to-spleen SUV ratio and maximum SUV ratio at baseline and 3 months after the first cycle of PRRT. They found a significant correlation with improvement in clinical symptoms.

Moreover, the decrease in tumor uptake predicted a longer time to progression. On the other hand, Gabriel et al. [58] found that an SUV analysis of individual lesions did not have an additional value in the prediction of individual responses to therapy compared with conventional anatomical imaging with CT. It is clear that further investigation is needed. A disadvantage of somatostatin-based imaging is that NETs may lose their receptors and become negative on these images. Therefore, it would be very interesting to measure the response with metabolic tracers like ^{18}F-DOPA or ^{11}C-5-HTP, which demonstrate metabolism within the tumor rather than expression of receptors. Unfortunately, there are so far no data available on the use of these tracers for response evaluation, but this type of response evaluation will become paramount within the next decade.

Conclusion

The initial diagnosis of NETs is made with radiological and histological methods. Nuclear imaging techniques are essential to estimate the total disease burden. Currently, the gold standard for the imaging of NETs is SRS with ^{111}In-DTPA-octreotide. It is almost certain that in the near future this will be replaced by ^{68}Ga-SSA PET imaging. ^{18}F-FDG PET has a limited role in the imaging of NETs, but may play a role in predicting the prognosis in G2/G3 tumor patients. ^{11}C-5-HTP and ^{18}F-DOPA PET show very promising results but are more difficult to produce and/or not widely available. ^{18}F-DOPA is commercially available in several European countries and its use may increase in the coming years. Besides, ^{18}F-DOPA has broader imaging applications than only NETs. Currently, selection for PRRT is based on SRS; further research needs to be done to translate the uptake on SRS to accumulation in the tumor on ^{68}Ga-SSA imaging. Subsequently, changes in tumor accumulation after therapy using metabolic tracers can have an additional value to the existing response criteria based on CT/MRI.

References

1 Townsend DW: Positron emission tomography/computed tomography. Semin Nucl Med 2008;38:152–166.

2 Cohade C, Wahl RL: Applications of positron emission tomography/computed tomography image fusion in clinical positron emission tomography – clinical use, interpretation methods, diagnostic improvements. Semin Nucl Med 2003;33:228–237.

3 Bosman FT, World Health Organization, International Agency for Research on Cancer: WHO Classification of Tumours of the Digestive System, ed 4. Lyon, IARC Press, 2010.

4 Araujo PB, Cheng S, Mete O, Serra S, Morin E, Asa SL, Ezzat S: Evaluation of the WHO 2010 grading and AJCC/UICC staging systems in prognostic behavior of intestinal neuroendocrine tumors. PLoS One 2013;8:e61538.

5 Krenning EP, Breeman WAP, Kooij PPM, Lameris JS, Bakker WH, Koper JW, Ausema L, Reubi JC, Lamberts SWJ: Localisation of endocrine-related tumours with radioiodinated analogue of somatostatin. Lancet 1989;333:242–244.

6 Reubi JC, Schär J-C, Waser B, Wenger S, Heppeler A, Schmitt JS, Macke HR: Affinity profiles for human somatostatin receptor subtypes SST1–SST5 of somatostatin radiotracers selected for scintigraphic and radiotherapeutic use. Eur J Nucl Med 2000;27:273–282.
7 Rinke A, Muller H-H, Schade-Brittinger C, Klose K-J, Barth P, Wied M, Mayer C, Aminossadati B, Pape U-F, Blaker M, Harder J, Arnold C, Gress T, Arnold R: Placebo-controlled, double-blind, prospective, randomized study on the effect of octreotide LAR in the control of tumor growth in patients with metastatic neuroendocrine midgut tumors: a report from the PROMID Study Group. J Clin Oncol 2009;27:4656–4663.
8 Balon HR, Brown TLY, Goldsmith SJ, Silberstein EB, Krenning EP, Lang O, Dillehay G, Tarrance J, Johnson M, Stabin MG: The SNM practice guideline for somatostatin receptor scintigraphy 2.0. J Nucl Med Technol 2011;39:317–324.
9 Kwekkeboom DJ, Kam BL, van Essen M, Teunissen JJM, van Eijck CHJ, Valkema R, de Jong M, de Herder WW, Krenning EP: Somatostatin receptor-based imaging and therapy of gastroenteropancreatic neuroendocrine tumors. Endocr Relat Cancer 2009;17: R53–R73.
10 Modlin IM, Kidd M, Latich I, Zikusoka MN, Shapiro MD: Current Status of Gastrointestinal Carcinoids. Gastroenterology 2005;128:1717–1751.
11 De Bruin C, Hofland LJ, Nieman LK, van Koetsveld PM, Waaijers AM, Sprij-Mooij DM, van Essen M, Lamberts SWJ, de Herder WW, Feelders RA: Mifepristone effects on tumor somatostatin receptor expression in two patients with Cushing's syndrome due to ectopic adrenocorticotropin secretion. J Clin Endocrinol Metab 2012;97:455–462.
12 Kwekkeboom DJ, de Herder WW, Kam BL, van Eijck CH, van Essen M, Kooij PP, Feelders RA, van Aken MO, Krenning EP: Treatment with the radiolabeled somatostatin analog [177Lu-DOTA0, Tyr3] octreotate: toxicity, efficacy, and survival. J Clin Oncol 2008;26:2124–2430.
13 Bombardieri E, Coliva A, Maccauro M, Seregni E, Orunesu E, Chiti A, Lucignani G: Imaging of neuroendocrine tumours with gamma-emitting radiopharmaceuticals. Q J Nucl Med Mol Imaging 2010; 54:3–15.
14 Gabriel M, Muehllechner P, Decristoforo C, von Guggenberg E, et al: ^{99m}Tc-EDDA/HYNIC-Tyr^{3}-octreotide for staging and follow-up of patients with neuroendocrine gastro-entero-pancreatic tumors. Q J Nucl Med Mol Imaging 2005;49:237–244.
15 Gabriel M, Decristoforo C, Donnemiller E, Ulmer H, Rychlinski CW, Mather SJ, Moncayo R: An intrapatient comparison of ^{99m}Tc-EDDA/HYNIC-TOC with ^{111}In-DTPA-octreotide for diagnosis of somatostatin receptor-expressing tumors. J Nucl Med 2003;44:708–716.
16 Geijer H, Breimer LH: Somatostatin receptor PET/CT in neuroendocrine tumours: update on systematic review and meta-analysis. Eur J Nucl Med Mol Imaging 2013;40:1770–1780.
17 Virgolini I, Ambrosini V, Bomanji JB, Baum RP, Fanti S, Gabriel M, Papathanasiou ND, Pepe G, Oyen W, Cristoforo C, Chiti A: Procedure guidelines for PET/CT tumour imaging with ^{68}Ga-DOTA-conjugated peptides: ^{68}Ga-DOTA-TOC, ^{68}Ga-DOTA-NOC, ^{68}Ga-DOTA-TATE. Eur J Nucl Med Mol Imaging 2010;37:2004–2010.
18 Gabriel M, Decristoforo C, Kendler D, Dobrozemsky G, Heute D, Uprimny C, Kovacs P, von Guggenberg E, Bale R, Virgolini IJ: ^{68}Ga-DOTA-Tyr^{3}-octreotide PET in neuroendocrine tumors: comparison with somatostatin receptor scintigraphy and CT. J Nucl Med 2007;48:508–518.
19 Buchmann I, Henze M, Engelbrecht S, Eisenhut M, Runz A, Schäfer M, Schilling T, Haufe S, Herrmann T, Haberkorn U: Comparison of ^{68}Ga-DOTATOC PET and ^{111}In-DTPAOC (Octreoscan) SPECT in patients with neuroendocrine tumours. Eur J Nucl Med Mol Imaging 2007;34:1617–1626.
20 Krausz Y, Freedman N, Rubinstein R, Lavie E, Orevi M, Tshori S, Salmon A, Glaser B, Chisin R, Mishani E, Gross DJ: ^{68}Ga-DOTA-NOC PET/CT imaging of neuroendocrine tumors: comparison with ^{111}In-DTPA-Octreotide (OctreoScan®). Mol Imaging Biol 2010;13:583–593.
21 Walker RC, Smith GT, Liu E, Moore B, Clanton J, Stabin M: Measured human dosimetry of ^{68}Ga-DOTATATE. J Nucl Med 2013;54:855–860.
22 Schreiter NF, Brenner W, Nogami M, Buchert R, Huppertz A, Pape U-F, Prasad V, Hamm B, Maurer MH: Cost comparison of ^{111}In-DTPA-octreotide scintigraphy and ^{68}Ga-DOTATOC PET/CT for staging enteropancreatic neuroendocrine tumours. Eur J Nucl Med Mol Imaging 2011;39:72–82.
23 Castellucci P, Pou Ucha J, Fuccio C, Rubello D, Ambrosini V, Montini GC, Pettinato V, Malizia C, Lodi F, Fanti S: Incidence of Increased ^{68}Ga-DOTANOC uptake in the pancreatic head in a large series of extrapancreatic NET patients studied with sequential PET/CT. J Nucl Med 2011;52:886–890.
24 Wang X, Zielinski MC, Misawa R, Wen P, Wang T-Y, Wang C-Z, Witkowski P, Hara M, Shi X: Quantitative analysis of pancreatic polypeptide cell distribution in the human pancreas. PLoS One 2013; 8:e55501.
25 Teunissen JJM, Kwekkeboom DJ, Valkema R, Krenning EP: Nuclear medicine techniques for the imaging and treatment of neuroendocrine tumours. Endocr Relat Cancer 2011;18:S27–S51.
26 Öberg K, Eriksson B: Nuclear medicine in the detection, staging and treatment of gastrointestinal carcinoid tumours. Best Pract Res Clin Endocrinol Metab 2005;19:265–276.

27 Modlin IM, Latich I, Zikusoka M, Kidd M, Eick G, Chan AK: Gastrointestinal carcinoids: the evolution of diagnostic strategies. J Clin Gastroenterol 2006;40: 572–582.

28 Adams S, Baum R, Rink T, Schumm-Dräger P-M, Usadel K-H, Hör G: Limited value of fluorine-18 fluorodeoxyglucose positron emission tomography for the imaging of neuroendocrine tumours. Eur J Nucl Med 1998;25:79–83.

29 Garin E, Le Jeune F, Devillers A, Cuggia M, de Lajarte-Thirouard A-S, Bouriel C, Boucher E, Raoul JL: Predictive value of ^{18}F-FDG PET and somatostatin receptor scintigraphy in patients with metastatic endocrine tumors. J Nucl Med 2009;50:858–864.

30 Severi S, Nanni O, Bodei L, Sansovini M, Ianniello A, Nicoletti S, Scarpi E, Matteucci F, Gilardi L, Paganelli G: Role of ^{18}FDG PET/CT in patients treated with ^{177}Lu-DOTATATE for advanced differentiated neuroendocrine tumours. Eur J Nucl Med Mol Imaging 2013;40:881–888.

31 Kayani I, Bomanji JB, Groves A, Conway G, Gacinovic S, Win T, Dickson J, Caplin M, Ell PJ: Functional imaging of neuroendocrine tumors with combined PET/CT using ^{68}Ga-DOTATATE (DOTA-DPhe1,Tyr^{3}-octreotate) and ^{18}F-FDG. Cancer 2008;112:2447–2455.

32 Naswa N, Sharma P, Gupta SK, Karunanithi S, Reddy RM, Patnecha M, Lata S, Kumar R, Malhotra A, Bal C: Dual tracer functional imaging of gastroenteropancreatic neuroendocrine tumors using ^{68}Ga-DOTA-NOC PET-CT and ^{18}F-FDG PET-CT: competitive or complimentary? Clin Nucl Med 2014;39:e27–e34.

33 Jager PL, Chirakal R, Marriott CJ, Brouwers AH, Koopmans KP, Gulenchyn KY: 6-L-^{18}F-fluorodihydroxyphenylalanine PET in neuroendocrine tumors: basic aspects and emerging clinical applications. J Nucl Med 2008;49:573–586.

34 Chondrogiannis S, Cristina Marzola M, Al-Nahhas A, Venkatanarayana TD, Mazza A, Opocher G, Rubello D: Normal biodistribution pattern and physiologic variants of ^{18}F-DOPA PET imaging. Nucl Med Commun 2013;34:1141–1149.

35 Rufini V, Baum RP, Castaldi P, Treglia G, Gaetano AM, Carreras C, Kaemmerer D, Hommann M, Horsch D, Bonomo L, Giordano A: Role of PET/CT in the functional imaging of endocrine pancreatic tumors. Abdom Imaging 2012;37:1004–1020.

36 Brown WD, Oakes TR, DeJesus OT, Taylor MD, Roberts AD, Nickles RJ, Holden JE: Fluorine-18-fluoro-L-DOPA dosimetry with carbidopa pretreatment. J Nucl Med 1998;39:1884–1891.

37 Timmers HJLM, Hadi M, Carrasquillo JA, Chen CC, Martiniova L, Whatley M, Ling A, Eisenhofer G, Adams KT, Pacak K: The Effects of carbidopa on uptake of 6-^{18}F-Fluoro-L-DOPA in PET of pheochromocytoma and extraadrenal abdominal paraganglioma. J Nucl Med 2007;48:1599–1606.

38 Kauhanen S, Seppänen M, Nuutila P: Premedication with carbidopa masks positive finding of insulinoma and β-cell hyperplasia in [^{18}F]-dihydroxy-phenylalanine positron emission tomography. J Clin Oncol 2008;26:5307–5308.

39 Kauhanen S, Seppanen M, Minn H, Nuutila P: Clinical PET imaging of insulinoma and β-cell hyperplasia. Curr Pharm Des 2010;16:1550–1560.

40 Balogova S, Talbot J-N, Nataf V, Michaud L, Huchet V, Kerrou K, Montravers F: ^{18}F-fluorodihydroxyphenylalanine vs other radiopharmaceuticals for imaging neuroendocrine tumours according to their type. Eur J Nucl Med Mol Imaging 2013;40:943–966.

41 Fiebrich H-B, Jong JR, Kema IP, Koopmans KP, Sluiter W, Dierckx RAJO, Walenkamp AM, Links TP, Brouwers AH, Vries EGE: Total ^{18}F-DOPA PET tumour uptake reflects metabolic endocrine tumour activity in patients with a carcinoid tumour. Eur J Nucl Med Mol Imaging 2011;38:1854–1861.

42 Tessonnier L, Sebag F, Ghander C, De Micco C, Reynaud R, Palazzo FF, Conte-Devolx B, Henry JF, Mundler O, Taieb D: Limited value of ^{18}F-F-DOPA PET to localize pancreatic insulin-secreting tumors in adults with hyperinsulinemic hypoglycemia. J Clin Endocrinol Metab 2010;95:303–307.

43 Orlefors H, Sundin A, Lu L, Oberg K, Långström B, Eriksson B, Bergstrom M: Carbidopa pretreatment improves image interpretation and visualisation of carcinoid tumours with ^{11}C-5-hydroxytryptophan positron emission tomography. Eur J Nucl Med Mol Imaging 2006;33:60–65.

44 Orlefors H: Whole-body ^{11}C-5-hydroxytryptophan positron emission tomography as a universal imaging technique for neuroendocrine tumors: comparison with somatostatin receptor scintigraphy and computed tomography. J Clin Endocrinol Metab 2005;90:3392–3400.

45 Orlefors H, Sundin A, Ahlström H, Bjurling P, Bergström M, Lilja A, Langstrom B, Oberg K, Eriksson B: Positron emission tomography with 5-hydroxytryprophan in neuroendocrine tumors. J Clin Oncol 1998;16:2534–2541.

46 Orlefors H, Sundin A, Eriksson B, Skogseid B, Oberg K, Akerström G, Hellman P: PET-guided surgery – high correlation between positron emission tomography with ^{11}C-5-hydroxytryptophane (5-HTP) and surgical findings in abdominal neuroendocrine tumours. Cancers 2012;4:100–112.

47 Koopmans KP, Neels OC, Kema IP, Elsinga PH, Sluiter WJ, Vanghillewe K, Brouwers AH, Jager PL, de Vries EGE: Improved staging of patients with carcinoid and islet cell tumors with ^{18}F-dihydroxy-phenyl-alanine and ^{11}C-5-hydroxy-tryptophan positron emission tomography. J Clin Oncol 2008;26:1489–1495.

48 Grant CS: Insulinoma. Best Pract Res Clin Gastroenterol 2005;19:783–798.

49 De Herder WW, Kwekkeboom DJ, Valkema R, Feelders RA, van Aken MO, Lamberts SWJ, van der Lely AJ, Krenning EP: Neuroendocrine tumors and somatostatin: imaging techniques. J Endocrinol Invest 2005;28:132–136.
50 Reubi JC, Waser B: Concomitant expression of several peptide receptors in neuroendocrine tumours: molecular basis for in vivo multireceptor tumour targeting. Eur J Nucl Med Mol Imaging 2003;30:781–793.
51 Christ E, Wild D, Forrer F, Brandle M, Sahli R, Clerici T, Gloor B, Martius F, Maecke H, Reubi JC: Glucagon-like peptide-1 receptor imaging for localization of insulinomas. J Clin Endocrinol Metab 2009;94:4398–4405.
52 Sowa-Staszczak A, Pach D, Mikołajczak R, Mäcke H, Jabrocka-Hybel A, Stefańska A, Tomaszuk M, Janota B, Gilis-Januszewska A, Malecki M, Kaminski G, Kowalska A, Kulig J, Matyja A, Osuch C, Hubalewska-Dydejczyk A: Glucagon-like peptide-1 receptor imaging with [Lys^{40}(Ahx-HYNIC-^{99m}Tc/EDDA)NH_2]-exendin-4 for the detection of insulinoma. Eur J Nucl Med Mol Imaging 2012;40:524–531.
53 Wild D, Christ E, Caplin ME, Kurzawinski TR, Forrer F, Brandle M, Seufert J, Weber WA, Bomanji J, Perren A, Ell PJ, Reubi JC: Glucagon-like peptide-1 versus somatostatin receptor targeting reveals 2 distinct forms of malignant insulinomas. J Nucl Med 2011;52:1073–1078.
54 Eisenhauer EA, Therasse P, Bogaerts J, Schwartz LH, Sargent D, Ford R, Dancey J, Arbuck S, Gwyther S, Mooney M, Rubinstein L, Shankar L, Dodd L, Kaplan R, Lacombe D, Verweij J: New response evaluation criteria in solid tumours: revised RECIST guideline (version 1.1). Eur J Cancer 2009;45:228–247.
55 van Vliet EI, Krenning EP, Teunissen JJ, Bergsma H, Kam BL, Kwekkeboom DJ: Comparison of response evaluation in patients with gastroenteropancreatic and thoracic neuroendocrine tumors after treatment with [^{177}Lu-DOTA^0, Tyr^3]octreotate. J Nucl Med 2013;54:1689–1696.
56 Sowa-Staszczak A, Chrzan R, Pach D, Stefańska A, Tomaszuk M, Buziak-Bereza M, Kolodziej M, Przybylik-Mazurek E, Hubalewska-Dydejczyk A: Are RECIST criteria sufficient to assess response to therapy in neuroendocrine tumors? Clin Imaging 2012;36:360–364.
57 Haug AR, Auernhammer CJ, Wangler B, Schmidt GP, Uebleis C, Goke B, Cumming P, Bartenstein P, Tiling R, Hacker M: ^{68}Ga-DOTATATE PET/CT for the early prediction of response to somatostatin receptor-mediated radionuclide therapy in patients with well-differentiated neuroendocrine tumors. J Nucl Med 2010;51:1349–1356.
58 Gabriel M, Oberauer A, Dobrozemsky G, Decristoforo C, Putzer D, Kendler D, Uprimny C, Kovacs P, Bale R, Virgolini IJ: ^{68}Ga-DOTA-Tyr^3-octreotide PET for assessing response to somatostatin-receptor-mediated radionuclide therapy. J Nucl Med 2009;50:1427–1434.

Tessa Brabander
Erasmus Medical Centre, Department of Nuclear Medicine, Room Cb206
Postbus 2040
NL–3000 CA Rotterdam (The Netherlands)
E-Mail t.brabander@erasmusmc.nl

Papotti M, de Herder WW (eds): Neuroendocrine Tumors: A Multidisciplinary Approach.
Front Horm Res. Basel, Karger, 2015, vol 44, pp 88–103 (DOI: 10.1159/000382062)

Endoscopy and Endoscopic Ultrasound in Assessing and Managing Neuroendocrine Neoplasms

Dermot O'Toole[a–c] • Laurent Palazzo[d]

[a]National Neuroendocrine Tumour Service, St. Vincent's University Hospital, [b]Department of Gastroenterology, St James's Hospital, and [c]Trinity College, Dublin, Ireland; [d]Service d'Endoscopie, Clinique du Trocadero, Paris, France

Abstract

Despite advances in radiological and metabolic imaging, standard axial endoscopy and endoscopic ultrasonography (EUS) still play a pivotal role in a number of neuroendocrine neoplasms (NENs) of the gastrointestinal and duodenopancreatic region. Upper gastrointestinal endoscopy is essential for the detection and characterization of NEN up to the angle of Treitz (esophageal, gastric and duodenal). Ileocolonoscopy allows the assessing and diagnosing of rectal, colonic and very occasionally distal ileal lesions. Endoscopic assessment is the mainstay for diagnosing gastric NENs associated with hypergastrinemia, but is also useful in detecting and diagnosing duodenal NENs (both functional and nonfunctional) and ampullary NENs. As rectal NENs are on the increase, standard colonoscopy (often combined with endorectal EUS) is also useful in detecting and treating small rectal NENs. EUS is the modality of choice for diagnosing pancreatic NENs and for locoregional staging of esophageal, gastric, duodenal, pancreatic and rectal NENs. This chapter will expand on the diagnostic and therapeutic role of endoscopy and EUS in the field of gastrointestinal and pancreatic NENs.

Gastrointestinal Neuroendocrine Neoplasms

Gastric Neuroendocrine Neoplasms

Gastric neuroendocrine neoplasms (NENs) have a varied spectrum with regard to histology, clinicopathologic background, stage and prognosis [1]. They are usually discovered incidentally and are for the most part benign. Two broad categories exist: (1) hypergastrinemia-related tumors – secondary to chronic atrophic gastritis (type 1

Table 1. Gastric and/or duodenal NENs: key factors for the endoscopist

	Comments
Atrophy?	Pernicious anemia or nonimmune-related chronic atrophic gastritis[1]
Hypertrophic gastric folds?	In cases of hypergastrinemia due to gastrinoma in ZES and MEN1
Association of gastric and duodenal nodules?	ZES and MEN1
Stigmata of hyperacidity?	ZES and MEN1
Gastric aspirate for random fasting pH!	If pH is high in a fasting patient, then suspect atrophic gastritis and achlorhydria[2]
Lesion assessment	Number, location, size, morphological aspect
Tumors approaching 1 cm	Perform EUS
Biopsy protocol (for gastric NENs)	
Predominant lesion(s)	++
Random biopsies	Gastric antrum Gastric body and fundus (check for atrophy and also for ECL-cell hyperplasia)
Check for metaplasia, adenomas, early neoplasia in chronic atrophic gastritis	Careful inspection using HRE and/or electronic chromoendoscopy and a proper sampling protocol

ZES = Zollinger-Ellison syndrome; HRE = high-resolution endoscopy.
[1] Antibodies to parietal cells or intrinsic factor antibodies are useful.
[2] pH is usually low in the setting of fasting for endoscopy.

gastric NENs) or more infrequently associated with Zollinger-Ellison syndrome as part of multiple endocrine neoplasia type 1 (MEN1; type 2 gastric NENs), and (2) sporadic or type 3 gastric NENs.

Type 1 Gastric NENs

Type 1 gastric NENs result from hypergastrinemia in chronic atrophic gastritis [either immune-related (pernicious anemia) or nonimmune] resulting in enterochromaffin-like (ECL) cell hyperplasia and eventually small gastric NENs. The natural history of type 1 gastric carcinoids is generally (>95%) favorable and simple surveillance is usually recommended for small (<1 cm) T1 tumors, with local (endoscopic or surgical) resection for larger lesions [1–3]. Larger tumors may require oncological resection or other forms of therapy (somatostatin analogs, gastrin receptor antagonists or chemotherapy, if stage IV). Rarely, gastric NENs have a malignant course and this is usually confined to type 2 and especially type 3 tumors; the latter mimic a biological course close to that of gastric adenocarcinoma and require radical oncological therapies.

Careful assessment with upper gastrointestinal endoscopy is required for gastric NENs (table 1). Biopsies should be obtained from the dominant tumor(s), but

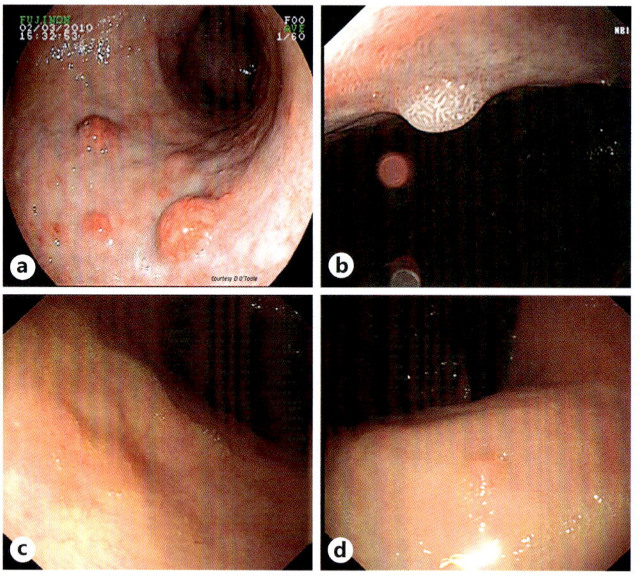

Fig. 1. Various endoscopic appearances of gastric NENs. **a** Gastroscopy revealing multiple sessile gastric NENs of various sizes located in the gastric body on a background to clearly define gastric atrophy. Note the rich vascular network on the surface of the two predominant lesions (gastric NENs with Ki-67 of 5%). Other smaller nodules <1 cm are also seen and correspond to either microcarcinoids or aggregates of ECL hyperplasia. **b** Polypoid gastric NENs on the anterior wall of the proximal gastric body (using narrow band imaging). **c** A flat and predominantly submucosal NEN. **d** A micropolyp.

in addition it is mandatory to sample the gastric antrum (2 biopsies) and body/fundus (4 biopsies) to establish a potential diagnosis of atrophic gastritis and ECL cell hyperplasia. In type 1 gastric NENs, careful inspection of the gastric cavity following full air insufflation usually reveals a lack of gastric folds and is often accompanied by a low volume of gastric mucus/acid pool. On-site pocket pH meters can be useful in confirming a high pH (thus confirming achlorhydria and 24-hour pH is rarely necessary to establish the diagnosis). Gastric NENs may take several forms (fig. 1), but are usually sessile and multiple and located in the gastric body and fundus. These tumors involve both mucosa and submucosa and occasionally display a rich vascular network on their surface (fig. 1a). Generous tumor sampling is necessary to look for standard histological features of NEN (and immunohistochemistry for chromogranin A, synaptophysin and Ki-67 proliferative marker). Random sampling from the gastric body/fundus mucosa should also be performed to search for associated ECL-like cell hyperplasia (the precursors of microcarcinoids and full tumors). Endoscopic ultrasonography (EUS; fig. 2) enables assessment of the degree of depth extension (invasion of the muscularis propria) and locoregional lymph node invasion (essential in patients with gastric tumors ≥1 cm) and is recommended before resection of polyps 1–2 cm in diameter [1–3] (fig. 2, 3).

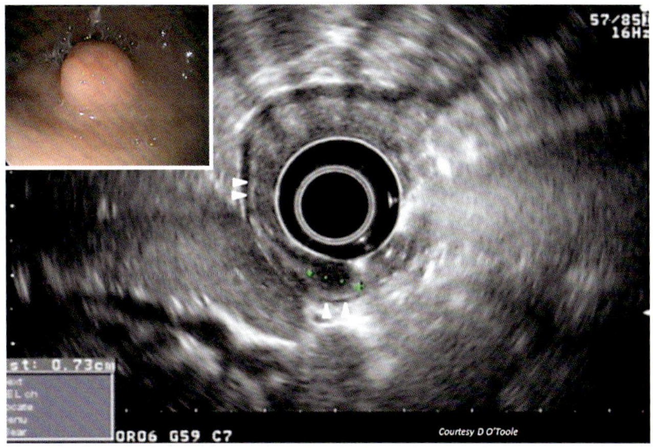

Fig. 2. EUS of a small 7-mm hypoechoic and homogeneous gastric neuroendocrine tumor. **insert** The corresponding axial endoscopic image of a small sessile nodule in the proximal gastric body. At EUS, the tumor is confined to the submucosa at a distance from the dark rim of the muscularis propria (arrow head) (uT1N0).

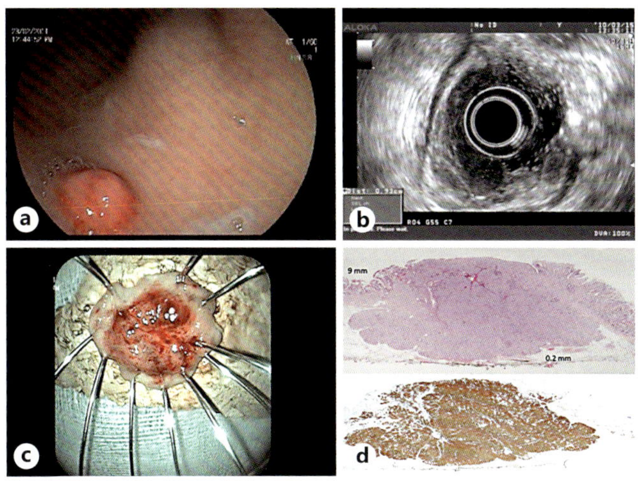

Fig. 3. Endoscopic evaluation of a gastric NEN (**a**) that is almost 1 cm in maximal diameter located in the gastric body and classified as uT1N0 on EUS (**b**). The tumor was fully excised using an EMR technique (**c**), pinned to spread the lesion before fixing in formalin and histology (**d**) revealing clear deep and peripheral margins: HE (upper image) and chromogranin A (lower image).

Finally, patients with chronic atrophic gastritis may harbor intestinal metaplasia or dysplasia and endoscopic assessment for mucosal field changes should be performed carefully using chromoendoscopy or electronic chromoendoscopy techniques and sampling.

Type 2 Gastric NENs

Patients with gastric NENs associated with hypergastrinemia from Zollinger-Ellison syndrome in the setting of MEN1 [4] can have tumors of similar distribution to type 1 tumors, but careful inspection of the duodenum is also required to search for duodenal NENs (gastrinomas) (fig. 4) [5, 6]. Type 2 gastric NENs can be multiple and can attain quite large sizes (fig. 4) and they are reported to have a malignant potential of up to 15%. At upper gastrointestinal endoscopy, the discerning endoscopist will also note the hypertrophied gastric folds (fig. 4c) and a large volume of gastric mu-

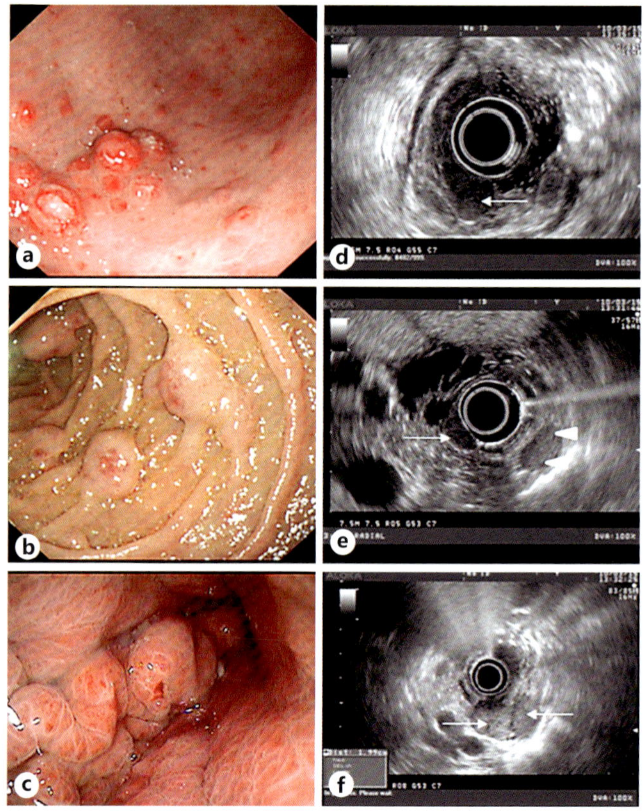

Fig. 4. Patient with type 2 gastric neuroendocrine tumors in the setting of Zollinger-Ellison syndrome and multiple endocrine neoplasia type 1. The patient has numerous gastric tumors of various sizes in the gastric body (**a**), some of which are ulcerated. There are also numerous duodenal NENs (**b**), some of which are responsible for the hypersecretion of gastrin that results in hypertrophic gastric folds (**c**). At EUS the gastric (**d**) and duodenal NENs (**e**, arrow) can be easily seen as well as periduodenal lymph nodes (**e**, arrow heads) and multiple sizable pancreatic NENs in the tail of the pancreas (**f**, arrows).

cus/acid: the secretory capacity is often quite heightened in these patients, such that following aspiration of a large volume of mucus/acid, this frequently replenishes by the end of the examinations. EUS in type 2 tumors needs to be meticulous and may take some time, as in addition to staging of the gastric tumors, evaluation is also required to assess for the presence of intraparietal duodenal gastrinoma (fig. 4d; often small, requiring a hyperinflated balloon, and occasionally the instillation of water to obtain better acoustic coupling) of pancreatic NENs and of adjacent lymphadenopathy (fig. 4).

Type 3 Gastric NENs

In cases of sporadic tumors (type 3 tumors), the tumors are usually sessile and located in the gastric antrum [7, 8]. They can be large (fig. 5), are usually single and may have a nonspecific aspect, but are distinguishable for their adenoma counterparts by the absence of a villiform mucosal pattern, which is easily recognizable using modern high-resolution endoscopy with electronic chromoendoscopy. Biopsies are required from the tumor site and also noninvolved mucosa (biopsies form mucosa more proximally reveals preservation of nonatrophic mucosa) and tumor grades here are often high. EUS is mandatory to aid staging (fig. 5) and, in addition,

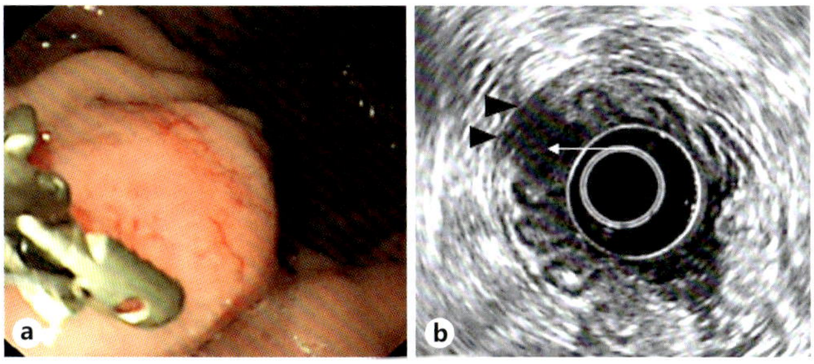

Fig. 5. A patient with a sporadic type 3 gastric neuroendocrine tumor. **a** The tumor is situated in the distal gastric body (junction with the antrum) and measures 2 cm in maximal dimension. **b** At EUS the tumor (arrow) is demonstrated to clearly involve the outer limits of the gastric wall (black arrow heads); surgery was performed with a partial gastrectomy and the tumor was confirmed to be pT3 with 1 of 13 lymph nodes positive.

a more extensive imaging protocol should be performed, such as a CT scan and somatostatin receptor scintigraphy (SRS) to assess for locoregional nodes and liver metastases.

Treatment of Gastric NENs

Management of gastric NENs is determined by subtype, and whether the disease is localized or metastatic. Since the most common subtype of gastric NENs is type 1, these usually display a benign and indolent clinical behavior; simple surveillance or localized endoscopic treatment modalities can be employed for small tumors [2]. For tumors <1 cm, surveillance can be recommended; for tumors between 1 and 2 cm confined to mucosa/submucosa (guided by careful EUS appraisal – uT1), endoscopic resection is recommended with an experienced endoscopist in this field and full endoscopic mucosal resection (EMR) or endoscopic submucosal dissection (ESD) techniques (fig. 3) should be employed to ensure complete resection. Endoscopic resection can be easily repeated provided tumors do not grow beyond uT1 [7, 8], and this strategy appears to be universally accepted now. Nonetheless, recurrences do occur. A recurrence rate in a recent series of patients treated endoscopically was 64% (21/33) at a median of 8 months and, of these, 67% (14/21) had a second recurrence [9]. A recent study in 82 patients demonstrated excellent recurrence-free and disease-free survival following endoscopic (n = 41) or surgical (n = 16) resections in patients with type I gastric NENs [10]. In our personal, nonpublished experience of more than 150 patients, EMR for lesions of 1 cm and above is infrequently required and the vast majority of patients have multiple small lesions that do not appear to grow over many years. The TNM staging system uses 1 cm in size as a cut-off to define T1/2 tumors, although there is inconsistency in the guidelines as to whether tumors between 1 and 2 cm should be treated with local resection. Surgery should be performed in the case of involvement beyond the submucosa (fig. 6), or positive margin after endoscopic resection and either a local resection (e.g. wedge resection)

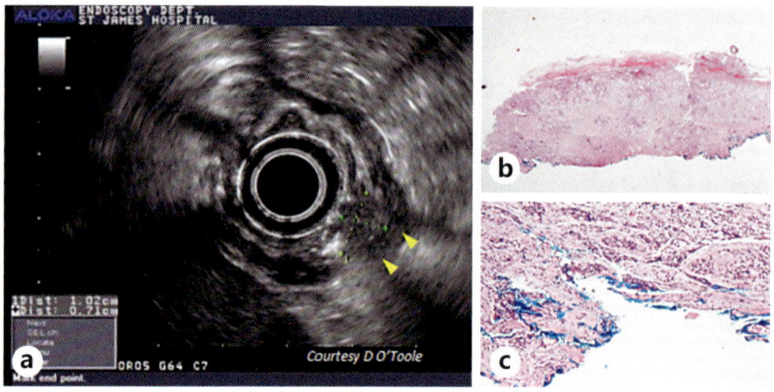

Fig. 6. A large (>1 cm) type 1 gastric NEN in a patient with pernicious anemia that clearly invades the muscularis propria on EUS (**a**) and in whom surgery was deemed a high-risk procedure. The lesion was resected using EMR and as predicted by EUS the deep margins were involved (**b**, **c**) and the patient went on to have a local gastrectomy with resection of the EMR scar site with one node involved (uT2N1).

and antrectomy or total gastrectomy (depending on tumor histological features, invasion and localization) have been recommended. While antrectomy has the theoretical advantage of removing the stimulus for gastrin secretion, this technique have become outdated by many expert groups [11] as the adequacy of antrectomy has been questioned in the past and a simple wedge or localized excision followed by endoscopic surveillance may be more appropriate [1, 11, 12].

Treatment of type 2 gastric NENs is dictated by the presence of other pancreatic and often duodenal NENs in the setting of MEN1 and Zollinger-Ellision syndrome. Endoscopic or surgical resection can be employed for large gastric NENs; however, given the complexity of the individual cases, this should be performed in a specialized center following careful multidisciplinary assessment [13].

While endoscopic resection of small (uT1) sporadic type 3 NENs is theoretically possible, these tumors often have a high proliferative capacity (whether well or poorly differentiated) and frequent nodal metastases. Oncological resection is therefore recommended after careful staging.

Duodenal NENs

Aside from the duodenal gastrinomas, other duodenal NENs are rare and can be summarized as nonfunctioning duodenal NENs (often incidentally discovered), somatostatinomas, poorly differentiated neuroendocrine carcinoma (including those of the ampulla of Vater) and duodenal paragangliomas [14]. Assessment is as for gastric NENs, axial endoscopy with biopsy is recommended and EUS to confirm the diagnosis and local stage of the disease [15, 16] (fig. 7, 8); the latter is especially important as their size is usually small and may be localized to the submucosa and not detected on axial endoscopy. In fact, duodenal gastrinomas are hard to detect even with the aid of EUS, and a combination with SRS or ^{68}Gallium PET-CT can increase detection rates.

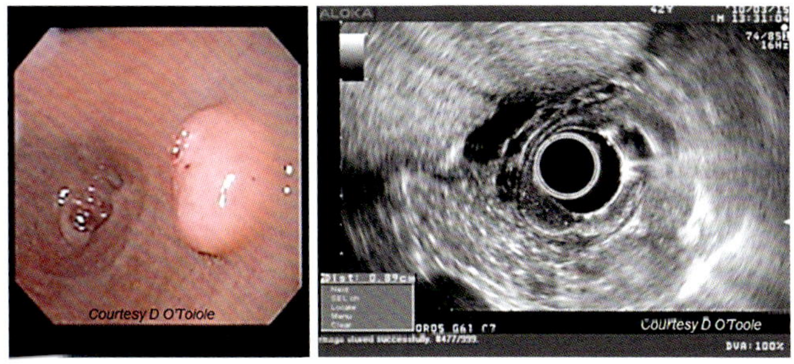

Fig. 7. Endoscopic view and EUS of a sporadic gastrinoma located in the duodenal bulb. At EUS the tumor is well defined and situated within the mucosal and submucosal space (uT1).

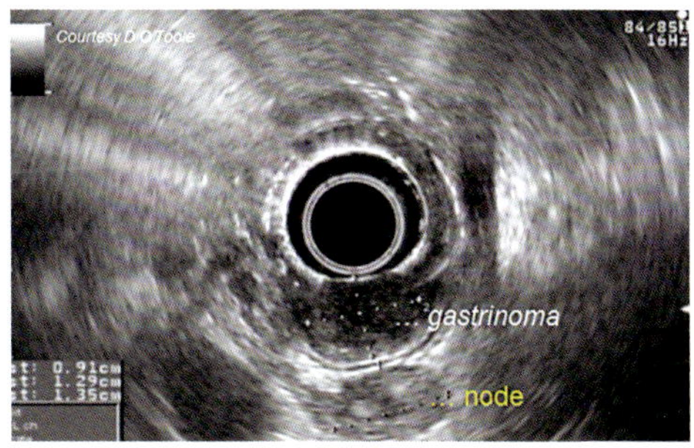

Fig. 8. EUS image using a radial probe of a duodenal gastrinoma (hypoechoic and homogeneous with clearly defined outlines) and a clearly demarcated local (periduodenal) lymph node (uT1N1).

Rectal NENs

Rectal NENs are increasing in incidence (0.2–0.9/100,000 from 1973 to 2004 in the SEER dataset) [17]. This rise – found not only in the USA, but also in Europe and Japan – may be due to a real increase in incidence, but might also be due to the larger number of incidentally discovered tumors at colonoscopy performed for unrelated reasons (especially colorectal screening programs). Some estimate that at least 50% are discovered incidentally [18] and, therefore, the majority are detected in a 'non-NEN expert' community. There are no accurate data pertaining to the site within the rectum, but they appear to localize to the mid or lower rectum. Their endoscopic aspect may vary (fig. 9–11) – the vast majority are small and are usually bland-appearing mucosa/submucosal firm bumps, often with a yellowish appearance. When evaluated using white light endoscopy and a high resolution endoscope and quality monitor they should not be mistaken for adenomatous or hyperplastic polyps as the mucosa covering these lesions is usually smooth and almost never villiform. They may have a predominant submucosal tumor aspect. In fact, general endoscopists are poor in reporting either the location or in marking rectal lesions that undergo resection, and this makes for follow-up analysis of incompletely resected rectal NENs very challenging [19]. The metastatic risk for rectal NENs is proportional to size: tumors <1 cm (3%), 1–2 cm (10–15%) and >2 cm (60% and more) [20]. In addition, special care must be taken with lesions demonstrating a centrally depressed zone, as they are often more advanced (fig. 10). Rectal NENs should be excised using

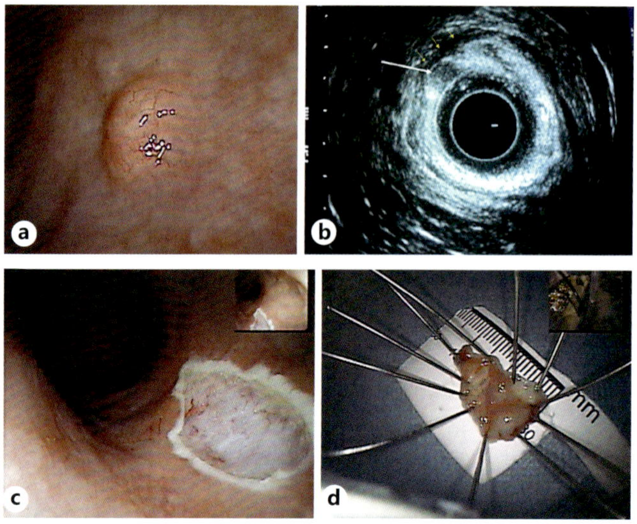

Fig. 9. Example of a rectal NEN incidentally discovered at screening colonoscopy for colorectal cancer. **a** At rectoscopy (endoscopic image) the lesion is a smooth sessile bump with a rich vascular network located in the mid rectum. **b** The tumor is also clearly seen on the rectal EUS (large arrow) as hypoechoic and well-defined within the mucosal and submucosal space, against the outer dark rim of muscularis propria (short arrows). In the same patient following EMR using a band EMR technique, the clear EMR scar site (**c**) and the pinned-down EMR resected margins prior to fixing for histology (**d**) are shown of the final well-differentiated NEN with a Ki-67 of 5% (grade 2) that was fully excised (0.3-mm-deep margins).

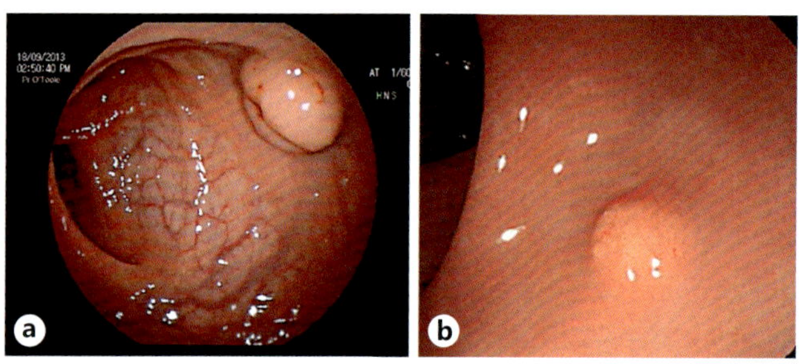

Fig. 10. Rectal neuroendocrine tumor measuring approximately 15 mm with a central depressed zone. **a** EUS revealed the lesion to be uT2 with involvement of the muscularis propria. Rectal resection (total mesorectal excision) confirmed a pT2 with 2 positive nodes. **b** Small 6-mm sessile rectal NEN with a predominantly submucosal aspect (faint yellow hue). Experienced endoscopists do not mistake this for a hyperplastic or adenomatous polyp and should perform a generous EMR and not a snare polypectomy.

a complete endoscopic resection technique. Selecting patients for treatment should always rely on accurate staging using EUS even for smaller tumors, as this has both an excellent correlation with tumor size, local staging and capacity to fully excise the tumors [21, 22]. EUS-guided biopsy can be performed on doubtful perirectal nodes (fig. 11).

Fig. 11. Perirectal lymph node in a patient who had an incomplete snare polypectomy excision of a 13-mm rectal NEN. The previous polypectomy scar site was not recognizable at rectoscopy but at EUS an 11-mm perirectal lymph node can be seen (dotted line) that was sampled using EUS-guided biopsy (the arrow indicates the 25-gauge needle) and smear cytology confirmed the neuroendocrine nature after staining positive for synaptophysin and CD56 (chromogranin A was negative). Ki-67 was 3% (not shown).

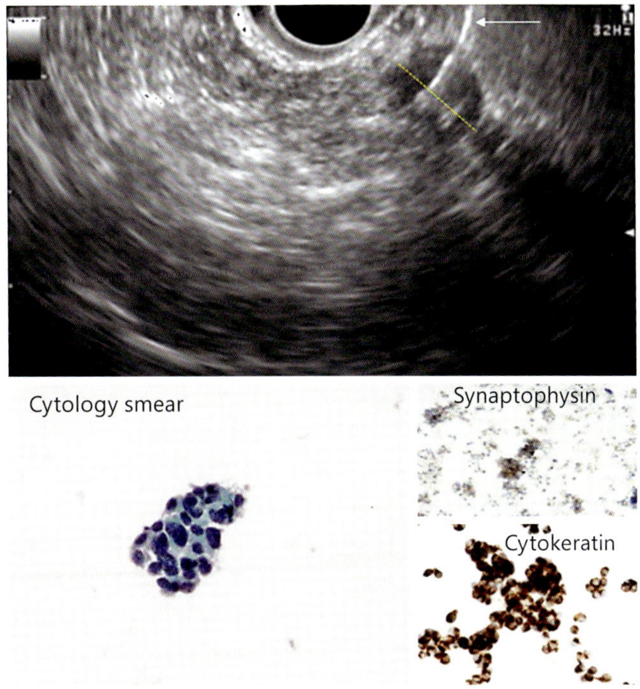

In treating small rectal NENs, snare polypectomy (unfortunately frequently employed by the general endoscopist) often results in incomplete excision (83% in some series) [23]. Even when performing EMR it has been shown that band-ligation EMR techniques are to be preferred to standard inject-lift-snare EMRs and several series have shown that ESD is better in terms of complete histological resection results (90 vs. 71% in one recent series) [24, 25]. In a pooled analysis or endoscopic techniques for resecting rectal NENs, Zhou et al. [25] demonstrated that ESD was superior to EMR (risk ratio 0.89, 0.79–0.99); they also found that modified EMRs (using band ligation techniques) was superior to standard EMR and equivalent to ESD. Complete local endoscopic excision yields excellent results but some patients may require additional local endoscopic resection (e.g. TEMS) or radical surgery.

Pancreatic Neuroendocrine Neoplasms

EUS has been the reference examination for accurate preoperative detection of duodenal and pancreatic NENs for over 30 years now. This is especially true for insulinomas and gastrinomas, two of the most frequent functional NENs of this region. EUS performs well due to the excellent resolution with accurate detection of small lesions (even <5 mm). Insulinomas are often small and hard to see on both CT scan

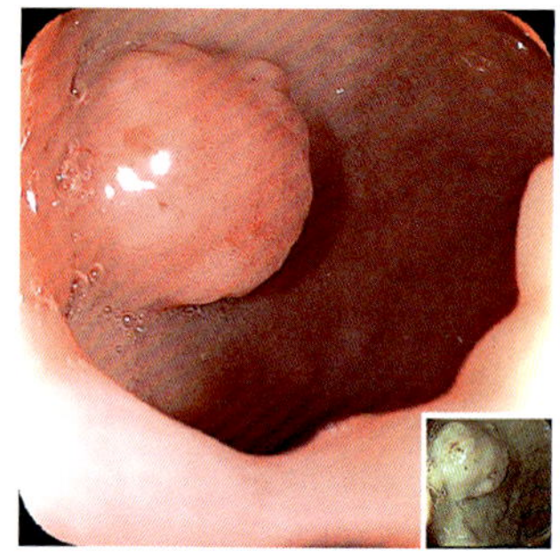

Fig. 12. Axial endoscopy showing a 10-mm postpyloric sporadic gastrinoma in the duodenal bulb. **insert** The same image using FICE.

and SRS (due to the absence of somatostatin receptor type 2), and gastrinomas are often very small and are predominantly found in the wall of the duodenum and, more rarely, the pancreas. In the past, nonfunctioning pancreatic NENs were often detected when the tumors were either large of metastatic, but now increasingly incidentally found small pancreatic NENs are a frequent occurrence (imaging for unrelated reasons) and EUS plays an integral role here [26]. When EUS is performed by an experienced operator (especially one versed in recognizing NENs), the diagnostic precision for detecting and localizing insulinomas is close to 95%; the diagnostic precision is lower for small duodenal gastrinomas, but remains high for gastrinomas of the pancreas and, when combined with SRS, overall gastrinoma detection exceeds 90% [27]. Standard axial endoscopy is also important in searching for sporadic or MEN1-related gastrinomas and should precede the EUS. Careful inspection of the entire duodenum should be performed, paying particular attention to the duodenal bulb (fig. 12) and postpyloric space where small tumors can be easily missed hiding behind the pyloric canal, and passing the scope several times via the pylorus is necessary to identify some lesions. EUS has also been shown to be a very sensitive method in the detection of pancreatic NENs as part of the MEN1 syndrome and indeed it is recommended in the follow-up of patients in detecting increases in size [28–30]. It is important to use methods capable of accurately determining size increases as guidelines have suggested surgical resection when tumors exceed 2 cm due to an enhanced metastatic risk [31].

The typical features of pancreatic NENs include hypoechoic and homogeneous, round, or oval-shaped, well-defined lesions (fig. 13). The tumors often display posterior enhancement with a hyperechoic rim corresponding to the rich vascularity (fig. 13–16). The tumors can be hard to detect once isoechoic with surrounding parenchyma, more infrequently hyperechoic to the pancreas and rarely cystic. Cystic spaces can also occur in larger lesions outgrowing their vascular supply. A smaller cystic pancreatic tumor is invariably imaged with a peripheral crest of solid tissue, often isoechoic and quite vascular in nature on Doppler; this feature is unique to cystic NENs. Overall, pancreatic NENs are often richly vascular on Doppler flow and the use of contrast-enhanced techniques can aid in determining the neuroendocrine tumor

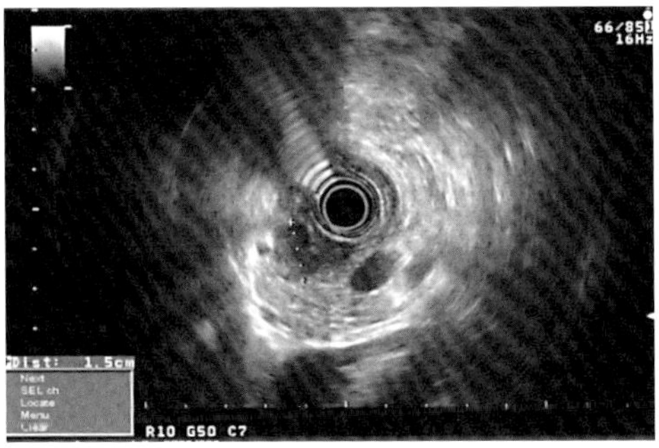

Fig. 13. Insulinoma on EUS measuring 15 mm in a 48-year-old patient, presenting classical symptoms of organic hyperinsulinism (hypoglycemic episodes with Whipple's triad over 12 years and in whom multiple CT scans and MRIs were normal). Calcium stimulation tests with venous sampling were positive, but failed to regionalize the lesion. EUS clearly identified the single hypoechoic tumor lying in the superior portion of the right body of the pancreas and at a distance from the main pancreatic duct that allowed a limited pancreatectomy with simple enucleation.

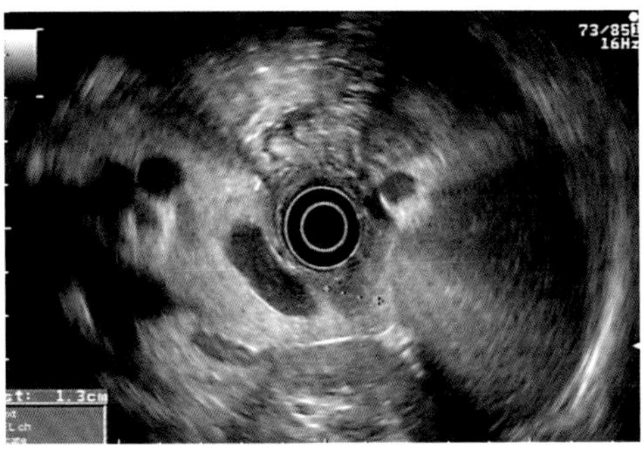

Fig. 14. Metastatic insulinoma in a pregnant 35-year-old lady complaining of episodes of significant hypoglycemia associated with documented low blood sugars (<1.8 mmol with high serum insulin and C-peptide). Transabdominal ultrasound and MRI demonstrated metastases in the liver, but the pancreas was normal. A single 1.2-cm, minimally hypoechoic, almost isoechoic, well-circumscribed tumor is seen to lie in the anterior portion of the pancreatic tail – just to the right of the junction body/tail and lies in front of the splenic vein and not far from the main pancreatic duct. The rest of the pancreatic parenchyma is well visualized and is normal.

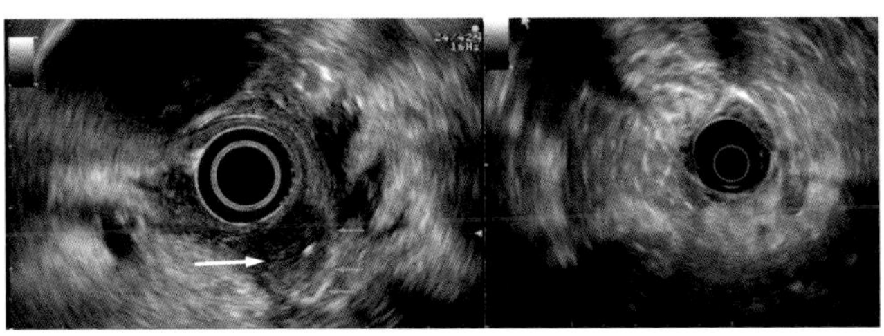

Fig. 15. Duodenal gastrinomas in a 35-year-old lady with MEN1 (with a history of parathyroidectomy at age 17 and peptic ulcer disease), presenting with 6 months of diarrhea and elevated serum gastrin (6 times the upper normal limit). No lesions were identified on CT scan or SRS, but EUS identified a well-defined 13-mm intraparietal duodenal tumor (large arrow) surrounded by a rim of hyperechoic submucosa (small arrows). Note also the intratumoral calcified spot. The adjacent image in the same patient shows two small (<10 mm) pancreatic NENs in the body and tail of the gland.

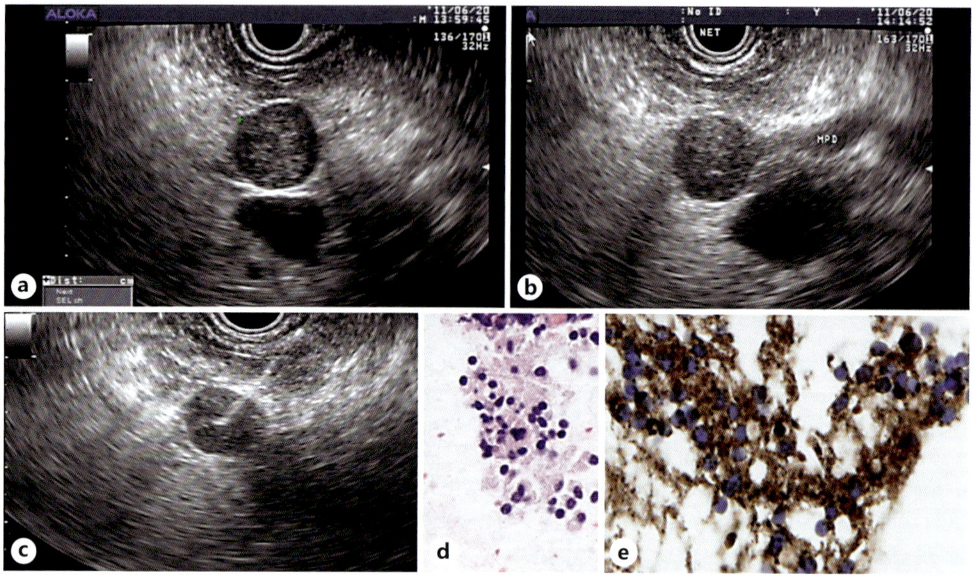

Fig. 16. EUS demonstrating a 10-mm incidentally discovered pancreatic neuroendocrine tumor in the right side of the body. **a** The tumor is hypoechoic and homogenous with a hyperechoic (slightly white periphery) attesting to its vascular nature. **b** The tumor is abutting the main pancreatic duct resulting in proximal dilatation of the duct (arrow), making it unresectable via enucleation. **c** EUS-FNAB with the needle (25 G) well centered in the tumor provided a fine core of tissue for cytology and immunohistochemistry. **d** ThinPrep cytosmear with characteristic cellular aspect of NEN. **e** Immunostaining for chromogranin A.

nature in cases of doubt. The presence of calcified spots (fig. 15), while not specific to NENs, can also give a clue to the diagnosis.

EUS is also essential in aiding to plan surgery. Attention to detail as to the precise localization within the pancreas, the possibility of regional nodal involvement, the proximity of main pancreatic and bile ducts and proximity to vascular structures are all vital in preoperative decision making. Surgery, especially for small lesions (non-functioning NENs or sporadic insulinomas) is encouraged to be as 'sparing' as possible and planning limited resections, enucleations or median pancreatectomies requires a solid symbiosis between the pancreatic EUS specialist and surgeon.

EUS-Guided Fine-Needle Aspiration and Biopsy, and Newer Techniques

EUS-guided fine-needle aspiration and biopsy (FNAB) of pancreatic NENs and locoregional nodes is also very sensitive in obtaining a cyto/histological proof of diagnosis. This technique not only provides cytology, but fine cores of tissue can be obtained in 90% of biopsies (EUS-FNAB) and this provides tissue for immunostaining that is invaluable in NENs [32]. The global sensitivity of FNAB is approximately 80%;

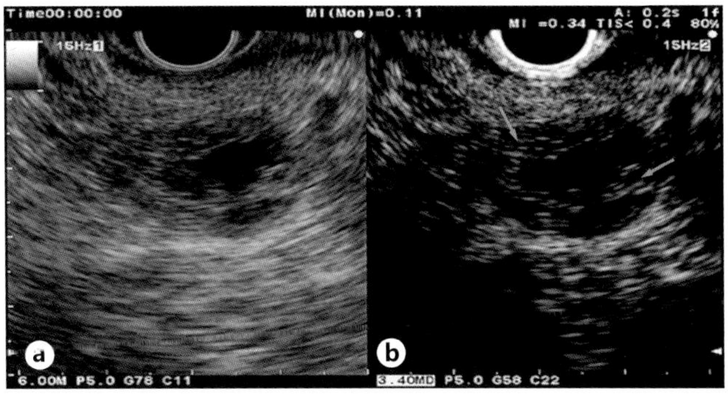

Fig. 17. a Contrast-enhanced EUS demonstrating a pancreatic neuroendocrine tumor with a cystic central zone. **b** The hypervascular nature is clearly visible with rapid incorporation of microbubbles after the injection of Sonovue© (arrows).

Table 2. Sensitivity of EUS-FNAB in the detection of pancreatic neuroendocrine tumors

First author and year	Sensitivity, %
Voss [35], 2000	75
Ardengh [36], 2004	83
Figueiredo [37], 2009	90
Atiq [38], 2012	91

this is higher in personal experience, especially with on-site pathology and careful processing with the aid of modern cytological techniques. EUS-FNAB is frequently requested in patients with incidental nonfunctioning small NENs; the biopsy permits the establishment of a certain diagnosis and avoids misdiagnosing a small adenocarcinoma or metastasis. Surveillance strategies are being employed more and more for small (<2 cm) pancreatic NENs [26] and, thus, getting the diagnosis correct at the outset is important. In addition, SRS using OctreoScan can be limited by tumor size, whilst EUS is highly performant regardless of size. Provision of fine cores of tissue can also aid in predicting the biological behavior as it is possible to obtain samples providing a clear cellular morphological aspect with immunostaining for Ki-67 to grade tumors. A recent series demonstrated good correlation between tissue obtained at EUS-FNAB and overall final pathological stage and outcome [33]. In another recent report, using a larger needle provided Ki-67 grading in up to 90% of patients [34]. In these authors' experience, EUS-FNAB for small nonfunctioning tumors is routine in helping to plan management algorithms; when tumors are small and well differentiated with a Ki-67% <5%, surveillance can be offered with more confidence.

Newer techniques – especially the use of contrast enhancement – have also been shown to help in detecting pancreatic NENs (table 2). Theses tumors rapidly incorporate the microbubbles following intravenous injection of contrast (e.g. Sonovue©; fig. 17), and impressive detection rates comparable with EUS-FANB have been reported [39]. In addition, a Japanese group demonstrated that EUS combined with contrast enhancement was useful in the differential diagnosis of malignant versus benign and preoperative localization of pancreatic NENs; this is similar to previous studies on the importance of vascular enhancement using contrast-enhanced CT [40].

References

1 Delle Fave G, Kwekkeboom DJ, van Cutsem E, Rindi G, Kos-Kudla B, Knigge U, et al: ENETS consensus guidelines for the management of patients with gastroduodenal neoplasms. Neuroendocrinology 2012; 95:74–87.

2 Schindl M, Kaserer K, Niederle B: Treatment of gastric neuroendocrine tumors: the necessity of a type-adapted treatment. Arch Surg 2001;136:49–54.

3 Ichikawa J, Tanabe S, Koizumi W, Kida Y, Imaizumi H, Kida M, et al: Endoscopic mucosal resection in the management of gastric carcinoid tumors. Endoscopy 2003;35:203–206.

4 Debelenko LV, Emmert-Buck MR, Zhuang Z, Epshteyn E, Moskaluk CA, Jensen RT, et al: The multiple endocrine neoplasia type I gene locus is involved in the pathogenesis of type II gastric carcinoids. Gastroenterology 1997;113:773–781.

5 Norton JA, Melcher ML, Gibril F, Jensen RT: Gastric carcinoid tumors in multiple endocrine neoplasia-1 patients with Zollinger-Ellison syndrome can be symptomatic, demonstrate aggressive growth, and require surgical treatment. Surgery 2004;136:1267–1274.

6 Norton JA, Warren RS, Kelly MG, Zuraek MB, Jensen RT: Aggressive surgery for metastatic liver neuroendocrine tumors. Surgery 2003;134:1057–1063, discussion 1063–1065.

7 Rindi G, Luinetti O, Cornaggia M, Capella C, Solcia E: Three subtypes of gastric argyrophil carcinoid and the gastric neuroendocrine carcinoma: a clinicopathologic study. Gastroenterology 1993;104:994–1006.

8 Rindi G, Azzoni C, La Rosa S, Klersy C, Paolotti D, Rappel S, et al: ECL cell tumor and poorly differentiated endocrine carcinoma of the stomach: prognostic evaluation by pathological analysis. Gastroenterology 1999;116:532–542.

9 Merola E, Sbrozzi-Vanni A, Panzuto F, D'Ambra G, Di Giulio E, Pilozzi E, et al: Type I gastric carcinoids: a prospective study on endoscopic management and recurrence rate. Neuroendocrinology 2011;95:207–213.

10 Sato Y, Imamura H, Kaizaki Y, Koizumi W, Ishido K, Kurahara K, et al: Management and clinical outcomes of type I gastric carcinoid patients: retrospective, multicenter study in Japan. Dig Endosc 2014;26: 377–384.

11 Gladdy RA, Strong VE, Coit D, Allen PJ, Gerdes H, Shia J, et al: Defining surgical indications for type I gastric carcinoid tumor. Ann Surg Oncol 2009;16: 3154–3160.

12 Delle Fave G, Capurso G, Annibale B, Panzuto F: Gastric neuroendocrine tumors. Neuroendocrinology 2004;80(suppl 1):16–19.

13 O'Toole D, Delle Fave G, Jensen RT: Gastric and duodenal neuroendocrine tumours. Best Pract Res Clin Gastroenterol 2013;26:719–735.

14 Modlin IM, Lye KD, Kidd M: A 5-decade analysis of 13,715 carcinoid tumors. Cancer 2003;97:934–959.

15 Dalenback J, Havel G: Local endoscopic removal of duodenal carcinoid tumors. Endoscopy 2004;36: 651–655.

16 Jensen RT, Rindi G, Arnold R, Lopes JM, Brandi ML, Bechstein WO, et al: Well-differentiated duodenal tumor/carcinoma (excluding gastrinomas). Neuroendocrinology 2006;84:165–172.

17 Yao JC, Hassan M, Phan A, Dagohoy C, Leary C, Mares JE, et al: One hundred years after 'carcinoid': epidemiology of and prognostic factors for neuroendocrine tumors in 35,825 cases in the United States. J Clin Oncol 2008;26:3063–3072.

18 Shields CJ, Tiret E, Winter DC: Carcinoid tumors of the rectum: a multi-institutional international collaboration. Ann Surg 2010;252:750–755.

19 Keller D, Jaffe J, Philp MM, Haluszka O, Khanna A: Should all endoscopically excised rectal polyps be tattooed? A plea for localization. Surg Endosc 2012; 26:3101–3105.

20 Caplin M, Sundin A, Nillson O, Baum RP, Klose KJ, Kelestimur F, et al: ENETS consensus guidelines for the management of patients with digestive neuroendocrine neoplasms: colorectal neuroendocrine neoplasms. Neuroendocrinology 2012;95:88–97.

21 Abe T, Kakemura T, Fujinuma S, Maetani I: Successful outcomes of EMR-L with 3D-EUS for rectal carcinoids compared with historical controls. World J Gastroenterol 2008;14:4054–4058.

22 Son HJ, Sohn DK, Hong CW, Han KS, Kim BC, Park JW, et al: Factors associated with complete local excision of small rectal carcinoid tumor. Int J Colorectal Dis 2012;28:57–61.
23 Kwaan MR, Goldberg JE, Bleday R: Rectal carcinoid tumors: review of results after endoscopic and surgical therapy. Arch Surg 2008;143:471–475.
24 Park HW, Byeon JS, Park YS, Yang DH, Yoon SM, Kim KJ, et al: Endoscopic submucosal dissection for treatment of rectal carcinoid tumors. Gastrointest Endosc 2010;72:143–149.
25 Zhou X, Xie H, Xie L, Li J, Fu W: Factors associated with lymph node metastasis in radically resected rectal carcinoids: a systematic review and meta-analysis. J Gastrointest Surg 2013;17:1689–1697.
26 Falconi M, Bartsch DK, Eriksson B, Kloppel G, Lopes JM, O'Connor JM, et al: ENETS consensus guidelines for the management of patients with digestive neuroendocrine neoplasms of the digestive system: well-differentiated pancreatic non-functioning tumors. Neuroendocrinology 2012;95:120–134.
27 Cadiot G, Lebtahi R, Sarda L, Bonnaud G, Marmuse JP, Vissuzaine C, et al: Preoperative detection of duodenal gastrinomas and peripancreatic lymph nodes by somatostatin receptor scintigraphy. Groupe D'etude Du Syndrome De Zollinger-Ellison. Gastroenterology 1996;111:845–854.
28 Kann PH, Balakina E, Ivan D, Bartsch DK, Meyer S, Klose KJ, et al: Natural course of small, asymptomatic neuroendocrine pancreatic tumours in multiple endocrine neoplasia type 1: an endoscopic ultrasound imaging study. Endocr Relat Cancer 2006;13: 1195–1202.
29 Triponez F, Dosseh D, Goudet P, Cougard P, Bauters C, Murat A, et al: Epidemiology data on 108 MEN 1 patients from the GTE with isolated nonfunctioning tumors of the pancreas. Ann Surg 2006;243:265–272.
30 Triponez F, Goudet P, Dosseh D, Cougard P, Bauters C, Murat A, et al: Is surgery beneficial for MEN1 patients with small (≤2 cm), nonfunctioning pancreaticoduodenal endocrine tumor? An analysis of 65 patients from the GTE. World J Surg 2006;30:654–662, discussion 663–664.
31 Jensen RT, Cadiot G, Brandi ML, de Herder WW, Kaltsas G, Komminoth P, et al: ENETS consensus guidelines for the management of patients with digestive neuroendocrine neoplasms: functional pancreatic endocrine tumor syndromes. Neuroendocrinology 2012;95:98–119.
32 Petrone MC, Poley JW, Bonzini M, Testoni PA, Abdulkader I, Biermann K, et al: Interobserver agreement among pathologists regarding core tissue specimens obtained with a new endoscopic ultrasound histology needle; a prospective multicentre study in 50 cases. Histopathology 2013;62:602–608.
33 Figueiredo FA, Giovannini M, Monges G, Bories E, Pesenti C, Caillol F, et al: EUS-FNA predicts 5-year survival in pancreatic endocrine tumors. Gastrointest Endosc 2009;70:907–914.
34 Larghi A, Capurso G, Carnuccio A, Ricci R, Alfieri S, Galasso D, et al: Ki-67 grading of nonfunctioning pancreatic neuroendocrine tumors on histologic samples obtained by EUS-guided fine-needle tissue acquisition: a prospective study. Gastrointest Endosc 2012;76:570–577.
35 Voss M, Hammel P, Molas G, Palazzo L, Dancour A, O'Toole D, et al: Value of endoscopic ultrasound guided fine needle aspiration biopsy in the diagnosis of solid pancreatic masses. Gut 2000;46:244–249.
36 Ardengh JC, de Paulo GA, Ferrari AP: EUS-guided FNA in the diagnosis of pancreatic neuroendocrine tumors before surgery. Gastrointest Endosc 2004;60: 378–384.
37 Figueiredo FA, Giovannini M, Monges G, Charfi S, Bories E, Pesenti C, et al: Pancreatic endocrine tumors: a large single-center experience. Pancreas 2009;38:936–940.
38 Atiq M, Bhutani MS, Bektas M, Lee JE, Gong Y, Tamm EP, et al: EUS-FNA for pancreatic neuroendocrine tumors: a tertiary cancer center experience. Dig Dis Sci 2012;57:791–800.
39 Gincul R, Palazzo M, Pujol B, Tubach F, Palazzo L, Lefort C, et al: Contrast-harmonic endoscopic ultrasound for the diagnosis of pancreatic adenocarcinoma: a prospective multicenter trial. Endoscopy 2014; 46:373–379.
40 Ishikawa T, Itoh A, Kawashima H, Ohno E, Matsubara H, Itoh Y, et al: Usefulness of EUS combined with contrast-enhancement in the differential diagnosis of malignant versus benign and preoperative localization of pancreatic endocrine tumors. Gastrointest Endosc 2010;71:951–959.

Dermot O'Toole, MD, FRCPI
National Neuroendocrine Tumour Service
St. Vincent's University Hospital, Elm Park
Dublin 4 (Ireland)
E-Mail otooled1@tcd.ie

Papotti M, de Herder WW (eds): Neuroendocrine Tumors: A Multidisciplinary Approach.
Front Horm Res. Basel, Karger, 2015, vol 44, pp 104–114 (DOI: 10.1159/000382135)

Pathology: Classification and Immunoprofile

Annika Blank · Anja Schmitt · Aurel Perren

Institute of Pathology, University of Bern, Switzerland

Abstract

The classification of neuroendocrine neoplasms (NENs) has been evolving steadily over the last decades. Important prognostic factors of NENs are their proliferative activity and presence/absence of necrosis. These factors are reported in NENs of all body sites; however, the terminology as well as the exact rules of classification differ according to the location of the primary tumor. Only in gastroenteropancreatic (GEP) NENs a formal grading is performed. This grading is based on proliferation assessed by the mitotic count and/or Ki-67 proliferation index. In the lung, NEN grading is an intrinsic part of the tumor designation with typical carcinoids corresponding to neuroendocrine tumor (NET) G1 and atypical carcinoids to NET G2; however, the presence or absence of necrotic foci is as important as proliferation for the differentiation between typical and atypical carcinoids. Immunohistochemical markers can be used to demonstrate neuroendocrine differentiation. Synaptophysin and chromogranin A are, to date, the most reliable and most commonly used for this purpose. Beyond this, other markers can be helpful, for example in the situation of a NET metastasis of unknown primary, where a hormonal profile or a panel of transcription factors can give hints to the primary site. Many immunohistochemical markers have been shown to correlate with prognosis but are not used in clinical practice, for example cytokeratin 19 and KIT expression in pancreatic NETs. There is no predictive biomarker in use, with the exception of somatostatin receptor (SSTR) 2 expression for predicting the amenability of a tumor to in vivo SSTR targeting for imaging or therapy.

Classification of Neuroendocrine Neoplasms in the Gastroenteropancreatic System

The histological diagnosis of neuroendocrine neoplasms (NENs) is based on morphological criteria and is confirmed by immunohistochemical staining. NENs are subdivided into well-differentiated tumors and poorly differentiated carcinomas, according to their histomorphologic appearance.

Table 1. Grading according to Rindi et al. [7] and UICC/AJCC 2010

Grade	Mitotic count (2 mm^2)	Ki-67, %
G1	<2	≤2
G2	2–20	3–20
G3	>20	>20

Well-Differentiated Neuroendocrine Tumors

Well-differentiated neuroendocrine tumors (NETs) are usually solitary, well-demarcated tumors which harbor a broad spectrum of possible growth patterns. Most commonly they show a solid, trabecular, gyriform or glandular pattern; less frequently they have a spindle cell, angiomatous, papillary or rhabdoid morphology [1, 2]. Occasionally, pancreatic NETs display cystic changes [3, 4].

The tumor cells are usually monomorphous with round to oval, centrally located nuclei and finely dispersed chromatin (so called 'salt and pepper'); however, they can also exhibit a striking variation in nuclear size and chromatin density. The cytoplasm has a granular, often eosinophilic aspect. Clear cell changes occur due to the storage of lipids [5].

The extent of the stromal component is very variable. The grading of gastroenteropancreatic (GEP)-NETs is either based on the mitotic count or on immunohistochemistry for Ki-67 [1, 6]. Mitoses are counted on hematoxylin and eosin (HE) staining in an area of 2 mm^2 in the area of highest mitotic count. The recommended Ki-67 antibody for assessment of the proliferation index is the clone MIB1. The proliferative index is determined in 2,000 tumor cells in the area of highest density of positive nuclear staining (the 'hot spot') with at least a 400-fold magnification (table 1).

Well-differentiated NETs are subdivided into two subgroups according to their proliferative activity. G1 NETs have a low proliferative activity (<2 mitoses/2 mm^2; MIB1 ≤2%) and an indolent clinical course with a prolonged survival. G2 NETs have an intermediate proliferative activity (≥2–20 mitoses/2 mm^2; MIB1 3–20%) and adverse outcome in comparison to G1 tumors, although they also have a prolonged clinical course [7, 8]. From a biological point of view, the actual strict separation into two prognostic groups can be questioned and in fact it seems that there might be a more gradual increase of the risk of malignancy with increase of the Ki-67 index [9].

Poorly Differentiated Neuroendocrine Carcinomas

Poorly differentiated neuroendocrine carcinomas (NECs) are characterized by a high degree of pleomorphism, irregular nuclei and hyperchromasia. The growth pattern is predominantly sheet-like or diffuse. Mitoses are frequently found as well as extensive geographic necrosis [5].

GEP-NECs [1, 6] have frequent mitoses, by definition more than 20 per 2 mm^2, and/or high proliferative indices of >20%, although most carcinomas exceed these thresholds by far. They are further subdivided into small and large cell NECs according to the size of their nuclei. Large cells are defined by a nuclear size of >3 lymphocytes. GEP-NECs are high-grade carcinomas with a rapid progression and short overall survival.

Mixed Adenoneuroendocrine Carcinoma
A mixed adenoneuroendocrine carcinoma (MANEC) is a neoplasm consisting of an exocrine and an endocrine component. By definition, each component should comprise at least 30% of the tumor volume, otherwise the tumor is referred to as adenocarcinoma with partial neuroendocrine differentiation [10]. An adenocarcinoma component is by far the most common for the exocrine element. An exception is represented by esophageal and anal MANEC, in which a squamous differentiation can also be found [11]. Each component should be graded separately, with the adenocarcinoma according to the guidelines for conventional adenocarcinomas of the affected organ, whereas the neuroendocrine component is graded according to the guidelines for GEP-NETs [11].

TNM Staging System
For GEP-NENs there are currently two staging systems in use, namely the UICC and the European Neuroendocrine Tumor Society (ENETS) systems [12, 13]. With the exception of pancreatic and appendiceal NETs, both systems are identical. While there are no data available yet for appendiceal NETs, for pancreatic NETs the ENETS staging system has repeatedly been shown to be superior in discriminating between prognostically meaningful different stages [7, 14–17]. To ensure the comparability of data and avoid confusion, both staging systems should be reported [18].

Classification in the Lung, Thymus and Genitourinary Tract

The nomenclature of pulmonary and thymic NENs differs from GEP-NENs. For these primary localizations, the term carcinoid is still in use. Carcinoids are distinguished from poorly differentiated NECs. Carcinoids correspond to well-differentiated NETs and are composed of bland, monomorphic cells. They show so-called differentiated growth patterns as in GEP-NETs. They are further subdivided according to the WHO classification (2004) into typical (TC) and atypical (AC) carcinoids; these groups show many similarities to G1 and G2 GEP-NETs, although they are not identical.

Typical Carcinoid
Carcinoid tumors share the same morphological criteria as well-differentiated NETs in other organ sites. Macroscopically, they are well-demarcated, tan to yellow tumors, often associated with bronchial mucosa. The histological diagnosis is based

on their cytological criteria and growth pattern. Monomorphic tumor cells with round to oval nuclei, finely dispersed chromatin and a moderate amount of eosinophilic cytoplasm are characteristic. The neoplastic cells often grow in a nested, trabecular or solid fashion. TC by definition have less than 2 mitoses per 2 mm^2 and no necrosis.

Atypical Carcinoid

By definition, AC have 2–10 mitoses per 2 mm^2 or necrosis. The necrotic areas are usually punctate. The morphological growth pattern and cytology are identical to TC.

Poorly Differentiated NECs

Pulmonary, thymic and urogenital NECs have more than 10 mitoses per 2 mm^2, although in most cases they exceed this number by far and show more than 50 mitoses per 2 mm^2. They do not show the differentiated growth patterns of NETs, but instead have a solid or sheet-like growth and frequently exhibit geographic necrosis. Also, for pulmonary NECs, a further subdivision into small and large cell variants corresponding to their nuclear size is recommended, with small cell variants having a cell size corresponding to less than three lymphocytes. Evaluation of the Ki-67 proliferative activity by MIB1 staining, which is an integral part of the assessment in GEP-NETs is, at least to date, not compulsory, although it seems to bear additional prognostic implications [19].

TNM Staging System

Pulmonary NENs are classified according to the 7th edition of the UICC/AJCC [6] as lung cancer, even if the prognostic value of this system has never been proven useful for NENs. Currently, there is also no specific TNM staging system for thymic and urogenital NENs.

Immunohistochemistry

Immunohistochemical Markers to Confirm Neuroendocrine Differentiation

Depending on the site of the tumor and the guideline used, immunohistochemistry is useful/mandatory to confirm the neuroendocrine differentiation. Today the most commonly used markers are synaptophysin and chromogranin A, which both have a cytoplasmic staining pattern. Chromogranin A is a component of large secretory granules. Its expression level depends on the number of secretory granules [20]; therefore, poorly differentiated NECs often show only focal staining or even a lack immunohistochemical positivity for chromogranin A [21].

Synaptophysin is a membrane protein of small vesicles of neuroendocrine cells [22]. It has a lower specificity but a higher sensitivity for neuroendocrine differentiation in comparison to chromogranin A. It is more likely to be preserved in poorly differentiated NENs.

Beyond this, neuron-specific enolase, CD56/NCAM and PGP9.5 are additional markers of neuroendocrine differentiation. Due to their lack of specificity their use is not recommended anymore [21].

Immunohistochemical Markers to Indicate the Primary Site

In the case of metastases, it is a challenge to identify the origin of the primary tumor on morphological grounds alone. A few markers have been shown to provide information regarding the primary site in such circumstances. They encompass either peptide hormones, enzymes involved in their biogenesis or transcription factors.

The vesicular monoamine transporter 2 (VMAT2) is expressed in gastric NENs [10]. A positive staining for serotonin suggests primarily an ileal origin, but can also be found in NETs from the jejunum or appendix and less frequently from other sites, such as the lung or pancreas [21]. Expression of somatostatin and gastrin points towards a duodenal or pancreatic primary. Cytoplasmic staining for NESP-55 (neuroendocrine secretory protein-55) seems to be restricted to tumors of pancreatic (or adrenal) origin [23], and the immunohistochemical expression of insulin, glucagon and pancreatic polypeptide points towards a pancreatic primary.

The transcription factor CDX2 is expressed in intestinal NETs. Nuclear staining for islet 1 strongly suggests a pancreatic origin [24]. Conflicting results have been published concerning the reliability of thyroid transcription factor 1 (TTF-1) for pulmonary NETs. Although a subset of carcinoids expresses this marker, there are other NETs, including medullary thyroid carcinoma, which express TTF-1. Therefore, immunohistochemical results must be interpreted with caution [24, 25]. Interestingly, 80–100% of rectal NETs express prostate-specific acid or prostate-specific acid phosphatase [26].

While all the above markers are of use in well-differentiated NETs, this is not the case for poorly differentiated NECs [27]. Immunohistochemistry here can be of help in the differential diagnosis between Merkel cell carcinomas and cutaneous metastases of pulmonary NECs: while Merkel cell carcinomas are usually positive for CK20, typically with a dot-like staining pattern, they are normally negative for TTF-1. In contrast, pulmonary NECs should be negative for CK20 and show TTF-1 expression in a proportion of cases.

Immunohistochemical Predictive Markers

The expression of somatostatin receptors (SSTR) is a typical feature of well-differentiated NENs with high expression levels, especially in tumors of GEP origin. In the absence of a preoperative SSTR imaging, immunohistochemistry is the best way to determine a potential receptor expression. Immunohistochemistry for SSTR subtype 2a has been shown repeatedly to be a reliable method by which to detect high receptor

Table 2. Discrimination between different types of gastric ECL cell carcinoids

	Type 1	Type 2	Type 3
Gastric mucosa	Chronic atrophic gastritis ECL cell hyperplasia (linear or micronodular) Multiple tumors	Hyperplasia of parietal cells ECL cell hyperplasia Multiple tumors	Normal
Grading	G1	G1–2	Often G3

expression levels. At least a moderate (noncircumferential) membranous staining [28] in at least 20% of tumor cells [29] correlates with in vivo SSTR-2 measurement. Markers predicting response to the wide range of therapeutic compounds applied to NENs have not yet been described.

Immunohistochemical Prognostic Markers

Estimation of the aggressiveness of NENs is a challenge since morphological characteristics, in contrast to other neoplasms, are of limited use. Proliferative activity measured by MIB1 staining has been proven in many studies to correlate with outcome. Beyond this, positive staining for cytokeratin 19 and KIT have been proven to be associated with an adverse outcome in pancreatic NENs [30, 31].

Important Organ-Specific Features

Gastric NENs

So-called ECL (enterochromaffin-like) cell carcinoids are the most frequent type of gastric NETs. They share phenotypes with normal ECL cells, such as the expression of VMAT2 [32]. Depending on the genetic and biological setting, three different types of gastric ECL cell carcinoids are defined. Even if the tumor tissue cannot be discriminated morphologically, the prognosis of ECL cell carcinoids and, therefore, the therapeutic approach depends strongly on this context. Examining biopsies of the surrounding nonneoplastic mucosa allows the pathologist to find hints to discriminate the three forms (table 2).

The most frequent form, type 1 ECL cell carcinoid [33], is associated with chronic atrophic gastritis. Hypergastrinemia is a driving factor of tumor development. ECL cell carcinoids are multiple and are accompanied by different stages of preneoplastic ECL cell lesions: linear, micronodular, adenomatoid hyperplasia and microcarcinoid. Recognition of the surrounding chronic atrophic gastritis, together with clinical/laboratory diagnosis of CAG, is diagnostic. The stages of preneoplastic lesions predict the risk of recurrence of type 1 ECL-cell carcinoids after endoscopic resection [34]. Most of these NETs are G1 and T1 (according to endoultrasonography), and in such cases therapy guidelines recommend endoscopic resection [35, 36].

Type 2 ECL cell carcinoids are associated with Zollinger-Ellison syndrome in the setting of a multiple endocrine neoplasia type 1 (MEN1). This rare variant is associated with hyperplasia of parietal cells in the surrounding gastric mucosa and is clinically more aggressive [35]. Biologically, these tumors have a loss of the wild-type MEN1 allele; however, this is not used for clinical diagnosis.

Type 3 ECL cell carcinoids of the stomach arise de novo and are solitary tumors. Frequently, they are poorly differentiated and show a high Ki-67 index corresponding to NEC G3.

All ECL cell carcinoids are characterized by the expression of VMAT2 [32]. The clinical significance of endocrine product expression, such as ghrelin or serotonin, in gastric NETs is unknown.

Duodenal, Jejunal and Ileal NENs

The predominant proportion of duodenal NENs are well differentiated with only 1–3% NECs [35]. Usually, they are small and solitary lesions. In 6% of cases they are associated with MEN1 and multiple tumors in particular should raise the suspicion of this hereditary condition, whereas the majority of NETs arising in a periampullary localization are associated with neurofibromatosis type 1 [35]. Ampullary NETs are often somatostatin-producing tumors, which characteristically contain psammoma bodies [35].

Jejunal and ileal NENs harbor a relatively high risk for an aggressive clinical course. In most cases, lymph node or distant metastases are present at the time of diagnosis [37]. Jejunal and ileal NENs only rarely arise in a hereditary setting [38].

Appendiceal NENs

Appendiceal NENs are the second most common neuroendocrine neoplasms, most of them being located at the tip of the appendix and found incidentally during appendectomy for appendicitis. Less than 5% of appendiceal NENs are MANECs, or so-called goblet cell carcinoids. Tumor cells have a signet-ring cell appearance with intracytoplasmic mucin and compressed nuclei at the periphery. These mixed tumors have been shown to be associated with an adverse clinical outcome compared to stage-matched ordinary NETs. Often they diffusely infiltrate into the appendiceal fat and show extensive perineural invasion (see also the section 'Mixed Adenoneuroendocrine Carcinoma') [37, 39].

Colonic and Rectal NENs

It is important to differentiate between colonic and rectal NENs as these neoplasms differ markedly from each other. The most common localization of colonic NENs is the cecum. They are often associated with adenomas or adenocarcinomas. In most cases of colonic NENs, metastases are present at the time of diagnosis, probably due

Table 3. Immunohistochemical hormonal markers with typical primary sites

Protein	Organ
Insulin	Pancreas
Glucagon	Pancreas
Somatostatin	Pancreas/duodenum
Gastrin	Duodenum/pancreas
Vasoactive intestinal polypeptide	Pancreas
Pancreatic polypeptide	Pancreas
Serotonin	Small intestine/pancreas
Adrenocorticotropic hormone	Pituitary/lung/pancreas
Calcitonin	Thyroid/pancreas/small intestine

to a long asymptomatic course, and therefore have the worst prognosis among GEP-NETs [24, 40].

In contrast, rectal NENs are more frequently diagnosed in a localized stage and are associated with a better prognosis. They often lack immunohistochemical expression of chromogranin A, while the expression of synaptophysin is retained [21]. Colonic and rectal NENs are not associated with hereditary disease.

Pancreatic NENs

Most pancreatic NENs are well-differentiated tumors. The recognizable growth patterns correspond to those seen in well-differentiated NENs. Beyond this, insulinomas often exhibit amyloid deposits, while psammoma bodies are frequently found in somatostatinomas [5].

Hormonal markers (table 3) are available and frequently expressed in pancreatic NETs. Their expression level does not imply information about the functional status. Functional tumors are exclusively defined by clinical symptoms due to inadequate hormonal secretion. Pancreatic NETs with a size <0.5 cm are classified as microadenomas. Pancreatic NETs can occur in the context of hereditary disease, with MEN1 being the most common, followed by von Hippel-Lindau disease and tuberous sclerosis [41].

Lung NENs

In contrast to other primary localizations, poorly differentiated NECs, which account for 20% of all lung tumors, are much more common than well-differentiated NETs, which represent 2% [42]. Small cell lung cancer (poorly differentiated NEC of the lung, small cell type) is heavily associated with smoking. Among carcinoids, TC forms are 8- to 10-times more frequent than AC.

A precondition, which has been shown to have the potential to progress to carcinoid tumors, is the so-called diffuse idiopathic pulmonary neuroendocrine cell hyperplasia. This is a very rare condition, which is defined by a diffuse proliferation of neuroendocrine cells, either in a linear or nodular fashion, in an otherwise unremarkable lung. If these aggregates of neuroendocrine cells extend beyond the basal membrane they are classified as tumorlets, which, by definition, are <5 mm in diameter. If the tumor is 0.5 cm or larger, it is classified as carcinoid. In 5% of the cases, carcinoid tumors arise in the context of MEN1 [43].

Thymic NENs

NETs of the thymus are rare tumors. They may arise in the setting of an inherited MEN1 syndrome. It is important to notice that, by definition, the whole tumor population must display an endocrine phenotype [44]. They are classified analogs to pulmonary NETs and the terms TC and AC are used for the well-differentiated thymic types (see also the section 'Lung NENs'). However, compared to the lung, a larger proportion of thymic NETs are categorized in the group of AC. Like their pulmonary counterparts, poorly differentiated thymic NENs are separated into small cell and large cell NECs.

Genitourinary NENs

The classification of genitourinary NENs is similar to that of pulmonary NENs. The well-differentiated forms arise most frequently in the ovary as ovarian carcinoids and can be associated with teratomas. Poorly differentiated NECs are reported in the ovaries and in the uterine cervix and endometrium, as well as in the urinary bladder and prostate.

Merkel Cell Carcinoma

The histological appearance of Merkel cell carcinomas corresponds to poorly differentiated NECs. Morphologically, Merkel cell carcinoma belongs to the group of small round blue cell tumors, which refers to the small nuclei size with sparse cytoplasm. There is no grading system for Merkel cell carcinomas. Several histopathologic features, such as a diffuse growth pattern, infiltration of the subcutis and pronounced lymphocytic infiltrate have been associated with an adverse outcome [45].

References

1 Kloppel G: Classification and pathology of gastroenteropancreatic neuroendocrine neoplasms. Endocr Relat Cancer 2011;18(suppl 1):S1–S16.

2 Asa SL: Pancreatic endocrine tumors. Mod Pathol 2011;24(suppl 2):S66–S77.

3 Ligneau B, Lombard-Bohas C, Partensky C, Valette PJ, Calender A, Dumortier J, Gouysse G, Boulez J, Napoleon B, Berger F, Chayvialle JA, Scoazec JY: Cystic endocrine tumors of the pancreas: clinical, radiologic, and histopathologic features in 13 cases. Am J Surg Pathol 2001;25:752–760.

4 Singhi AD, Chu LC, Tatsas AD, Shi C, Ellison TA, Fishman EK, Kawamoto S, Schulick RD, Wolfgang CL, Hruban RH, Edil BH: Cystic pancreatic neuroendocrine tumors: a clinicopathologic study. Am J Surg Pathol 2012;36:1666–1673.

5 DeLellis R, Heitz P, Lloyd R, Eng C: Pathology and Genetics of Tumours of Endocrine Organs. Lyon, IARC Press, 2004.

6 Edge S, Byrd DR, Compton CC, Fritz AG, Greene FL, Trotti A (eds): American Joint Committee on Cancer Staging Manual, ed 7. Springer, New York, 2010.

7 Rindi G, Falconi M, Klersy C, Albarello L, Boninsegna L, Buchler MW, Capella C, Caplin M, Couvelard A, Doglioni C, Delle Fave G, Fischer L, Fusai G, de Herder WW, Jann H, Komminoth P, de Krijger RR, La Rosa S, Luong TV, Pape U, Perren A, Ruszniewski P, Scarpa A, Schmitt A, Solcia E, Wiedenmann B: TNM staging of neoplasms of the endocrine pancreas: results from a large international cohort study. J Natl Cancer Inst 2012;104:764–777.

8 Klimstra DS: Pathology reporting of neuroendocrine tumors: essential elements for accurate diagnosis, classification, and staging. Semin Oncol 2013;40:23–36.
9 Panzuto F, Boninsegna L, Fazio N, Campana D, Pia Brizzi M, Capurso G, Scarpa A, De Braud F, Dogliotti L, Tomassetti P, Delle Fave G, Falconi M: Metastatic and locally advanced pancreatic endocrine carcinomas: analysis of factors associated with disease progression. J Clin Oncol 2011;29:2372–2377.
10 Anlauf M: Neuroendocrine neoplasms of the gastroenteropancreatic system: pathology and classification. Horm Metab Res 2011;43:825–831.
11 La Rosa S, Marando A, Sessa F, Capella C: Mixed adenoneuroendocrine carcinomas (MANECs) of the gastrointestinal tract: an update. Cancers 2012;4:11–30.
12 Rindi G, Kloppel G, Alhman H, Caplin M, Couvelard A, de Herder WW, Erikssson B, Falchetti A, Falconi M, Komminoth P, Korner M, Lopes JM, McNicol AM, Nilsson O, Perren A, Scarpa A, Scoazec JY, Wiedenmann B: TNM staging of foregut (neuro)endocrine tumors: a consensus proposal including a grading system. Virchows Arch 2006;449:395–401.
13 Rindi G, Kloppel G, Couvelard A, Komminoth P, Korner M, Lopes JM, McNicol AM, Nilsson O, Perren A, Scarpa A, Scoazec JY, Wiedenmann B: TNM staging of midgut and hindgut (neuro) endocrine tumors: a consensus proposal including a grading system. Virchows Arch 2007;451:757–762.
14 Ekeblad S, Skogseid B, Dunder K, Oberg K, Eriksson B: Prognostic factors and survival in 324 patients with pancreatic endocrine tumor treated at a single institution. Clin Cancer Res 2008;14:7798–7803.
15 Fischer L, Kleeff J, Esposito I, Hinz U, Zimmermann A, Friess H, Buchler MW: Clinical outcome and long-term survival in 118 consecutive patients with neuroendocrine tumours of the pancreas. Br J Surg 2008;95:627–635.
16 Pape UF, Jann H, Muller-Nordhorn J, Bockelbrink A, Berndt U, Willich SN, Koch M, Rocken C, Rindi G, Wiedenmann B: Prognostic relevance of a novel TNM classification system for upper gastroenteropancreatic neuroendocrine tumors. Cancer 2008;113:256–265.
17 La Rosa S, Klersy C, Uccella S, Dainese L, Albarello L, Sonzogni A, Doglioni C, Capella C, Solcia E: Improved histologic and clinicopathologic criteria for prognostic evaluation of pancreatic endocrine tumors. Hum Pathol 2009;40:30–40.
18 Kloppel G, Rindi G, Perren A, Komminoth P, Klimstra DS: The ENETS and AJCC/UICC TNM classifications of the neuroendocrine tumors of the gastrointestinal tract and the pancreas: a statement. Virchows Arch 2010;456:595–597.
19 Pelosi G, Rindi G, Travis WD, Papotti M: Ki-67 antigen in lung neuroendocrine tumors: unraveling a role in clinical practice. J Thorac Oncol 2014;9:273–284.
20 Modlin IM, Oberg K, Chung DC, Jensen RT, de Herder WW, Thakker RV, Caplin M, Delle Fave G, Kaltsas GA, Krenning EP, Moss SF, Nilsson O, Rindi G, Salazar R, Ruszniewski P, Sundin A: Gastroenteropancreatic neuroendocrine tumours. Lancet Oncol 2008;9:61–72.
21 Kloppel G, Couvelard A, Perren A, Komminoth P, McNicol AM, Nilsson O, Scarpa A, Scoazec JY, Wiedenmann B, Papotti M, Rindi G, Plockinger U, et al: ENETS consensus guidelines for the standards of care in neuroendocrine tumors: towards a standardized approach to the diagnosis of gastroenteropancreatic neuroendocrine tumors and their prognostic stratification. Neuroendocrinology 2009;90:162–166.
22 Wiedenmann B, Franke WW, Kuhn C, Moll R, Gould VE: Synaptophysin: a marker protein for neuroendocrine cells and neoplasms. Proc Natl Acad Sci U S A 1986;83:3500–3504.
23 Srivastava A, Padilla O, Fischer-Colbrie R, Tischler AS, Dayal Y: Neuroendocrine secretory protein-55 (NESP-55) expression discriminates pancreatic endocrine tumors and pheochromocytomas from gastrointestinal and pulmonary carcinoids. Am J Surg Pathol 2004;28:1371–1378.
24 Schmitt AM, Riniker F, Anlauf M, Schmid S, Soltermann A, Moch H, Heitz PU, Kloppel G, Komminoth P, Perren A: Islet 1 (Isl1) expression is a reliable marker for pancreatic endocrine tumors and their metastases. Am J Surg Pathol 2008;32:420–425.
25 Cheuk W, Kwan MY, Suster S, Chan JK: Immunostaining for thyroid transcription factor 1 and cytokeratin 20 aids the distinction of small cell carcinoma from Merkel cell carcinoma, but not pulmonary from extrapulmonary small cell carcinomas. Arch Pathol Lab Med 2001;125:228–231.
26 Ramage JK, Goretzki PE, Manfredi R, Komminoth P, Ferone D, Hyrdel R, Kaltsas G, Kelestimur F, Kvols L, Scoazec JY, Garcia MI, Caplin ME, et al: Consensus guidelines for the management of patients with digestive neuroendocrine tumours: well-differentiated colon and rectum tumour/carcinoma. Neuroendocrinology 2008;87:31–39.
27 Agaimy A, Erlenbach-Wunsch K, Konukiewitz B, Schmitt AM, Rieker RJ, Vieth M, Kiesewetter F, Hartmann A, Zamboni G, Perren A, Kloppel G: ISL1 expression is not restricted to pancreatic well-differentiated neuroendocrine neoplasms, but is also commonly found in well and poorly differentiated neuroendocrine neoplasms of extrapancreatic origin. Mod Pathol 2013;26:995–1003.
28 Papotti M, Bongiovanni M, Volante M, Allia E, Landolfi S, Helboe L, Schindler M, Cole SL, Bussolati G: Expression of somatostatin receptor types 1–5 in 81 cases of gastrointestinal and pancreatic endocrine tumors: a correlative immunohistochemical and reverse-transcriptase polymerase chain reaction analysis. Virchows Arch 2002;440:461–475.

29 Korner M, Waser B, Schonbrunn A, Perren A, Reubi JC: Somatostatin receptor subtype 2A immunohistochemistry using a new monoclonal antibody selects tumors suitable for in vivo somatostatin receptor targeting. Am J Surg Pathol 2012;36:242–252.

30 Zhang L, Lohse CM, Dao LN, Smyrk TC: Proposed histopathologic grading system derived from a study of KIT and CK19 expression in pancreatic endocrine neoplasm. Hum Pathol 2011;42:324–331.

31 Schmitt AM, Anlauf M, Rousson V, Schmid S, Kofler A, Riniker F, Bauersfeld J, Barghorn A, Probst-Hensch NM, Moch H, Heitz PU, Kloeppel G, Komminoth P, Perren A: WHO 2004 criteria and CK19 are reliable prognostic markers in pancreatic endocrine tumors. Am J Surg Pathol 2007;31:1677–1682.

32 Rindi G, Paolotti D, Fiocca R, Wiedenmann B, Henry JP, Solcia E: Vesicular monoamine transporter 2 as a marker of gastric enterochromaffin-like cell tumors. Virchows Arch 2000;436:217–223.

33 Rindi G, Luinetti O, Cornaggia M, Capella C, Solcia E: Three subtypes of gastric argyrophil carcinoid and the gastric neuroendocrine carcinoma: a clinicopathologic study. Gastroenterology 1993;104:994–1006.

34 La Rosa S, Inzani F, Vanoli A, Klersy C, Dainese L, Rindi G, Capella C, Bordi C, Solcia E: Histologic characterization and improved prognostic evaluation of 209 gastric neuroendocrine neoplasms. Hum Pathol 2011;42:1373–1384.

35 Delle Fave G, Kwekkeboom DJ, van Cutsem E, Rindi G, Kos-Kudla B, Knigge U, Sasano H, Tomassetti P, Salazar R, Ruszniewski P, et al: ENETS consensus guidelines for the management of patients with gastroduodenal neoplasms. Neuroendocrinology 2012;95:74–87.

36 Salazar R, Wiedenmann B, Rindi G, Ruszniewski P: ENETS 2011 consensus guidelines for the management of patients with digestive neuroendocrine tumors: an update. Neuroendocrinology 2012;95:71–73.

37 Boudreaux JP, Klimstra DS, Hassan MM, Woltering EA, Jensen RT, Goldsmith SJ, Nutting C, Bushnell DL, Caplin ME, Yao JC, et al: The NANETS consensus guideline for the diagnosis and management of neuroendocrine tumors: well-differentiated neuroendocrine tumors of the jejunum, ileum, appendix, and cecum. Pancreas 2010;39:753–766.

38 Eriksson B, Kloppel G, Krenning E, Ahlman H, Plockinger U, Wiedenmann B, Arnold R, Auernhammer C, Korner M, Rindi G, Wildi S, et al: Consensus guidelines for the management of patients with digestive neuroendocrine tumors: well-differentiated jejunal-ileal tumor/carcinoma. Neuroendocrinology 2008;87:8–19.

39 Plockinger U, Couvelard A, Falconi M, Sundin A, Salazar R, Christ E, de Herder WW, Gross D, Knapp WH, Knigge UP, Kulke MH, Pape UF, et al: Consensus guidelines for the management of patients with digestive neuroendocrine tumours: well-differentiated tumour/carcinoma of the appendix and goblet cell carcinoma. Neuroendocrinology 2008;87:20–30.

40 Caplin M, Sundin A, Nillson O, Baum RP, Klose KJ, Kelestimur F, Plockinger U, Papotti M, Salazar R, Pascher A, et al: ENETS consensus guidelines for the management of patients with digestive neuroendocrine neoplasms: colorectal neuroendocrine neoplasms. Neuroendocrinology 2012;95:88–97.

41 Falconi M, Plockinger U, Kwekkeboom DJ, Manfredi R, Korner M, Kvols L, Pape UF, Ricke J, Goretzki PE, Wildi S, Steinmuller T, Oberg K, Scoazec JY, et al: Well-differentiated pancreatic nonfunctioning tumors/carcinoma. Neuroendocrinology 2006;84:196–211.

42 Horsch D, Schmid KW, Anlauf M, Darwiche K, Denecke T, Baum RP, Spitzweg C, Grohe C, Presselt N, Stremmel C, Heigener DF, Serke M, Kegel T, Pavel M, Waller CF, Deppermann KM, Arnold R, Huber RM, Weber MM, Hoffmann H: Neuroendocrine tumors of the bronchopulmonary system (typical and atypical carcinoid tumors): current strategies in diagnosis and treatment – conclusions of an expert meeting February 2011 in Weimar, Germany. Oncol Res Treat 2014;37:266–276.

43 Sachithanandan N, Harle RA, Burgess JR: Bronchopulmonary carcinoid in multiple endocrine neoplasia type 1. Cancer 2005;103:509–515.

44 Rosai J, Sobin LH: Histological Typing of Tumours of the Thymus. Berlin, Springer, 1999.

45 Mott RT, Smoller BR, Morgan MB: Merkel cell carcinoma: a clinicopathologic study with prognostic implications. J Cutan Pathol 2004;31:217–223.

Aurel Perren
Institute of Pathology
University of Bern
Murtenstrasse 31, CH–3010 Bern (Switzerland)
E-Mail aurel.perren@pathology.unibe.ch

Papotti M, de Herder WW (eds): Neuroendocrine Tumors: A Multidisciplinary Approach.
Front Horm Res. Basel, Karger, 2015, vol 44, pp 115–138 (DOI: 10.1159/000382138)

Genetics and Epigenetics of Pancreatic Neuroendocrine Tumors and Pulmonary Carcinoids

Koen M.A. Dreijerink[a] • Jules L. Derks[b] • Ivana Cataldo[d] • Aldo Scarpa[d] • Gerlof D. Valk[a] • Ernst-Jan M. Speel[c]

[a]Department of Endocrine Oncology, University Medical Centre Utrecht, Utrecht, and Departments of [b]Respiratory Diseases and [c]Pathology, GROW-School of Oncology and Developmental Biology, Maastricht University Medical Centre, Maastricht, The Netherlands; [d]Department of Pathology and Diagnostics, University and Hospital Trust of Verona, Verona, Italy

Abstract

In this chapter, we give an overview of the genetic and epigenetic background of neuroendocrine tumors (NETs), in particular pancreatic and pulmonary NETs. Studying the mechanism of disease of the inherited syndromes that feature NETs has provided valuable insights that have revolutionized the therapeutic options for these tumor types: both inhibition of mTOR (mammalian target of rapamycin) signaling and inhibition of angiogenesis have become standard treatments. Although sporadic NETs harbor relatively few somatic gene mutations, these somatic mutations often affect genes that encode epigenetic regulators. Restoring the aberrant epigenetic characteristics may be an attractive approach for future treatment.

Neuroendocrine tumors (NETs) include a variety of tumor types that can arise at many anatomic sites in the body. Categorizing these tumors has historically been challenging. Classically, NETs were subdivided based on the embryonic origin of the tumor cells in foregut, midgut and hindgut carcinoid tumors. More recently, the World Health Organization classification for gastrointestinal and pancreatic (p)NETs was modified and is now based on tumor differentiation and grade, irrespective of the

K.M.A.D., J.L.D., G.D.V. and E.-J.M.S. contributed equally to this work.

Table 1. Hereditary tumor syndromes associated with NETs

Syndrome	NET location	Frequency
MEN1	Pancreas	50–80%
	Thymus (mostly male)	2–5%
	Pulmonary	2–8%
	Gastric, type 2 NETs	5–35%
VHL	Pancreas	15%
NF1	Pancreas (periampullary)	Cases
TSC	Pancreas	Cases
MEN4	Pancreas	Cases

organ or cell of origin [1, 2]. Pulmonary NETs should be classified as carcinoids (typical/atypical) and grading differs from pNETs and gastrointestinal NETs with regard to the use of Ki-67 and the mitotic index.

Several types of NETs, in particular pancreatic, gastric, pulmonary and thymic NETs, occur in the spectrum of multisystem autosomal dominant genetic disorders (table 1). Studying the mechanisms of disease in these syndromes has provided valuable insight into NET development.

The two endocrine tumor syndromes that feature NETs most frequently are multiple endocrine neoplasia type 1 (MEN1) and von Hippel-Lindau (VHL) disease. Less commonly, endocrine tumors of the pancreas are observed in neurofibromatosis type 1 (NF1), tuberous sclerosis complex (TSC) and in families with germline mutations in cyclin-dependent kinase inhibitor (CDKI) genes (table 1). In addition, reports on genetic changes in nonfamilial NETs have increased our understanding of the complete mutational landscape of neuroendocrine tumorigenesis.

There is emerging evidence that epigenetic changes contribute significantly to NET development. Epigenetics can be defined as the study of heritable changes in gene expression without alteration of the underlying DNA sequence, such as DNA methylation and histone modifications. In recent years, studies examining the molecular basis of disease have increased enormously due to the development of next-generation DNA and RNA sequencing methods. Genome-wide approaches may contribute to define a molecular classification for NETs and pave the road for personalized targeted diagnostic and therapeutic approaches.

In this chapter, we provide an overview of the inherited syndromes that feature NETs and we review the genetic and epigenetic studies that have been performed in sporadic NETs. We discuss the state-of-the-art of current NET treatment and give our perspective on how the increasing knowledge of genetic and epigenetic aspects may further change the therapeutic arsenal for NETs.

Inherited Neuroendocrine Tumor Predisposition Syndromes

Multiple Endocrine Neoplasia Type 1

MEN1 (MIM 131100) is an autosomal dominantly inherited genetic disorder, typically characterized by parathyroid hyperplasia/adenoma, NETs of the pancreas and duodenum (dpNETs) and adenomas of the anterior pituitary. In addition, MEN1 patients may develop NETs of the thymus, stomach and lungs, and adenomas of the adrenal cortex [3, 4]. The prevalence of MEN1 is approximately 1 in 20,000–40,000 individuals [3, 4]. The clinical prevalence of dpNETs in MEN1 is over 50% in recent large series [5, 6]. The penetrance of clinically manifest dpNETs at the age of 80 years is more than 80% [7]. In patients with MEN1-related dpNETs the estimated 10-year survival is 75% [8, 9]. The life expectancy of MEN1 patients is thus influenced significantly by the development of NETs. Monitoring of MEN1 patients and gene mutation carriers is expected to reduce the disease burden and mortality from MEN1.

Unlike sporadic dpNETs, MEN1-related dpNETs are characterized by multifocality and multiplicity. MEN1 dpNETs are usually diagnosed a decade earlier in life than sporadic dpNETs [4]. About 70% of MEN1 dpNETs are clinically active, i.e. producing an excess of one or more peptides/hormones, which can cause distinct clinical syndromes [9]. Gastrinomas represent more than half of all functional MEN1 dpNETs, are a major cause of morbidity and mortality in MEN1 patients, and are associated with a poor prognosis. In MEN1 patients, the majority of gastrinomas (>90%) are located in the duodenum and may manifest with the typical symptoms of Zollinger-Ellison syndrome before the age of 40 years [10, 11]. Insulinomas in MEN1 patients are usually also diagnosed before the age of 40 years, which is earlier than the diagnosis of sporadic insulinomas [12]. Glucagonomas are rare but have been reported in MEN1.

Except in a Japanese cohort, thymic NETs almost exclusively occur in male patients with MEN1. Their prevalence is about 2–5% [3, 4, 13, 14]. Among the manifestations of the MEN1 syndrome, thymic NETs carry the highest risk of death with an estimated 10-year survival of 30–36% [13, 14]. Pulmonary carcinoids occur in 2–8% of MEN1 patients and are not associated with an increased risk of death in MEN1 patients [3, 4, 15, 16]. Gastric NETs in MEN1 patients almost exclusively develop in the presence of Zollinger-Ellison syndrome. They are generally characterized as type 2 enterochromaffin-like tumors or gastric carcinoids. These generally well-differentiated lesions usually have an indolent clinical course [17].

MEN1 is caused by inactivating germline mutations of the MEN1 tumor suppressor gene on chromosome 11q13 and encodes the protein menin [18]. In accordance with the Knudson two-hit hypothesis, tumorigenesis is caused by the inherited inactivation of growth suppressor genes and subsequent loss of expression of the wild-type allele [19]. More than 450 germline MEN1 gene mutations and more than 160 somatic inactivating mutations have been identified [20]. There is no clear genotype/

phenotype relation among germline and somatic MEN1 mutations [20]. Loss of heterozygosity (LOH) of MEN1 has been demonstrated in most reported MEN1-related pNETs [21]. LOH of chromosome 11q13 has also been shown in MEN1-related pulmonary and gastric NETs [22, 23]. Intriguingly, no LOH was found in thymic NETs [24, 25].

The MEN1 gene product menin interacts with many other proteins involved in various cellular processes. Most interacting proteins point towards a function for menin in the regulation of gene transcription [26]. Menin has been found to be a component of protein complexes that have histone lysine methyltransferase (KMT) activity directed at trimethylation of lysine 4 (K4) of histone H3 (H3K4me3); menin interacts with the mixed lineage leukemia (MLL) proteins MLL1 (KMT2A) and MLL2 (KMT2B; fig. 1a) [27, 28]. Menin-H3K4me3 complexes are considered to play a role in NET development [29]. Menin-MLL1 complexes stimulate the expression of the CDKN1Band CDKN2C genes encoding the $p27^{Kip1}$ and $p18^{Ink4c}$ CDKI proteins, respectively, in certain cell types [30, 31]. Loss of function of menin or MLL1 results in downregulation of $p27^{Kip1}$ and $p18^{Ink4c}$ [30]. Downregulation of CDKI genes can lead to tumorigenesis and MEN1 pancreatic tumor formation (fig. 1a) [31, 32]. Inhibiting H3K4me3 demethylases could restore the loss of H3K4me3 in MEN1 models; indeed, synchronous genetic knockout of the H3K4me3 demethylase (Rbp2/Jarid1a/Kdm5a) in a MEN1 mouse model has been shown to slow pNET development [33].

VHL Disease

VHL (MIM 193300) is an autosomal dominantly inherited genetic disorder that predisposes affected individuals to a number of benign and malignant highly vascularized tumor types. The VHL spectrum includes retinal angiomas, central nervous system (CNS) hemangioblastomas, clear cell renal carcinomas, pheochromocytomas, nonfunctional pancreatic lesions, endolymphatic sac tumors of the middle ear, and papillary cystadenomas of the epididymis and broad ligament [34]. The prevalence of VHL is approximately 1 per 36,000 [35]. Pancreatic lesions are rarely the presenting manifestation of VHL. In a recent report on a large cohort of patients affected by VHL, 60% of VHL patients had pancreatic involvement including solitary or multiple cysts, serous cystadenomas and pNETs (in 15%) [36]. In contrast to MEN1 tumors, VHL-related pNETs are mostly nonfunctional. Two percent of VHL patients (13% of VHL patients with pNETs) had metastatic disease [36].

Germline mutations of the VHL gene are now identified in more than 95% of the patients with clinical manifestations of VHL disease. About 200 distinct mutations have been identified. Loss of the wild-type allele has been demonstrated in VHL-associated NETs [37].

The VHL gene is a tumor-suppressor gene located on chromosome 3p25–26 [38]. The VHL protein (pVHL) plays a major role in the regulation of the oxygen-sensing pathway by targeting the alpha subunits of the hypoxia-inducible factor (HIF) for

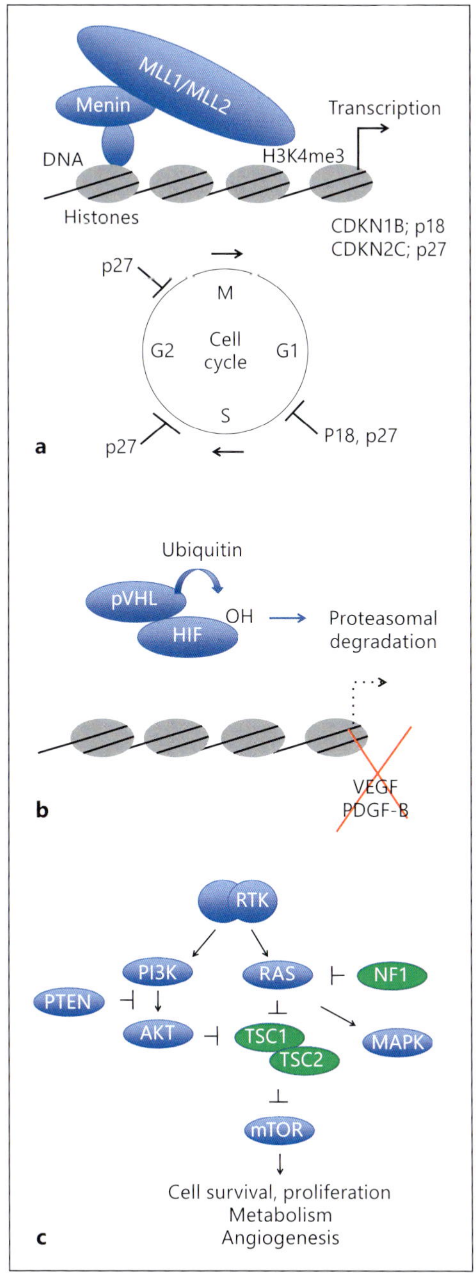

Fig. 1. Molecular mechanisms of inherited pNETs and pulmonary carcinoids. **a** The MEN1 gene product menin is an integral part of protein complexes containing MLL proteins that have histone methyltransferase activity specifically directed at trimethylation of lysine 4 (K4) of histone H3 (H3K4me3). This is a chromatin mark of active gene transcription. Among the target genes of the menin H3K4me3 complexes are the CDKI genes CDKN1B and CDKN2C, encoding the $p18^{Ink4c}$ and $p27^{Kip1}$ proteins, respectively. The absence of menin (in MEN1) or $p27^{Kip1}$ (in MEN4) can lead to uninterrupted cell cycle progression and, thus, cell proliferation. **b** Under normoxic conditions, the transcription factor HIF is hydroxylated and subsequently undergoes proteasomal degradation after ubiquitilation by pVHL. This prevents transcription of HIF target genes, such as VEGF and PDGF-β. Inactivation of pVHL leads to increased transcription of these genes and results in angiogenesis. **c** Signaling by receptor tyrosine kinases (RTK) results in activation of the PI3K and RAS pathways. Neurofibromin (NF1), hamartin (TSC1) and tuberin (TSC2) interfere with these pathways and block the activity of the mTOR. Loss of inhibition (in NF1 and TSC) leads to increased cell survival, cell proliferation, metabolism and angiogenesis. PTEN = Phosphatase and tensin homolog.

degradation (fig. 1b) [reviewed in 39]. Under conditions of normoxia the transcription factor HIF is hydroxylated and subsequently degraded. In the absence of pVHL, lack of degradation of HIF results in increased transcription of HIF target genes mimicking hypoxia. HIF target genes control angiogenesis, metabolism and apoptosis. Moreover, the most prominent HIF1 target genes include the genes encoding vascular endothelial growth factor (VEGF) and platelet-derived growth factor-β (PDGF-β). Both VEGF and PDGF-β are strong stimulators of angiogenesis. Additionally, pVHL has several HIF-independent functions that are also relevant to tumor development, such as maintenance of the primary cilium, regulation of extracellular matrix formation and turnover, and regulation of apoptosis [39]. The discovery of the mechanism of disease in VHL has contributed to the development of angiogenesis inhibitors as a therapeutic strategy in pNETs.

Neurofibromatosis Type 1

NF1 (von Recklinghausen disease; MIM 162200) is an autosomal-dominant genetic disorder characterized by neurofibromas, cafe-au-lait spots, axillary and inguinal freckling, iris hematomas (Lisch nodules), skeletal abnormalities, CNS gliomas, pheochromocytomas and paragangliomas, and occasionally periampullary somatostatinomas [40–42]. The clinical diagnosis is based on criteria established by the National Institutes of Health Consensus Development Conference in 1988 [43].

The prevalence of NF1 is about 1 in 3,000 individuals. Approximately 40% of periampullary somatostatinomas are associated with NF1 [41]. The most common localizations are the ampulla of Vater and the appendix. However, these NETs can develop at any site in the gastrointestinal tract. Although metastatic disease has been reported, NF1-related NETs have an indolent course, with a 5-year survival rate of 95% and low prevalence of metastatic disease for tumors smaller than 2 cm [40, 44].

The NF1 tumor suppressor gene is located on chromosome 17q11.2 [45, 46]. Only 50% of patients have a first-degree relative with NF1; the other 50% of patients have a de novo mutation. Variety in clinical expression is a characteristic of NF1 depending on the nature, timing, location, type of mutations and somatic mutations in modifier genes [42]. The NF1 gene encodes the cytoplasmic protein neurofibromin that controls cellular proliferation by inactivating the p21 RAS protein [47]. Loss of NF1 leads to increased activity of the mitogen-activated protein kinase (MAPK) and phosphoinositide 3-kinase (PI3K)-AKT-mTOR signal transduction pathways (fig. 1c) [48].

Tuberous Sclerosis Complex

TSC (OMIM 191100) is an autosomal dominant genetic disorder that is characterized by a heterogeneous presentation of hamartomas in various organs, including tubers and subependymal giant-cell astrocytomas in the brain and tumors in the heart, skin, eyes, kidneys, lungs and liver. The diagnosis of definite or possible TSC is based on the presence of a combination of major and/or minor features of the disease [49]. The live-birth prevalence of TSC is approximately 10–16 cases per 100,000 individuals [50].

NETs have been observed in patients with TSC. However, reports are limited to case reports and, thus, appear to be very rare [51]. In particular, pNETs producing insulin appear to be more frequent in TSC patients than in the general population. Current clinical recommendations for TSC do not include a routine investigation for pNETs [52].

TSC is caused by inactivating mutations in either the gene TSC1 (located on chromosome 9q34 and encoding the protein hamartin) or TSC2 (located on chromosome 16p13.3 and encoding the gene product tuberin) [53, 54]. More than 300 mutations have been reported for TSC, including missense, nonsense, frameshift deletions/insertions and splice junction mutations [55, 56]. Although TSC is a genetic disorder the majority of cases occur de novo: only 20% of patients have a positive family history of TSC, and 70–80% of TSC patients present as sporadic cases [50]. Most 'second hits' are large deletions involving loss of surrounding loci and LOH in TSC1 or TSC2, which have been reported in angiomyolipomas, rhabdomyomas and lymphangioleiomyomatosis (LAM) cells [57]. Although the incidence of NETs appears to be low, in two TSC-related insulinomas and in one pulmonary NET from a patient with LAM only, LOH of the wild-type TSC allele was found [58–60].

The TSC1 and TSC2 products hamartin and tuberin form heterodimers in the cytoplasm, which explains the common phenotype of TSC (fig. 1c). The hamartin-tuberin complex is a critical negative regulator of mTOR [61]. In TSC-associated tumors, loss of TSC1 or TSC2 results in unregulated autonomous mTOR-dependent signaling. Activation of mTOR leads to increased cell survival and proliferation as well as changes in cellular metabolism and angiogenesis [62]. The inhibition of mTOR has proved to be a successful treatment modality for many TSC-associated lesions [63].

Multiple Endocrine Neoplasia Type 4

Inherited mutations in the CDKN1B gene, encoding the CDKI $p27^{Ink4a}$, have been found in families with a MEN-like phenotype [64]. This very rare syndrome has been named MENX or MEN4 (MIM 610755). Although hyperparathyroidism and pituitary tumors are the most commonly described manifestations, NETs have also been described in association with CDKN1B mutations [65, 66]. Molatore at al. [67] found LOH in a pulmonary NET of a patient with a CDKN1B germline mutation. Based on these studies, $p27^{kip1}$ may play a role in inherited NET development.

Genetic and Epigenetic Studies in Sporadic Neuroendocrine Tumors

Pancreatic NETs

pNETs are commonly encountered in clinical syndromes related to the previously described germline mutations MEN1/VHL/NF1 and TSC. However, these germline mutations and associated clinical syndromes merely represent 10% of all pNETs. The remaining 90% occur due to sporadic genetic alterations, but the exact mechanisms of pathogenesis in sporadic pNETs have yet to be fully unraveled.

Comparative genomic hybridization (CGH) of pNETs has been extensively reviewed [68, 69]. These papers summarized that in nonfunctioning pNETs, among others, loss of chromosome 11q (containing the genes MEN1, BRCA2 and ATM), 6q and 11p, as well as gains in 17q (NEU/ERB2), 7q and 20q (AURKA, cMET) are common. In insulinomas, loss of 11q and 22q, and gain of 9q is found in over 50% of cases. Moreover, loss of 6q and gains of 17q are common in malignant insulinomas. Early events in the development of insulinomas are a gain of chromosome 9q and loss of 22q along with 11q, whereas telomeric loss is recognized during disease progression. Chromosomal aberrations in gastrinomas are common at 3p (loss) and 9p (gain).

LOH in pNETs has been reported for chromosome location 3p23 (74%), 6p22 (62%), 10q23 (50%; PTEN), 11q13 (67%; MEN1) and 22q12.1 (75%), among others [68, 69]. Recently, the PHLDA3 gene (1q31) was identified as a possible tumor suppressor in pNETs [69, 70]. LOH of PHLDA3 was found in 72% of cases along with promoter DNA methylation of the retained allele. Loss of Phlda3 in mice diminishes its repressing effect on AKT expression, increasing the PI3K/AKT/mTOR pathway activity, which leads to increased islet cell activity and hyperplasia.

From conventional DNA sequencing studies it was known that somatic inactivating mutations in the MEN1 tumor suppressor gene are common in sporadic pNETs [71]. In addition to MEN1 mutations, sporadic mutations have been found in the VHL and PTEN genes [72]. Yet mutations found frequently in pancreatic adenocarcinomas, such as KRAS, TP53, CDKN2A and SMAD3, are uncommon in sporadic pNETs [68]. A report by Jiao et al. [73] in 2011 was among the first to describe next-generation DNA sequencing in tumor samples. The authors studied a set of 10 nonfunctioning pNETs by exome sequencing in combination with a validation cohort of 58 additional pNETs that was Sanger sequenced. In addition to MEN1 gene mutations (in 44% of cases), loss of function mutations in DAXX (death-domain-associated protein) and ATRX (alpha thalassemia/mental retardation syndrome X-linked) genes were found frequently (43%), as well as mutations activating the PI3K-AKT-mTOR signal transduction cascade (14%; table 2). A single study investigated 35 kinase genes commonly mutated in cancer. Direct sequencing revealed that both ATM (5.5%) and KIT (2.7%) were mutated in sporadic pNETs [74].

The functional importance of MEN1 and mTOR has been discussed previously. The exact role of DAXX/ATRX in normal and tumor cells is less clear, but has been extensively reviewed [75, 76]. Relevant mechanisms by which DAXX/ATRX mutations may effect pNET development are discussed here (fig. 2). Both DAXX and ATRX function as chromatin remodelers and are involved in the incorporation of the histone variant H3.3 at the telomeres and pericentric heterochromatin [77, 78]. Thus, mutational activation/inactivation may affect the epigenetic regulation of several genes. Moreover, the DAXX-ATRX-H3.3 complex is linked to alternative telomerase lengthening (ALT); a mechanism by which cells may escape from senescence or cell crisis (immortalization). In a series of pNETs and tumors from the CNS, mutations

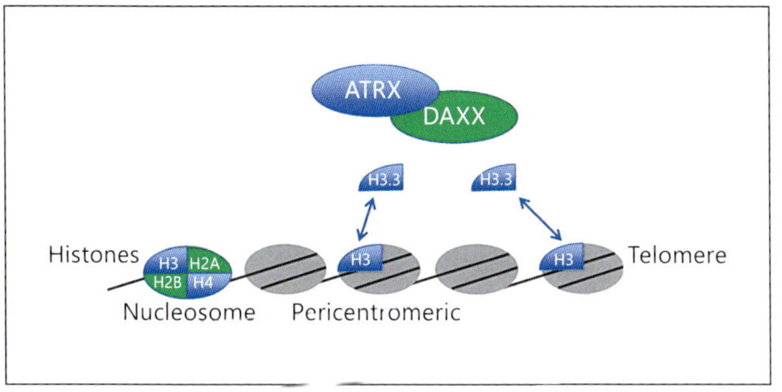

Fig. 2. A regular nucleosome consists of an octamer of four histone pairs of histone H2A, H2B, H3 and H4, and roughly 150 bp of DNA. The DAXX and ATRX proteins are involved in incorporation of the histone H3.3 variant at the pericentromeric and telomeric regions. The exchange of H3.3 and the canonical H3 affects gene transcription and is linked to ALT.

Table 2. Pathways most frequently mutated (>5%) and affected genes in sporadic pNETs and pulmonary carcinoids in next-generation sequencing studies

pNETs	
Nonfunctional [73]	
Chromatin modifying enzymes (62%)	MEN1 (44%), DAXX/ATRX (43%)
PI3K-AKT-mTOR pathway (15%)	PTEN (7.3%), TSC2 (8.8%), PIK3CA (1.4%)
Insulinoma [86]	
PI3K-AKT-mTOR pathway	YY1 (30%)
Pulmonary carcinoid [103]	
Covalent chromatin modification (40%)	MEN1 (8.9%), PSIP1 (8.9%), HDAC5 (2.2%), BRWD3 (2.2%), BCL11A, SETDB1, SETD1B, NSD1, KDM4A, PHF8, JMJD1C, Polycomb repressive complex (11.1%), (CDX61, EZH1, YY1)
SWI/SNF complexes (22.2%)	ARID1A, SMARCA1, SMARCA2, SMARCA4, ARID2, SMARCC2, SMARCB1
Sister chromatid cohesion (8.9%)	STAG1, NIBPL, DICER, ERCC6L
siNETs [119, 120]	
Cell cycle	CDKN1B (8%)
TGF-β pathway	SMAD4 (46%)
PI3K-AKT-mTOR pathway (29%)	

in DAXX or ATRX were strongly correlated with the ALT phenotype [79]. Besides ALT and chromatin remodeling, DAXX has both proapoptotic and antiapoptotic effects by p53 modulation, i.e. it regulates p53 through the DAXX/Axin/HIPK2/p53 complex as well as the DAXX/Hausp/MDM2 complex [80–82]. Additionally, ATM activation may deregulate the DAXX-MDM2 complex [83].

Jiao et al. [73] found that mutations of the MEN1 and DAXX/ATRX genes were associated with a better prognosis of pNETs. However, a recent study of 149 pNETs provided contradicting results, suggesting that patients with loss of DAXX or ATRX expression had a poorer prognosis compared to normal DAXX-ATRX expression. Additionally, loss of DAXX or ATRX was associated with chromosome instability (CIN) indicative of a more aggressive subtype [84]. Furthermore, in MEN1 germline-affected patients DAXX/ATRX mutations were only found in large tumors [85]. These combined results suggest that ATRX or DAXX inactivation is a late event in sporadic pNET development where ALT induces CIN, eventually leading towards tumor metastasis.

In 2013, a study of 10 whole-exome sequenced sporadic insulinomas showed a recurrent T372R gain of function mutation of the Ying Yang 1 (YY1) transcription factor gene (table 2). These results were validated in a series of 113 tumors, of which 30% were affected [86]. MEN1 and ATRX/DAXX mutations were investigated in 39 tumors and a mutation was found in 2.5 and 2.5/0%, respectively. Previously, YY1 was shown to function as a target of mTOR signaling and can be a component of Polycomb repressive histone modification complexes. In this capacity, YY1 is a metabolic regulator through regulation of mitochondrial gene expression [87, 88].

Thus far, no genome-wide DNA methylation studies in pNETs have been performed. Candidate approaches have revealed aberrant DNA methylation of the promoter of the Ras-association domain family 1 tumor suppressor gene RASSF1A in 75% of nonfunctioning pNETs and of the cyclin-dependent kinase (CDK) gene CDKN2A (encoding $p16^{Ink4a}$) in a number of tumors, although not in insulinomas [89–92]. Aberrant methylation of RASSF1A may be of interest, as RASSF1A is known to function by disrupting the DAXX-MDM2-HAUSP complex, thereby stabilizing p53 and inhibiting cell cycle progression upon DNA damage [93]. Nested DNA methylation-specific PCR analysis of 14 tumor suppressor genes in 18 pNETs showed that the promoters of APC/p73/RARβ (33%), $p16^{INK4a}/p15^{INK4b}/hMLH1/p14^{ARF}$ (39%) and BRCA1 (50%) were commonly hypermethylated [94].

Several studies have published gene expression data comparing pNETs with normal pancreas tissue or islets. The majority of these studies reported heterogeneous results due to differences in analysis platforms and group composition. The largest study thus far analyzed 72 primary pNETs (insulinomas and nonfunctioning tumors). Expression profiling revealed that inhibitors of the AKT-mTOR pathway, i.e. PTEN and TSC2, were downregulated and associated with a poor survival [69, 95]. In a cohort of 152 patients with sporadic pNETs, the hypoxia signaling genes HIF-1α, CA-9 and GLUT 1, previously found to be upregulated in pNETs of patients with a hereditary VHL mutation, were shown to be downregulated by VHL promoter hypermethylation (6%) or chromosomal deletion (18%). Moreover, protein expression of CA-9 was associated with poor survival, although the observed activation of hypoxia signaling genes may also be related to tumor progression [96].

Table 3. Results of miR profiling studies in pulmonary, pancreatic and small intestinal NETs

Author	Patients	NET type	Method	Comparison	MiR down- and upregulations	Overlapping miRs	Conclusions
Rapa [109], 2014	37 (22 TC/ 15 AC)	Pulmonary	qPCR-array	Metastatic vs. nonmetastatic AC vs. TC	Downregulated: 129-5p, 409-3p, 409-5p and 431-5p Downregulated: 129-5p, 409-3p and 409-5p	129-5p ↓ 409-3p ↓	Mir 129-5p, 409-3p, 409-5p and 431-5p are associated with malignant behavior
Mairinger [108], 2014	12 (3 TC/3 AC/ 3 LCNEC/ 3 SCLC)	Pulmonary	qPCR-array	TC vs. AC vs. LCNEC vs. SCLC	29a, 29b, 29c, 367, 504, 513c and 1200 negatively associated with tumor grade 18a, 15b, 335 and 1201 associated positively with tumor grade increase		PI3K and MAPK signaling pathway genes mostly targeted by identified miRs
Deng [107], 2014	47 (44 TC/3 AC)	Pulmonary	Illumina miRNA arrays	NET vs. normal tissue	Top upregulated miRs: 129, 323-3p, 487b, 410, 369-3p, 376a, 432, 129-3p, 409-3p, 494, 376a, 136, 370, 127-3p and 154 Top downregulated miRs 203, 224, 155, 302, 34b, 181b, 193a-5p, 34b, 222, 30a-3p, 938, 218, 511, 34c-3p, 10a, 146a and 1	155 ↓ 222 ↓ 409-3p ↑	No miR correlated with disease-free survival mRNA expression of CREB5 and PTPRB significantly associated with disease-free survival
Lee [110], 2012	63 (19 TC/6 AC/19 LCNEC/ 19 SCLC)	Pulmonary	Targeted qPCR miRNA 21, 155 and let-7a	TC/AC vs. LCNEC/ SCLC Lymph metastasis vs. no lymph metastasis	Tumor grade positively associated with miR-21 and 155 miR-21 positively associated with lymph node disease in TC/AC	155 ↑ 21 ↑	miR-21 expression is associated with lymph node metastasis in carcinoid
Roldo [97], 2006	40 (12 insulinomas, 28 nonfunctioning pNETs)	Pancreatic	Customized microRNA array	Normal tissue vs. tumor Insulinomas vs. NF-PET Liver vs. no liver metastasis	Upregulated: 107, 103, 23a, 26b, 192 and 342 Downregulated: 155 Upregulated: 204, 211 and 203 Upregulated: 21	21 ↑ 155 ↓	miR-204 expression correlates with insulinomas Liver metastatic disease is associated with high miR-21 expression. High miR-103/107 and lack of miR-155 expression is associated pancreatic tumors
Li [124], 2013	24 (8 primary, 8 liver metastases, 8 lymph node metastases)	Small intestinal	Affymetrix miRNA 1.0 array	Progression	Upregulated miRs: 96, 182, 183, 196a and 200a Downregulated miRs: 31, 129-5p, 133a and 215	129-5p ↓	Several miRNAs are differently expressed during tumor progression in siNETs
Ruebel [123], 2010	8 (8 primary; 7 liver, 1 lymph node)	Small intestinal	qPCR-array	Metastasis vs. primary tumor	Downregulated: 133a, 145, 156, 222 and 10b Upregulated: 183, 488, 19a and 19b	222 ↓	Several miRNAs are differently expressed during tumor progression in siNETs

Interpretation of commonly expressed miRs: downregulation of miR-129-5p and upregulation of miR-21 during tumor progression has been observed in siNETs and pulmonary NETs. miR-409-3p is upregulated in a cohort of pulmonary NETs compared to normal tissue; however, it has also been observed that miR 409-3p is downregulated during disease progression. Both up- and downregulation of miR-155 has been observed in pulmonary NETs; downregulation has been observed in pNETs. miR-222 is downregulated in pulmonary NETs; however, downregulation has also been observed during tumor progression in siNETs. TC = Typical carcinoids; AC = atypical carcinoids; LCNEC = large cell neuroendocrine carcinoma; SCLC = small cell lung cancer.

Studies investigating the effect of microRNAs (miR) in pNETs are scarce (table 3). The global miR expression in a series of pancreatic cancers and normal tissue showed that miR-103 and miR-107 were upregulated and miR-155 was downregulated in pNETs compared to normal tissue. In insulinomas, miR-204 was overexpressed compared to nonfunctioning pNETs. miR-21 expression was associated with liver metastatic disease and tumor grade (i.e. Ki-67 index), similar to what was observed in pulmonary carcinoids (see below). No significant differences in miR expression could be identified between pancreatic acinar cell carcinoma and pNETs [97].

In general, nonfunctioning pNETs show 60% fewer gene mutations compared to pancreatic adenocarcinomas [73]. As the majority of mutations are found in genes regulating either chemical chromatin modification or chromatin remodeling, it seems likely that the epigenome is the major tumorigenic driver in nonfunctioning pNETs, with a special role for MEN1, DAXX and ATRX. Additionally, the PI3K/AKT/mTOR signaling cascade and the VHL gene with subsequent HIF-pathway signaling is affected in several pNETs. In insulinomas, alterations in this cascade may be more dominant with recurrent mutations in YY1, a target of mTOR signaling. During progression, an accumulation of genetic alterations (CIN) is observed, probably induced by telomere loss and/or ALT as a result of inactivation of DAXX/ATRX.

Pulmonary NETs (Carcinoids)

Most likely, the majority of pulmonary carcinoids are sporadic, though somatic MEN1 gene mutations are known to be present in approximately 13–18% of pulmonary carcinoids [98]. MEN1 has been shown to occur more frequently in atypical carcinoids and is associated with a poor prognosis [99].

Major chromosomal alterations are relatively rare in sporadic pulmonary carcinoids with an average of 2.8- and 6.1-Mb chromosomal alterations in typical/atypical carcinoids compared to 18.8-Mb alterations in small cell lung cancer [100]. Genome-wide CGH analysis has revealed recurrent chromosomal losses of 11q and 13q [100]. At 11q, areas of loss cluster at 11q13, known for the location of MEN1, 11q22-q23 and 11q24 [100]. Deletion of chromosome 13q is mostly present in atypical carcinoids and is known for the location of the tumor suppressor gene retinoblastoma (*RB*; 13q14) [100, 101].

A recently published whole-genome/exome sequencing study of 69 pulmonary carcinoids revealed somatic mutations in several other genes in addition to the MEN1 gene. Forty percent of all pulmonary NETs carried a mutually exclusive histone covalent modifying gene mutation. These histone covalent modifying genes could be subdivided into the menin-binding protein PSIP1, the histone methyltransferases SETD1B, SETDB1 and NSD1, the histone demethylases KDM4A, PHF8 and JMJD1C, as well as members of the Polycomb repressive histone H3K27 methyltransferase complexes CBX6, EZH1 and also YY1 [102]. In addition, mutations were detected in the histone modifiers BRWD3 and HDAC5. Moreover, numerous mutations were found in ATP-dependent chromatin remodeling SWI/SNF complex members ARID1, SMARCA1, SMARCA2, SMARCA4, ARID2, SMARCC2, SMARCB1 and BCL11A. Another recurrently affected pathway was sister chromatid cohesion – the process by which sister chromosomes are paired and held together during cell cycle progression – with the following genes mutated: STAG1,

NIPBL16, DICER and ERCC6L. Additionally, statistically significant mutations were found in the WDR26, EIF1AX and SEC31 genes and in several E3 ubiquitin ligases. Overall, only the MEN1, PSIP1 and ARID1A genes were recurrently mutated. The genes TP53 and RB that are commonly mutated in high-grade lung neuroendocrine carcinomas were affected in none of the typical carcinoids and in 2/5 atypical carcinoids. Another study, investigating PIK3CA exon 9 and 20 mutations, revealed that 13.3% of typical and 39.1% of atypical carcinoids harbored a missense mutation affecting the PI3K/Akt/mTOR pathway [103].

The field of DNA methylation still has to be thoroughly investigated in pulmonary carcinoids. Methylation analysis has revealed RASSF1A as the most frequently hypermethylated promoter [101]. Additionally, the gene encoding the p15Ink4b CDKI, CDKN2B, was found to be methylated in 15% of lung NET cases [104]. MEN1 gene methylation analysis revealed no correlation between low mRNA levels of MEN1 and the frequency of methylation [99].

Similar to pNETs, gene expression in pulmonary carcinoids is heterogeneous. To date, a single study has specifically investigated carcinoids, focusing on different pathways involved in carcinoid progression. In total, 10 tumors were screened with gene arrays and the results were validated in a cohort of 65 pulmonary NETs. The RET proto-oncogene was strongly upregulated in patients with poor survival. In addition, the OTP (orthopedia homeobox) gene was strongly downregulated in these patients. Pathway analysis revealed alterations in the cell cycle, DNA damage detection and repair pathways. Other specific pathways affected were the mitotic spindle checkpoint, the chromosomal passenger complex (CPC), mitotic kinase CDC2 and the BRCA-Fanconi anemia (FA) pathway. An in-depth analysis of the CPC pathway revealed that the genes Aurora B kinase and BIRC5 (Survivin) were expressed at higher levels in high-grade neuroendocrine carcinomas and upregulation of the Aurora B kinase was associated with poor survival. Other individual genes predictive for survival in carcinoid disease were CD44, IL20RA, KLK12 and the already mentioned OTP [105]. A complete overview of gene expression covering both low-grade NETs and high-grade neuroendocrine carcinomas is provided by Swarts [106].

A number of recent studies have examined microRNA expression in pulmonary carcinoids using different profiling platforms (table 3) and reported differences between normal lung tissue and tumor, carcinoids and high-grade neuroendocrine carcinomas, and localized and metastatic disease [107–110]. Although these studies are difficult to compare, some recurrent deregulated miRs in lung NET progression were identified, including miR-129–5p, miR-409–3p and miR-155. In addition, miR-21 upregulation was correlated with metastatic disease, which was also observed in pNETs [111]. This miR was previously shown to deregulate PTEN [112], involved in the mTOR pathway, and ANP32A/SMARCA4 [113], two genes that are involved in chromatin remodeling.

The available literature on the (epi)genetic background of tumorigenic drivers in sporadic pulmonary carcinoids indicates that chromatin modification and remodeling is of key essence. Yet, contrary to pNETs, there is so far no evidence for ALT and DAXX/ATRX involvement in pulmonary carcinoids [114]. Similar to observations in pNETs, a small subgroup of pulmonary carcinoids shows activation of the PI3K/AKT/mTOR pathway.

Small Intestinal NETs

NETs of the small intestine (siNETs) are not known to occur in the context of a genetic syndrome (see above). A family history of carcinoid disease was present in 0.5% of patients with siNETs that were registered in a Swedish population-based study [115]. In addition, germline single nucleotide polymorphisms in the genes IL12A (involved in inflammation and angiogenesis) and DAD1 (involved in apoptosis) have been associated with the occurrence of siNETs [116].

Chromosomal alterations in siNETs have been extensively studied and reviewed [117]. CGH and LOH analyses revealed a common loss of chromosome 18q (common regions of deletions 18q21.1-q21.31, 18q22.1-q22.2 and 18q22.3-q23) associated with early onset disease. Other chromosomal losses and LOH is located at chromosomes 3, 9, 11, 13 and 16. Gains are frequently found at chromosomes 4, 5, 14 and 20. Candidate genes located at these chromosomes are SMAD2 and 4, CDKN2A, ADHD/CASP, DAD1 and RYBP, the latter being an encoder of YY1 and RING1 previously found altered in insulinomas.

Thus far, two comprehensive sequencing studies have been published on siNETs (table 2). Banck et al. [118] exome sequenced 48 mainly primary well-differentiated siNETs, which showed a low mean exome mutation rate [an average of 0.1 somatic single nucleotide variations (SNV)/10^6 bp]. This rate is comparable with pulmonary carcinoids. A heterogeneous mixture of mutations in well-known tumor-associated genes was identified including the FGF receptor 2 (FGFR2), MEN1, HOOK3, the H3K27 histone methyltransferase EZH2, MLF1, CARD11, VHL, NONO, FANCD2 and BRAF. However, no recurrent mutations were detected. Commonly amplified oncogenes (in 14–20% of siNETs) were SRC, AURKA, MAP2K2, PDGFR and AKT1/AKT2. SMAD4 was recurrently mutated or deleted in 46% of cases, indicating a role in tumorigenesis. Combining mutations and CNVs in an integrative analysis of biological processes revealed several cell signaling pathways to be affected, such as TGFβ-Wnt (in 48% of patients), ECM/Adhesion/SRC (33%), PI3K/AKT/mTOR (29%) and ERK/MAPK (27%). Furthermore, mitosis/spindle formation (27%), DNA damage (19%), chromatin remodeling (17%), apoptosis (15%), axon guidance (10%) and E3 ligase ubiquitin (6%) were affected.

Francis et al. [119] performed an exome/genome sequencing study on 50 sporadic siNETs. The mean SNV/10^6 bp was 0.77, which was 7.7-fold higher than in the above-described study, possibly due to the analyses of more metastatic samples. The most frequently mutated gene was the CDK inhibitor gene CDKN1B (MEN4). CDKN1B regulates cell cycle progression at G1-S, through phosphorylation of the RB gene; dissociation of p27 from the cyclin E/CDK2 complex activates CDK2, which phosphorylates RB. Its role in NET tumorigenesis has been reviewed previously [120]. CDKN1B was affected in 8% of cases (mostly insertions and deletions leading to frame shifts). Moreover, the gene was hemizygously deleted in 14% of cases, indicating deregulation of the cell cycle in the etiology of siNETs. Loss of chromosome 18 was observed in 78% of cases. In-depth analysis of growth inhibitory or STOP genes revealed no recurrent mutations, yet haploinsufficiency of specific genes located at chromosome 18 may be one of the underlying mechanisms of siNET tumorigenesis. Remarkably, there was no significant overlap in observed mutations with the study by Banck et al. [118], as well as with the pNET study by Jiao et al. [73], suggesting that many of the mutations in NETs are passengers and not drivers.

Only a few methylation studies are reported for siNETs. In 16 siNETs, promoter hypermethylation of RASSF1A (69%), p14 (69%) and p16 (25%) was observed [121]. In another cohort of 33 siNETs, RASSF1A promoter hypermethylation was found in 85% of metastatic and 61% of primary tumor tissue, whereas normal enterochromaffin cells showed no methylation. A similar pattern was found for the CTNNB1 gene (58 vs. 27%). Other commonly methylated genes were LAMB3, LAMC2 and CDH1. RASSF1A hypermethylation was accompanied by downregulation of protein expression, as assessed by Western blotting analyses [122].

Two microRNA profiling studies have been conducted on 24 and 8 siNETs, respectively [123, 124]. Several miRs were found to be deregulated during tumor progression (see table 3). miR-133a, located on chromosome 18q11.2, was found to be downregulated in both studies and validated by in situ hybridization and Northern blot analysis. miR-133a may function as a tumor suppressor and has been described in lung cancer and osteosarcomas as a repressor of cell growth through repression of insulin growth factor 1 receptor and AKT signaling [125, 126].

Several gene expression studies have been reported [117]. From these studies it became clear that siNETs could be categorized into three distinct groups based on gene expression, i.e. upregulation of BANP/CDK5R2, upregulation of RUNX1 and TGFBR2, and upregulation of TPH1, CDH6 and TUSC2 mRNA. Deregulated cellular processes included cell cycle control, apoptosis, cell adhesion, extracellular matrix formation and migration. Furthermore, besides miR133a, upregulation of APLP1 and downregulation of CXCL14, NKX2–3, ACTG2, GREM2 and REG3A were also associated with metastatic disease.

The genetic background of somatic siNETs is heterogeneous with few recurrent mutations. Up to three quarters of siNETs harbor chromosome 18 losses, pointing to involvement of one or more genes in tumorigenesis. Because no recurrent mutations are found in genes on this chromosome, haploinsufficiency has been suggested to be the mechanism involved, although the exact genes are unclear. Furthermore, the identification of CDKN1B mutations (encoding p27) and methylation of p16 and p14 implicate deregulation of the cell cycle to be important in siNETs. Similar to pNETs and pulmonary carcinoids, somatic mutation and SNV analyses point to chromatin remodeling and the PI3K-Akt-mTOR signaling pathways being affected in siNETs.

Therapeutic Consequences of Genetic and Epigenetic Studies in Neuroendocrine Tumors

Several therapeutic options are currently adopted for NETs according to the biological and clinical characteristics of the individual patient. According to guidelines for the management of NETs, surgery remains the only curative option for NETs of any site [127, 128]. For GEP-NETs, surgical resection of both primary tumor and locoregional nodal metastasis is recommended whenever possible. The presence of liver metastasis is not an absolute contraindication per se for surgery if radical removal can be guaranteed. In functioning NETs associated with liver metastasis, a first-line treatment with somatostatin analogs can anticipate surgical resection. Medical therapy as well as polypeptide radionuclide receptor therapy can also be considered in a nonresectable tumor as a chance to downstage the neoplasm and make resection feasible [127, 129–133]. In selected patients, an incomplete debulking surgery, although with limited indications, may improve the quality of life [132]. In the presence of extrahepatic disease, palliative care consists in medical control of symptoms through local and/or systemic therapies, including surgery, local ablative interventions, systemic chemotherapy and biological approaches such as polypeptide radionuclide receptor therapy. Somatostatin and its analogs (e.g. lanreotide, octreotide) have been successfully implemented into clinical practice. These agents act through a family of 5 G-protein-coupled receptors (sst1–sst5) to perform a variety of functions, including inhibition of endocrine and exocrine secretions and of tumor cell growth [134]. However, patients treated with somatostatin analogs may develop resistance over time [135]. This has been partially explained by the recent finding of novel truncated sst5 receptor variants, one of which (sst5TMD4) is upregulated in tumors, while barely expressed in normal tissues. For example, the expression of sst5TMD4 in pituitary adenomas causing acromegaly is related to the reduced ability of octreotide at normalizing hormone secretion in poorly responsive tumors [136]. In patients with well-differentiated metastatic midgut NETs systemic chemotherapy has shown poor results, thus in these patients it has to be considered only after the failure of all the other therapeutic options [132].

In recent years, the advent of next-generation sequencing technologies has accelerated our understanding of the complexity of cancer genetics. The identification of genetic signatures and driver mutations has provided evidence for the detection of biomarkers for diagnosis, subclassification and targets for therapy [137], which holds promise for the development of personalized care.

mTOR Inhibition

From the TSC and NF1 models, and later gene expression profiling and sequencing studies in NETs, it has become clear that PI3K-AKT-mTOR signaling is affected in a major proportion of NETs [138–141]. The mTOR inhibitor everolimus has been shown to be effective as a treatment for patients with TSC [63, 142, 143]. Combined mTOR and MAPK inhibition is effective in preclinical NF1 nerve sheath tumor models [144].

The RADIANT (RAD001 in Advanced Neuroendocrine Tumors) 2 and RADIANT-3 clinical trials showed that the mTOR inhibitor everolimus had significant antitumor efficacy in NETs [145–147]. Currently accepted guidelines consider its use only in progressive disease [131, 148–150].

The median progression-free survival in the RADIANT-3 phase III trial was 11 months with everolimus as compared to 4.6 months with placebo with an acceptable toxicity profile [145]. In the RADIANT-2 study, patients with any type of advanced low- or intermediate-grade NETs were recruited, including patients with pNETs and also pulmonary carcinoids and siNETs [147]. Patients were treated with somatostatin analogs or somatostatin analogs combined with everolimus. Progression-free survival was 16.4 months in the combination therapy group and 11.3 months in the control group.

Inhibition of Angiogenesis

NETs are highly vascularized tumors and the VEGF signaling pathway has been reported to be deregulated [151]. Strong mRNA expression of VEGFA and its encoded protein receptors (VEGFR1 and VEGFR2) were observed in sporadic and VHL-related pNETs [152]. The VEGF inhibitor bevacizumab and the VEGF receptor inhibitors pazopanib and sorafenib have shown clinical activity [146, 153]. Cabozantinib (a small molecule inhibitor of the c-Met and VEGFR2 tyrosine kinases) and sunitinib (a multitargeted receptor tyrosine kinase including PDGFRs, VEGFRs, CD117 and RET) are promising new drugs for advanced disease [149, 154]. In 2011, results from a phase III randomized clinical trial were published on the effects of the VEGF tyrosine kinase inhibitor sunitinib in patients with advanced, well-differentiated pNETs. Patients who used sunitinib had a progression-free survival of 11.4 months versus 5.5 months in the control group [153]. Sunitinib has been approved for use in patients with advanced pNETs.

CDK Inhibition

Alterations in CDK function seem to play a role in every NET type. Aberrant expression of the CDKN1B and CDKN2C genes is observed in MEN1 model systems. Inherited mutations in CDKN1B lead to MEN4, which appears to include NETs as a manifestation. In sporadic pNETs high amounts of CDK4 or its partner protein cyclin D1 have been found leading to high amounts of phosphorylated retinoblastoma protein [155]. Promoter methylation of CDKN2A and CDKN2B has been reported in pNETs and pulmonary carcinoids. Somatic CDKN1B mutations were present in a significant proportion of siNETs. Synthetic CDK inhibitors are currently under investigation as therapeutic agents in various types of cancer, e.g. the CDK4/6 inhibitors that have entered clinical trials. These agents could be of use for the treatment of NETs [156].

DNA Methyltransferase and Histone Demethylase Inhibitors
As gene mutations are observed relatively infrequently in NETs, and epigenetic changes may be major drivers of NET development, compounds that target epigenetic alterations may be effective for patients with NETs [157]. DNA methylation and histone modifications are attractive therapeutic targets as these modifications are reversible, which is in contrast to DNA mutations. DNA methyltransferase-inhibiting compounds such as 5-AZA-deoxycytidine have only been investigated in NET cell lines [158]. MEN1 gene mutations are present in most NET subtypes. Aberrant H3K4me3 is thought to be causal to MEN1 tumorigenesis. Inhibiting H3K4me3 demethylases increases H3K4me3 levels. A novel class of compounds that inhibit H3K4me3 demethylases from the KDM5 family is currently being developed. Indeed, in a MEN1 knockout pNETs mouse model tumor development was attenuated significantly by synchronous knockout of the H3K4me3 demethylase Kdm5A [33]. Inhibition of KDM5 proteins could be an attractive future strategy to restore H3K4me3 on menin target genes in NETs with alterations in histone methyltransferase activity [159].

Over the last decades, studying the mechanisms of disease of inherited and sporadic pNETs and pulmonary carcinoids has provided valuable insight into NET development and contributed significantly to the recent development of revolutionary therapeutic approaches. Genome-wide analysis of genetic and epigenetic characteristics of these tumor types is likely to further innovate the treatment options for patients with advanced NETs.

References

1 Klimstra DS, Modlin IR, Coppola D, Lloyd RV, Suster S: The pathologic classification of neuroendocrine tumors: a review of nomenclature, grading, and staging systems. Pancreas 2010;39:707–712.

2 Bosman FT, Carneiro F, Hruban RH, Theisse ND: WHO Classification of Tumours of the Digestive System. Lyon, IARC, 2010.

3 Brandi ML, Gagel RF, Angeli A, et al: Guidelines for diagnosis and therapy of MEN type 1 and type 2. J Clin Endocrinol Metab 2001;86:5658–5671.

4 Thakker RV, Newey PJ, Walls GV, et al: Clinical practice guidelines for multiple endocrine neoplasia type 1 (MEN1). J Clin Endocrinol Metab 2012;97: 2990–3011.

5 Goudet P, Bonithon-Kopp C, Murat A, et al: Gender-related differences in MEN1 lesion occurrence and diagnosis: a cohort study of 734 cases from the Groupe d'Etude des Tumeurs Endocrines. Eur J Endocrinol 2011;165:97–105.

6 Sakurai A, Suzuki S, Kosugi S, et al: Multiple endocrine neoplasia type 1 in Japan: establishment and analysis of a multicentre database. Clin Endocrinol 2012;76:533–539.

7 Triponez F, Goudet P, Dosseh D, et al: Is surgery beneficial for MEN1 patients with small (≤2 cm), nonfunctioning pancreaticoduodenal endocrine tumor? An analysis of 65 patients from the GTE. World J Surg 2006;30:654–662, discussion 663–654.

8 Carty SE, Helm AK, Amico JA, et al: The variable penetrance and spectrum of manifestations of multiple endocrine neoplasia type 1. Surgery 1998;124: 1106–1113, discussion 1113–1104.

9 Kouvaraki MA, Shapiro SE, Cote GJ, et al: Management of pancreatic endocrine tumors in multiple endocrine neoplasia type 1. World J Surg 2006;30:643–653.

10 Jensen RT: Management of the Zollinger-Ellison syndrome in patients with multiple endocrine neoplasia type 1. J Intern Med 1998;243:477–488.

11 Doherty GM: Multiple endocrine neoplasia type 1: duodenopancreatic tumors. Surg Oncol 2003;12: 135–143.

12 de Herder WW, Niederle B, Scoazec JY, et al: Well-differentiated pancreatic tumor/carcinoma: insulinoma. Neuroendocrinology 2006;84:183–188.

13 Goudet P, Murat A, Cardot-Bauters C, et al: Thymic neuroendocrine tumors in multiple endocrine neoplasia type 1: a comparative study on 21 cases among a series of 761 MEN1 from the GTE (Groupe des Tumeurs Endocrines). World J Surg 2009;33:1197–1207.
14 Sakurai A, Imai T, Kikumori T, et al: Thymic neuroendocrine tumour in multiple endocrine neoplasia type 1: female patients are not rare exceptions. Clin Endocrinol 2013;78:248–254.
15 Goudet P, Murat A, Binquet C, et al: Risk factors and causes of death in MEN1 disease: a GTE (Groupe d'Etude des Tumeurs Endocrines) cohort study among 758 patients. World J Surg 2010;34:249–255.
16 de Laat JM, Pieterman CR, van den Broek MF, et al: Natural course and survival of neuroendocrine tumors of thymus and lung in MEN1 patients. J Clin Endocrinol Metab 2014;99:3325–3333.
17 Delle Fave G, Kwekkeboom DJ, van Cutsem E, et al: ENETS consensus guidelines for the management of patients with gastroduodenal neoplasms. Neuroendocrinology 2012;95:74–87.
18 Chandrasekharappa SC, Guru SC, Manickam P, et al: Positional cloning of the gene for multiple endocrine neoplasia-type 1. Science 1997;276:404–407.
19 Knudson AG Jr: Mutation and cancer: statistical study of retinoblastoma. Proc Natl Acad Sci U S A 1971;68:820–823.
20 Lemos MC, Thakker RV: Multiple endocrine neoplasia type 1 (MEN1): analysis of 1,336 mutations reported in the first decade following identification of the gene. Hum Mutat 2008;29:22–32.
21 Lubensky IA, Debelenko LV, Zhuang Z, et al: Allelic deletions on chromosome 11q13 in multiple tumors from individual MEN1 patients. Cancer Res 1996;56: 5272–5278.
22 Debelenko LV, Emmert-Buck MR, Zhuang Z, et al: The multiple endocrine neoplasia type I gene locus is involved in the pathogenesis of type II gastric carcinoids. Gastroenterology 1997;113:773–781.
23 Dong Q, Debelenko LV, Chandrasekharappa SC, et al: Loss of heterozygosity at 11q13: analysis of pituitary tumors, lung carcinoids, lipomas, and other uncommon tumors in subjects with familial multiple endocrine neoplasia type 1. J Clin Endocrinol Metab 1997;82:1416–1420.
24 Gibril F, Chen YJ, Schrump DS, et al: Prospective study of thymic carcinoids in patients with multiple endocrine neoplasia type 1. J Clin Endocrinol Metab 2003;88:1066–1081.
25 Teh BT: Thymic carcinoids in multiple endocrine neoplasia type 1. J Intern Med 1998;243:501–504.
26 Matkar S, Thiel A, Hua X: Menin: a scaffold protein that controls gene expression and cell signaling. Trends Biochem Sci 2013;38:394–402.
27 Hughes CM, Rozenblatt-Rosen O, Milne TA, et al: Menin associates with a trithorax family histone methyltransferase complex and with the hoxc8 locus. Mol Cell 2004;13:587–597.
28 Yokoyama A, Wang Z, Wysocka J, et al: Leukemia proto-oncoprotein MLL forms a SET1-like histone methyltransferase complex with menin to regulate *Hox* gene expression. Mol Cell Biol 2004;24:5639–5649.
29 Pieterman CR, Conemans EB, Dreijerink KM, et al: Thoracic and duodenopancreatic neuroendocrine tumors in multiple endocrine neoplasia type 1. Endocr Relat Cancer 2014;21:R121–R142.
30 Milne TA, Hughes CM, Lloyd R, et al: Menin and MLL cooperatively regulate expression of cyclin-dependent kinase inhibitors. Proc Natl Acad Sci U S A 2005;102:749–754.
31 Karnik SK, Hughes CM, Gu X, et al: Menin regulates pancreatic islet growth by promoting histone methylation and expression of genes encoding $p27^{Kip1}$ and $p18^{INK4c}$. Proc Natl Acad Sci U S A 2005;102:14659–14664.
32 Besson A, Dowdy SF, Roberts JM: CDK inhibitors: cell cycle regulators and beyond. Dev Cell 2008;14: 159–169.
33 Lin W, Cao J, Liu J, et al: Loss of the retinoblastoma binding protein 2 (RBP2) histone demethylase suppresses tumorigenesis in mice lacking Rb1 or Men1. Proc Natl Acad Sci U S A 2011;108:13379–13386.
34 Maher ER, Neumann HP, Richard S: Von Hippel-Lindau disease: a clinical and scientific review. Eur J Hum Genet 2011;19:617–623.
35 Hes FJ, Hoppener JW, Luijt RB, Lips CJ: Von Hippel-Lindau disease. Hered Cancer Clin Pract 2005;3: 171–178.
36 Charlesworth M, Verbeke CS, Falk GA, Walsh M, Smith AM, Morris-Stiff G: Pancreatic lesions in von Hippel-Lindau disease? A systematic review and meta-synthesis of the literature. J Gastrointest Surg 2012;16:1422–1428.
37 Lott ST, Chandler DS, Curley SA, et al: High frequency loss of heterozygosity in von Hippel-Lindau (VHL)-associated and sporadic pancreatic islet cell tumors: evidence for a stepwise mechanism for malignant conversion in VHL tumorigenesis. Cancer Res 2002;62:1952–1955.
38 Latif F, Tory K, Gnarra J, et al: Identification of the von Hippel-Lindau disease tumor suppressor gene. Science 1993;260:1317–1320.
39 Kaelin WG Jr: The von Hippel-Lindau tumour suppressor protein: O2 sensing and cancer. Nat Rev Cancer 2008;8:865–873.
40 Basile U, Cavallaro G, Polistena A, et al: Gastrointestinal and retroperitoneal manifestations of type 1 neurofibromatosis. J Gastrointest Surg 2010;14:186–194.

41 Relles D, Baek J, Witkiewicz A, Yeo CJ: Periampullary and duodenal neoplasms in neurofibromatosis type 1: two cases and an updated 20-year review of the literature yielding 76 cases. J Gastrointest Surg 2010;14:1052–1061.
42 Pasmant E, Vidaud M, Vidaud D, Wolkenstein P: Neurofibromatosis type 1: from genotype to phenotype. J Med Genet 2012;49:483–489.
43 National Institutes of Health Consensus Development Conference: Neurofibromatosis. Conference statement. Arch Neurol 1988;45:575–578.
44 Lodish MB, Stratakis CA: Endocrine tumours in neurofibromatosis type 1, tuberous sclerosis and related syndromes. Best Pract Res Clin Endocrinol Metab 2010;24:439–449.
45 Wallace MR, Marchuk DA, Andersen LB, et al: Type 1 neurofibromatosis gene: identification of a large transcript disrupted in three NF1 patients. Science 1990;249:181–186.
46 Xu GF, O'Connell P, Viskochil D, et al: The neurofibromatosis type 1 gene encodes a protein related to GAP. Cell 1990;62:599–608.
47 Martin GA, Viskochil D, Bollag G, et al: The GAP-related domain of the neurofibromatosis type 1 gene product interacts with ras p21. Cell 1990;63:843–849.
48 Brems H, Beert E, de Ravel T, Legius E: Mechanisms in the pathogenesis of malignant tumours in neurofibromatosis type 1. Lancet Oncol 2009;10:508–515.
49 Northrup H, Krueger DA: Tuberous sclerosis complex diagnostic criteria update: recommendations of the 2012 international tuberous sclerosis complex consensus conference. Pediatr Neurol 2013;49:243–254.
50 Osborne JP, Fryer A, Webb D: Epidemiology of tuberous sclerosis. Ann N Y Acad Sci 1991;615:125–127.
51 Dworakowska D, Grossman AB: Are neuroendocrine tumours a feature of tuberous sclerosis? A systematic review. Endocr Relat Cancer 2009;16:45–58.
52 Yates JR, Maclean C, Higgins JN, et al: The Tuberous Sclerosis 2000 Study: presentation, initial assessments and implications for diagnosis and management. Arch Dis Child 2011;96:1020–1025.
53 van Slegtenhorst M, de Hoogt R, Hermans C, et al: Identification of the tuberous sclerosis gene TSC1 on chromosome 9q34. Science 1997;277:805–808.
54 Xu L, Sterner C, Maheshwar MM, et al: Alternative splicing of the tuberous sclerosis 2 (TSC2) gene in human and mouse tissues. Genomics 1995;27:475–480.
55 Astrinidis A, Henske EP: Tuberous sclerosis complex: linking growth and energy signaling pathways with human disease. Oncogene 2005;24:7475–7481.
56 Sancak O, Nellist M, Goedbloed M, et al: Mutational analysis of the TSC1 and TSC2 genes in a diagnostic setting: genotype – phenotype correlations and comparison of diagnostic DNA techniques in tuberous sclerosis complex. Eur J Hum Genet 2005;13:731–741.
57 Jozwiak J, Jozwiak S, Wlodarski P: Possible mechanisms of disease development in tuberous sclerosis. Lancet Oncol 2008;9:73–79.
58 Verhoef S, van Diemen-Steenvoorde R, Akkersdijk WL, et al: Malignant pancreatic tumour within the spectrum of tuberous sclerosis complex in childhood. Eur J Pediatr 1999;158:284–287.
59 Francalanci P, Diomedi-Camassei F, Purificato C, et al: Malignant pancreatic endocrine tumor in a child with tuberous sclerosis. Am J Surg Pathol 2003;27:1386–1389.
60 Sato T, Seyama K, Kumasaka T, et al: A patient with TSC1 germline mutation whose clinical phenotype was limited to lymphangioleiomyomatosis. J Int Med 2004;256:166–173.
61 Huang J, Manning BD: The TSC1-TSC2 complex: a molecular switchboard controlling cell growth. Biochem J 2008;412:179–190.
62 Lebwohl D, Anak O, Sahmoud T, et al: Development of everolimus, a novel oral mTOR inhibitor, across a spectrum of diseases. Ann N Y Acad Sci 2013;1291:14–32.
63 Franz DN, Weiss BD: Molecular therapies for tuberous sclerosis and neurofibromatosis. Curr Neurol Neurosci Rep 2012;12:294–301.
64 Pellegata NS, Quintanilla-Martinez L, Siggelkow H, et al: Germ-line mutations in p27Kip1 cause a multiple endocrine neoplasia syndrome in rats and humans. Proc Natl Acad Sci U S A 2006;103:15558–15563.
65 Agarwal SK, Mateo CM, Marx SJ: Rare germline mutations in cyclin-dependent kinase inhibitor genes in multiple endocrine neoplasia type 1 and related states. J Clin Endocrinol Metab 2009;94:1826–1834.
66 Occhi G, Regazzo D, Trivellin G, et al: A novel mutation in the upstream open reading frame of the CDKN1B gene causes a MEN4 phenotype. PLoS Genet 2013;9:e1003350.
67 Molatore S, Marinoni I, Lee M, et al: A novel germline CDKN1B mutation causing multiple endocrine tumors: clinical, genetic and functional characterization. Hum Mutat 2010;31:E1825–E1835.
68 Jonkers YM, Ramaekers FC, Speel EJ: Molecular alterations during insulinoma tumorigenesis. Biochim Biophys Acta 2007;1775:313–332.
69 Capurso G, Festa S, Valente R, et al: Molecular pathology and genetics of pancreatic endocrine tumours. J Mol Endocrinol 2012;49:R37–R50.
70 Ohki R, Saito K, Chen Y, et al: PHLDA3 is a novel tumor suppressor of pancreatic neuroendocrine tumors. Proc Natl Acad Sci U S A 2014;111:E2404–E2413.
71 Zhuang Z, Vortmeyer AO, Pack S, et al: Somatic mutations of the MEN1 tumor suppressor gene in sporadic gastrinomas and insulinomas. Cancer Res 1997;57:4682–4686.

72 Schmitt AM, Schmid S, Rudolph T, et al: VHL inactivation is an important pathway for the development of malignant sporadic pancreatic endocrine tumors. Endocr Relat Cancer 2009;16:1219–1227.
73 Jiao Y, Shi C, Edil BH, et al: DAXX/ATRX, MEN1, and mTOR pathway genes are frequently altered in pancreatic neuroendocrine tumors. Science 2011; 331:1199–1203.
74 Corbo V, Beghelli S, Bersani S, et al: Pancreatic endocrine tumours: mutational and immunohistochemical survey of protein kinases reveals alterations in targetable kinases in cancer cell lines and rare primaries. Ann Oncol 2012;23:127–134.
75 Salomoni P: The PML-interacting protein DAXX: histone loading gets into the picture. Front Oncol 2013;3:152.
76 Clynes D, Higgs DR, Gibbons RJ: The chromatin remodeller ATRX: a repeat offender in human disease. Trends Biochem Sci 2013;38:461–466.
77 Lewis PW, Elsaesser SJ, Noh KM, Stadler SC, Allis CD: Daxx is an H3.3-specific histone chaperone and cooperates with ATRX in replication-independent chromatin assembly at telomeres. Proc Natl Acad Sci U S A 2010;107:14075–14080.
78 Wong LH, McGhie JD, Sim M, et al: ATRX interacts with H3.3 in maintaining telomere structural integrity in pluripotent embryonic stem cells. Genome Res 2010;20:351–360.
79 Heaphy CM, de Wilde RF, Jiao Y, et al: Altered telomeres in tumors with ATRX and DAXX mutations. Science 2011;333:425.
80 Li Q, Wang X, Wu X, et al: Daxx cooperates with the Axin/HIPK2/p53 complex to induce cell death. Cancer Res 2007;67:66–74.
81 Tang J, Qu LK, Zhang J, et al: Critical role for Daxx in regulating Mdm2. Nat Cell Biol 2006;8:855–862.
82 Michaelson JS, Bader D, Kuo F, Kozak C, Leder P: Loss of Daxx, a promiscuously interacting protein, results in extensive apoptosis in early mouse development. Genes Dev 1999;13:1918–1923.
83 Tang J, Agrawal T, Cheng Q, et al: Phosphorylation of Daxx by ATM contributes to DNA damage-induced p53 activation. PloS One 2013;8:e55813.
84 Marinoni I, Kurrer AS, Vassella E, et al: Loss of DAXX and ATRX are associated with chromosome instability and reduced survival of patients with pancreatic neuroendocrine tumors. Gastroenterology 2014;146:453–460.
85 de Wilde RF, Heaphy CM, Maitra A, et al: Loss of ATRX or DAXX expression and concomitant acquisition of the alternative lengthening of telomeres phenotype are late events in a small subset of MEN-1 syndrome pancreatic neuroendocrine tumors. Mod Pathol 2012;25:1033–1039.
86 Cao Y, Gao Z, Li L, et al: Whole exome sequencing of insulinoma reveals recurrent T372R mutations in YY1. Nat Commun 2013;4:2810.
87 Cunningham JT, Rodgers JT, Arlow DH, Vazquez F, Mootha VK, Puigserver P: mTOR controls mitochondrial oxidative function through a YY1-PGC-1α transcriptional complex. Nature 2007;450:736–740.
88 Brown JL, Mucci D, Whiteley M, Dirksen ML, Kassis JA: The Drosophila Polycomb group gene pleiohomeotic encodes a DNA binding protein with homology to the transcription factor YY1. Mol Cell 1998;1:1057–1064.
89 Bartsch DK, Kersting M, Wild A, et al: Low frequency of *p16*^{INK4a} alterations in insulinomas. Digestion 2000;62:171–177.
90 House MG, Herman JG, Guo MZ, et al: Prognostic value of hMLH1 methylation and microsatellite instability in pancreatic endocrine neoplasms. Surgery 2003;134:902–908, discussion 909.
91 Dammann R, Schagdarsurengin U, Liu L, et al: Frequent RASSF1A promoter hypermethylation and K-ras mutations in pancreatic carcinoma. Oncogene 2003;22:3806–3812.
92 Karpathakis A, Dibra H, Thirlwell C: Neuroendocrine tumours: cracking the epigenetic code. Endocr Relat Cancer 2013;20:R65–R82.
93 Song MS, Song SJ, Kim SY, Oh HJ, Lim DS: The tumour suppressor RASSF1A promotes MDM2 self-ubiquitination by disrupting the MDM2-DAXX-HAUSP complex. Embo J 2008;27:1863–1874.
94 Guo M, Jia Y, Yu Z, et al: Epigenetic changes associated with neoplasms of the exocrine and endocrine pancreas. Discov Med 2014;17:67–73.
95 Missiaglia E, Dalai I, Barbi S, et al: Pancreatic endocrine tumors: expression profiling evidences a role for AKT-mTOR pathway. J Clin Oncol 2010;28:245–255.
96 Schmitt AM, Schmid S, Rudolph T, et al: VHL inactivation is an important pathway for the development of malignant sporadic pancreatic endocrine tumors. Endocr Relat Cancer 2009;16:1219–1227.
97 Roldo C, Missiaglia E, Hagan JP, et al: MicroRNA expression abnormalities in pancreatic endocrine and acinar tumors are associated with distinctive pathologic features and clinical behavior. J Clin Oncol 2006;24:4677–4684.
98 Debelenko LV, Brambilla E, Agarwal SK, et al: Identification of MEN1 gene mutations in sporadic carcinoid tumors of the lung. Hum Mol Genet 1997;6: 2285–2290.
99 Swarts DR, Scarpa A, Corbo V, et al: MEN1 gene mutation and reduced expression are associated with poor prognosis in pulmonary carcinoids. J Clin Endocrinol Metab 2014;99:E374–E378.

100 Swarts DR, Ramaekers FC, Speel EJ: Molecular and cellular biology of neuroendocrine lung tumors: evidence for separate biological entities. Biochim Biophys Acta 2012;1826:255–271.
101 Pelosi G, Fumagalli C, Trubia M, et al: Dual role of RASSF1 as a tumor suppressor and an oncogene in neuroendocrine tumors of the lung. Anticancer Res 2010;30:4269–4281.
102 Fernandez-Cuesta L, Peifer M, Lu X, et al: Frequent mutations in chromatin-remodelling genes in pulmonary carcinoids. Nat Commun 2014;5:3518.
103 Capodanno A, Boldrini L, Ali G, Pelliccioni S, Mussi A, Fontanini G: Phosphatidylinositol-3-kinase alpha catalytic subunit gene somatic mutations in bronchopulmonary neuroendocrine tumours. Oncol Rep 2012;28:1559–1566.
104 Chaussade L, Eymin B, Brambilla E, Gazzeri S: Expression of p15 and p15.5 products in neuroendocrine lung tumours: relationship with $p15^{INK4b}$ methylation status. Oncogene 2001;20:6587–6596.
105 Swarts DR, van Neste L, Henfling ME, et al: An exploration of pathways involved in lung carcinoid progression using gene expression profiling. Carcinogenesis 2013;34:2726–2737.
106 Swarts DR: Molecular profiling of pulmonary carcinoids: Insight into tumor biology and identification of prognostic markers; PhD thesis, Maastricht University, 2013.
107 Deng B, Molina J, Aubry MC, et al: Clinical biomarkers of pulmonary carcinoid tumors in never smokers via profiling miRNA and target mRNA. Cell Biosci 2014;4:35.
108 Mairinger FD, Ting S, Werner R, et al: Different micro-RNA expression profiles distinguish subtypes of neuroendocrine tumors of the lung: results of a profiling study. Mod Pathol 2014;27:1632–1640.
109 Rapa I, Votta A, Felice B, et al: PS-09–030 Identification of microRNAs differentially expressed in lung carcinoid subtypes and progression (abstract). Virchows Archiv 2014;465(suppl 1):S1–S379.
110 Lee HW, Lee EH, Ha SY, et al: Altered expression of microRNA miR-21, miR-155, and let-7a and their roles in pulmonary neuroendocrine tumors. Pathol Int 2012;62:583–591.
111 Roldo C, Missiaglia E, Hagan JP, et al: MicroRNA expression abnormalities in pancreatic endocrine and acinar tumors are associated with distinctive pathologic features and clinical behavior. J Clin Oncol 2006;24:4677–4684.
112 Meng F, Henson R, Wehbe-Janek H, Ghoshal K, Jacob ST, Patel T: MicroRNA-21 regulates expression of the PTEN tumor suppressor gene in human hepatocellular cancer. Gastroenterology 2007;133: 647–658.
113 Schramedei K, Morbt N, Pfeifer G, et al: MicroRNA-21 targets tumor suppressor genes ANP32A and SMARCA4. Oncogene 2011;30:2975–2985.
114 Zaffaroni N, Villa R, Pastorino U, et al: Lack of telomerase activity in lung carcinoids is dependent on human telomerase reverse transcriptase transcription and alternative splicing and is associated with long telomeres. Clin Cancer Res 2005;11: 2832–2839.
115 Hiripi E, Bermejo JL, Sundquist J, Hemminki K: Familial gastrointestinal carcinoid tumours and associated cancers. Ann Oncol 2009;20:950–954.
116 Ter-Minassian M, Wang Z, Asomaning K, et al: Genetic associations with sporadic neuroendocrine tumor risk. Carcinogenesis 2011;32:1216–1222.
117 Nilsson O: Profiling of ileal carcinoids. Neuroendocrinology 2013;97:7–18.
118 Banck MS, Kanwar R, Kulkarni AA, et al: The genomic landscape of small intestine neuroendocrine tumors. J Clin Invest 2013;123:2502–2508.
119 Francis JM, Kiezun A, Ramos AH, et al: Somatic mutation of CDKN1B in small intestine neuroendocrine tumors. Nat Genet 2013;45:1483–1486.
120 Marinoni I, Pellegata NS: p27kip1: a new multiple endocrine neoplasia gene? Neuroendocrinology 2011;93:19–28.
121 Liu L, Broaddus RR, Yao JC, et al: Epigenetic alterations in neuroendocrine tumors: methylation of RAS-association domain family 1, isoform A and p16 genes are associated with metastasis. Mod Pathol 2005;18:1632–1640.
122 Zhang HY, Rumilla KM, Jin L, et al: Association of DNA methylation and epigenetic inactivation of RASSF1A and β-catenin with metastasis in small bowel carcinoid tumors. Endocrine 2006;30:299–306.
123 Ruebel K, Leontovich AA, Stilling GA, et al: MicroRNA expression in ileal carcinoid tumors: downregulation of microRNA-133a with tumor progression. Mod Pathol 2010;23:367–375.
124 Li SC, Essaghir A, Martijn C, et al: Global microRNA profiling of well-differentiated small intestinal neuroendocrine tumors. Mod Pathol 2013;26:685–696.
125 Zhao H, Li M, Li L, Yang X, Lan G, Zhang Y: MiR-133b is downregulated in human osteosarcoma and inhibits osteosarcoma cells proliferation, migration and invasion, and promotes apoptosis. PloS One 2013;8:e83571.
126 Wang LK, Hsiao TH, Hong TM, et al: MicroRNA-133a suppresses multiple oncogenic membrane receptors and cell invasion in non-small cell lung carcinoma. PloS One 2014;9:e96765.

127 Horsch D, Schmid KW, Anlauf M, et al: Neuroendocrine tumors of the bronchopulmonary system (typical and atypical carcinoid tumors): current strategies in diagnosis and treatment. Conclusions of an expert meeting February 2011 in Weimar, Germany. Oncol Res Treat 2014;37:266–276.
128 Salazar R, Wiedenmann B, Rindi G, Ruszniewski P: ENETS 2011 consensus guidelines for the management of patients with digestive neuroendocrine tumors: an update. Neuroendocrinology 2012;95:71–73.
129 Caplin M, Sundin A, Nillson O, et al: ENETS consensus guidelines for the management of patients with digestive neuroendocrine neoplasms: colorectal neuroendocrine neoplasms. Neuroendocrinology 2012;95:88–97.
130 Falconi M, Bartsch DK, Eriksson B, et al: ENETS consensus guidelines for the management of patients with digestive neuroendocrine neoplasms of the digestive system: well-differentiated pancreatic non-functioning tumors. Neuroendocrinology 2012;95:120–134.
131 Pape UF, Perren A, Niederle B, et al: ENETS consensus guidelines for the management of patients with neuroendocrine neoplasms from the jejuno-ileum and the appendix including goblet cell carcinomas. Neuroendocrinology 2012;95:135–156.
132 Pavel M, Baudin E, Couvelard A, et al: ENETS consensus guidelines for the management of patients with liver and other distant metastases from neuroendocrine neoplasms of foregut, midgut, hindgut, and unknown primary. Neuroendocrinology 2012;95:157–176.
133 Weinstock B, Ward SC, Harpaz N, Warner RR, Itzkowitz S, Kim MK: Clinical and prognostic features of rectal neuroendocrine tumors. Neuroendocrinology 2013;98:180–187.
134 Patel YC: Somatostatin and its receptor family. Front Neuroendocrinol 1999;20:157–198.
135 Hofland LJ, Lamberts SW: The pathophysiological consequences of somatostatin receptor internalization and resistance. Endocr Rev 2003;24:28–47.
136 Duran-Prado M, Gahete MD, Martinez-Fuentes AJ, et al: Identification and characterization of two novel truncated but functional isoforms of the somatostatin receptor subtype 5 differentially present in pituitary tumors. J Clin Endocrinol Metab 2009;94:2634–2643.
137 Lawrence MS, Stojanov P, Mermel CH, et al: Discovery and saturation analysis of cancer genes across 21 tumour types. Nature 2014;505:495–501.
138 Capurso G, Fazio N, Festa S, Panzuto F, De Braud F, Delle Fave G: Molecular target therapy for gastroenteropancreatic endocrine tumours: biological rationale and clinical perspectives. Crit Rev Oncol Hematol 2009;72:110–124.
139 Kasajima A, Pavel M, Darb-Esfahani S, et al: mTOR expression and activity patterns in gastroenteropancreatic neuroendocrine tumours. Endocr Relat Cancer 2011;18:181–192.
140 Missiaglia E, Dalai I, Barbi S, et al: Pancreatic endocrine tumors: expression profiling evidences a role for AKT-mTOR pathway. J Clin Oncol 2010;28:245–255.
141 Shida T, Kishimoto T, Furuya M, et al: Expression of an activated mammalian target of rapamycin (mTOR) in gastroenteropancreatic neuroendocrine tumors. Cancer Chemother Pharmacol 2010;65:889–893.
142 Krueger DA, Care MM, Holland K, et al: Everolimus for subependymal giant-cell astrocytomas in tuberous sclerosis. N Engl J Med 2010;363:1801–1811.
143 Bissler JJ, Kingswood JC, Radzikowska E, et al: Everolimus for angiomyolipoma associated with tuberous sclerosis complex or sporadic lymphangioleiomyomatosis (EXIST-2): a multicentre, randomised, double-blind, placebo-controlled trial. Lancet 2013;381:817–824.
144 Watson AL, Anderson LK, Greeley AD, et al: Co-targeting the MAPK and PI3K/AKT/mTOR pathways in two genetically engineered mouse models of Schwann cell tumors reduces tumor grade and multiplicity. Oncotarget 2014;30:1502–1514.
145 Yao JC, Shah MH, Ito T, et al: Everolimus for advanced pancreatic neuroendocrine tumors. N Engl J Med 2011;364:514–523.
146 Oberg K, Casanovas O, Castano JP, et al: Molecular pathogenesis of neuroendocrine tumors: implications for current and future therapeutic approaches. Clin Cancer Res 2013;19:2842–2849.
147 Pavel ME, Hainsworth JD, Baudin E, et al: Everolimus plus octreotide long-acting repeatable for the treatment of advanced neuroendocrine tumours associated with carcinoid syndrome (RADIANT-2): a randomised, placebo-controlled, phase 3 study. Lancet 2011;378:2005–2012.
148 Noel-Savina E, Descourt R: Focus on treatment of lung carcinoid tumor. Onco Targets Ther 2013;6:1533–1537.
149 Reid MD, Balci S, Saka B, Adsay NV: Neuroendocrine tumors of the pancreas: current concepts and controversies. Endocr Pathol 2014;25:65–79.
150 Yao JC, Phan AT, Chang DZ, et al: Efficacy of RAD001 (everolimus) and octreotide LAR in advanced low- to intermediate-grade neuroendocrine tumors: results of a phase II study. J Clin Oncol 2008;26:4311–4318.
151 Zhang J, Francois R, Iyer R, Seshadri M, Zajac-Kaye M, Hochwald SN: Current understanding of the molecular biology of pancreatic neuroendocrine tumors. J Natl Cancer Inst 2013;105:1005–1017.

152 Speisky D, Duces A, Bieche I, et al: Molecular profiling of pancreatic neuroendocrine tumors in sporadic and von Hippel-Lindau patients. Clin Cancer Res 2012;18:2838–2849.
153 Raymond E, Dahan L, Raoul JL, et al: Sunitinib malate for the treatment of pancreatic neuroendocrine tumors. N Engl J Med 2011;364:501–513.
154 Raut CP, Kulke MH: Targeted therapy in advanced well-differentiated neuroendocrine tumors. Oncologist 2011;16:286–295.
155 Tang LH, Contractor T, Clausen R, et al: Attenuation of the retinoblastoma pathway in pancreatic neuroendocrine tumors due to increased cdk4/cdk6. Clin Cancer Res 2012;18:4612–4620.
156 Canavese M, Santo L, Raje N: Cyclin dependent kinases in cancer: potential for therapeutic intervention. Cancer Biol Ther 2012;13:451–457.
157 Larsson C: Epigenetic aspects on therapy development for gastroenteropancreatic neuroendocrine tumors. Neuroendocrinology 2013;97:19–25.
158 Alexander VM, Roy M, Steffens KA, Kunnimalaiyaan M, Chen H: Azacytidine induces cell cycle arrest and suppression of neuroendocrine markers in carcinoids. Int J Clin Exp Med 2010;3:95–102.
159 Hojfeldt JW, Agger K, Helin K: Histone lysine demethylases as targets for anticancer therapy. Nat Rev Drug Discov 2013;12:917–930.

Koen M.A. Dreijerink
Department of Endocrine Oncology, University Medical Centre Utrecht
Heidelberglaan 100
NL–3584 CX Utrecht (The Netherlands)
E-Mail k.m.a.dreijerink@umcutrecht.nl

Papotti M, de Herder WW (eds): Neuroendocrine Tumors: A Multidisciplinary Approach.
Front Horm Res. Basel, Karger, 2015, vol 44, pp 139–148 (DOI: 10.1159/000382143)

Pancreatic Surgery

Angela Maurizi · Stefano Partelli · Massimo Falconi

Pancreatic Surgery Unit, AOUI Ospedali Riuniti – Università Politecnica delle Marche, Ancona, Italy

Abstract

Pancreatic neuroendocrine tumors (pNETs) are rare and clinically demanding diseases. They are clinically defined as functioning or nonfunctioning depending on the presence of a syndrome related to inappropriate hormone secretion. Functioning pNETs are often small in size and localization may be difficult also due to their possible extraduodenal-pancreatic origin in the jejunum, stomach, mesentery, spleen and ovaries. The improvement and the widespread use of cross-sectional imaging techniques has significantly increased the detection of small, nonfunctioning pNETs. The European Neuroendocrine Tumor Society (ENETS) guidelines now suggest a 'wait and see' policy for these small, incidentally discovered tumors, which are smaller than 2 cm. On the other hand, surgery still always represents the treatment of choice for pNETs >2 cm and/or for symptoms. A large proportion of patients with pNETs have locally advanced disease at diagnosis. Radical surgery of pNETs includes both typical and atypical pancreatic resections. At diagnosis, between 25 and 93% of patients with pNETs have synchronous neuroendocrine tumor liver metastases. Radical resection of the primary tumor, associated with complete, eventually multistep, resection of the liver metastases, can be considered in selected cases. In recent years minimally invasive approaches, either laparoscopic or robotic, have played an increasing role in the treatment of pNETs.

Pancreatic neuroendocrine tumors (pNETs) are rare and clinically demanding diseases. They consist of single or multiple benign or malignant neoplasms and in 10–20% of patients they can be associated with inherited syndromes, such as MEN1 (multiple endocrine neoplasia type 1) [1]. pNETs are clinically defined as functioning or nonfunctioning depending on the presence of a syndrome related to inappropriate hormone secretion [2]. The heterogeneous presentation and their varied biological behavior pose a complicated set of questions about surgical management. Radical surgery for pNETs includes both typical and atypical pancreatic resections. Typical resections differ according to the tumor site: lesions of the pancreatic head are treated with a pancreaticoduodenectomy, while lesions of the body and tail with a distal pancreatectomy. Pancreatic typical resections performed in high-volume centers have an acceptable mortality rate (less than 5%), even though the percentage of complications is still significant, ranging from 40 to 50% [3]. Typical pancreatic resections are also associated with a high incidence of exocrine and endocrine insufficiency. These short- and long-term complications, as well as the increasingly incidental recognition of small and asymptomatic lesions, have increased the use of parenchyma-sparing techniques or atypical resections such as enucleation and middle pancreatectomy. The main advantage for atypical resections is that they are associated with a lower risk of long-term endocrine/exocrine impairment when compared to standard resections [4]. On the other hand, atypical resections are associated with a high rate of pancreatic fistulas, although they are mostly transient and have a low clinical impact [5]. Moreover, if the lesion is not very well capsulated, negative margins cannot be obtained after enucleation, and in both enucleation and intermediate resection a lymphadenectomy is not usually performed.

Surgical Approaches for Primary Tumor with Clinical Endocrine Syndrome

Functioning pNETs are often small in size and localization may be difficult also due to their possible extraduodenal-pancreatic origin (for gastrinomas) in the jejunum, stomach, mesentery, spleen and ovaries. When a clinical syndrome is present and the tumor cannot be assessed preoperatively, a careful abdominal inspection of the liver, the stomach and the mesentery is always the first step of surgical exploration. After the Kocher maneuver, the pancreatic gland should be well exposed, and both the superior and the inferior margins of the gland and splenic ligament accurately dissected. The whole pancreatic gland is then accessible for a bidigital manual examination and the entire parenchyma can be examined by intraoperative ultrasound.

Insulinomas

Insulinoma is one of the most frequent functional neoplasms and, after localizing the tumor, one must decide whether the insulinoma can be safely enucleated or a formal pancreatic resection, either pancreaticoduodenectomy or distal pancreatectomy, is indicated. After enucleation, it is essential to evaluate any exocrine secretion leak. Rather than over sewing the enucleation site, a drain should be placed in its location. Most insulinomas can be enucleated [6]. However, if a plane between the tumor capsule and the pancreatic parenchyma cannot be easily identified, resection is indicated. As more than 90% of insulinomas are benign, in case of a tail location, a spleen-preserving distal pancreatectomy is generally preferred to an en bloc resection of the tail of the pancreas and spleen. If metastases are absent, the only evidence of malignancy is often provided by local infiltration or the size of the tumor. When resection is indicated on this basis, malignant insulinomas located in the body or tail of the pancreas are effectively treated by distal pancreatectomy with splenectomy and lymphadenectomy. In case of tumors located in the head of the gland, the preferred resection is pancreaticoduodenectomy.

Gastrinomas
Most gastrinomas are located in the 'gastrinoma triangle', which comprises the head of the pancreas and the first and second parts of the duodenum [7]. Gastrinomas are classified according to the World Health Organization classification (2010) and malignancy is defined by infiltrating growth, lymph node metastases or distant metastases. Most gastrinomas grow slowly but show aggressive growth. Although they are often small in size, 60–90% of them are malignant with nodal and/or hepatic metastases at diagnosis [8]. Surgical management is directed at identification and resection of the primary tumor and lymph nodes or liver metastases to prevent progression of the disease [9]. Before a duodenotomy is performed, the duodenum should be carefully palpated from the pylorus to the level of the superior mesenteric vein. Generally, only gastrinomas larger than 0.5 cm are palpable without opening the duodenum [10]. In the setting of Zollinger-Ellison syndrome, after the pancreas is carefully explored, a duodenal transillumination followed by a 3-cm longitudinal duodenal incision should be performed. This maneuver allows a complete examination of the entire mucosal surface, including the medial wall. If it is necessary to open the duodenum, an excision of the tumor with a full-thickness margin of the duodenal wall is required [10]. The lymphadenectomy should include peripancreatic lymph nodes as well as the lymph nodes of the celiac trunk and hepatic ligament, in order to rule out the presence of a primary lymph node gastrinoma [11].

The extent of surgery is a highly controversial issue in gastrinoma [8]. This is especially true for duodenal gastrinomas. Several groups have suggested that duodenotomy with excision of duodenal wall gastrinomas, enucleation of any head gastrinomas and peripancreatic lymph node dissection with or without distal pancreatic resection is the adequate procedure for duodenal gastrinoma. However, other groups – including ourselves – choose pancreaticoduodenectomy as the first-line procedure for duodenal gastrinoma, because it is very likely that proliferative gastrin cells in the normal duodenal mucosa are the precursors of these tumors, and, for this reason, long-term cure is only possible if the organ of origin is removed. Another reason is that pancreaticoduodenectomy allows radical treatment of the all peripancreatic nodal lesions. In addition, cephalic macroscopic gastrinomas can also be treated by pancreaticoduodenectomy by extending the procedure to include part of the pancreatic body. Finally, a simple enucleation can be added to pancreaticoduodenectomy, if gastrinomas are found more distally in the pancreatic tail. Regarding the pancreaticoduodenectomy procedures, both the pylorus-preserving and the classical variant with antrectomy (according to Whipple) procedures can be considered. The latter is the most radical operation, but with a potential higher risk of long-term nutritional complications, such as dumping syndrome, maldigestion and malabsorption, when compared to the former. However, the major concern about the pylorus-preserving procedure is the risk of recurrence or persistence of gastrinomas in the residual 1- to 2-cm duodenal mucosa that will be preserved.

Other Syndromic Neoplasms

Also in the case of tumors secreting hormones such as somatostatin, adrenocorticotrophin, parathyroid hormone-related protein and pancreatic polypeptide, the treatment recommendations are similar [12]. Small (<2 cm) and peripheral tumors can be enucleated with or without the removal of regional nodes, and distal pancreatectomy can be performed with or without the removal of regional nodes and with or without splenectomy. Deeper, larger (>2 cm) or invasive tumors are treated with pancreaticoduodenectomy if they are located in the head of the pancreas, and with distal pancreatectomy and splenectomy if they are distally located. Resection of larger or malignant-appearing tumors should include total removal of the tumor with negative margins (including adjacent organs) and regional lymph nodes.

In the setting of unidentified disease, an intraoperative frozen section is always recommended in order to check if the lesion removed is compatible with an endocrine neoplasm. In addition, a so-called 'blind resection' for undiscovered gastrinomas or insulinomas is inadequate and must be avoided. When a laparotomy fails to localize the tumor, a strict follow-up of the patient is recommended until the lesion is recognized.

Localized Nonfunctioning Pancreatic Neuroendocrine Tumors

The improvement and the widespread use of cross-sectional imaging techniques significantly increased the detection of small, nonfunctioning pNETs. The choice of surgery should always be carefully balanced with the patients' age and comorbidities [13].

The European Neuroendocrine Tumor Society (ENETS) guidelines now recommend a 'wait and see' policy for these small, incidentally discovered tumors, <2 cm [14]. On the other hand, surgery still always represents the treatment of choice for pNETs >2 cm and/or for symptomatic forms [15, 16].

Locally Advanced Pancreatic Neuroendocrine Tumors

A large proportion of patients with pNETs have locally advanced disease at diagnosis. The surgical removal of the tumor mass is mandatory and the major goal is a potentially curative resection with improved survival for patients [7]. The criteria for surgical resection of pNETs also include the extent of the resection to nearby eventually invaded organs (such as the stomach, spleen, colon, kidney and adrenal gland) or the invasion of vascular structures. The treatment of choice is always a typical resection combined with lymphadenectomy. Splenectomy is routinely performed in left pancreatectomy. A pancreatic head mass involving the stomach can be removed by a Whipple procedure, while tumors infiltrating the colon require standard or segmental colon resection. A total pancreatectomy should be considered when multiple frozen sections demonstrate an involvement of the whole pancreas. When a portal or superior mesenteric vein infiltration occurs, the surgeon must achieve negative resection margins, performing, if necessary, segmental resection of the superior mesenteric vein or splenomesenteric portal vein confluence, occasionally with the use of a vein graft. On the other hand, an arterial resection is rarely performed when the mesenteric-celiac arterial axis is involved. Palliative surgery is indicated in those patients who complain of symptoms associated with biliary and/or gastrointestinal obstruction. In this context, surgical interventions such as biliojejunostomy and gastrojejunostomy should be preferred to endoscopic treatment, considering the usually long life expectancy of these patients.

Metastatic Disease

Between 25 and 93% of patients diagnosed with pNETs have synchronous liver metastases [17]. Radical resection of the primary tumor, associated with complete, eventually multistep, resection of the liver metastases can be considered in selected cases.

Nevertheless, a radical liver resection is possible in less than 20% of patients due to the high incidence of multifocal and bilateral metastases [18]. There are some criteria that should be met before proposing surgery for metastatic pNETs: (1) the absence of extra-abdominal disease, (2) the finding of low proliferative index (Ki-67) by fine-needle biopsy and (3) the existence of somatostatin receptors in order to deliver radiolabeled therapies as they are effective after cytoreductive surgery [19]. The type of hepatic resection depends on the number of liver metastases and the site and hepatic reserve itself. It can range from simple enucleation to segmental resection or to hepatectomy. The 3- and 5-year survival rates in patients who undergo radical liver surgery for neuroendocrine tumor metastases are 95 and 79%, respectively. An alternative option for multifocal liver metastases can be ablative and embolization techniques or an integrated approach of partial hepatectomy combined with radiofrequency ablation. As regards to primary tumor resection, cytoreductive surgery is helpful to control hormonal secretion-related symptoms in functioning metastatic endocrine carcinoma. In metastatic nonfunctioning neoplasms, a clear advantage in terms of survival after primary tumor resection has not been demonstrated, although it seems to be associated with a trend toward a better survival [18, 19]. In nonfunctioning tumors, a pancreatic resection could be justified to prevent life-threatening and obstructive complications, including bleeding or acute pancreatitis, jaundice or gastric obstruction [18, 19]. Liver transplantation has been proposed as a potentially curative treatment in patients free of extra hepatic metastases, for whom standard surgical and medical therapies have failed.

Surgical Techniques

Typical Resection

Pancreaticoduodenectomy

Once metastatic disease is excluded, the pancreaticoduodenal block is exposed to mobilize the hepatic flexure of the colon and to perform the Kocher maneuver to the left side of the aorta. The omental cavity is accessed after sectioning the gastrocolic ligament, and the gastrocolic trunk is transected at the level of the superior mesenteric vein. Retrograde cholecystectomy is performed, and the hepatic pedicle is dissected with skeletonization of the vessels. The gastroduodenal artery is transected through clamping, following confirmation of no obstruction in the celiac trunk. The bile duct is sectioned below the main biliary convergence. Hepatic pedicle lymphadenectomy extends from the biliary convergence to the origin of the hepatic artery. The gastric antrum is then resected and removed en bloc with the pancreatic head if a Whipple procedure is performed, whereas it is preserved if a Traverso-Longmire resection is performed. The pancreas is sectioned to the left of the portal vein, and pulsatile bleeding on the sectioned edge of the pancreatic body is monitored. An intraoperative biopsy of the pancreatic and biliary transection margins is performed in case of malignant tumor. The jejunum is transected approximately 15 cm from the ligament of Treitz and transposed to the right side of the mesenteric axis. Finally, the retroportal pancreatic lamina is sectioned to the right side of the superior mesenteric artery to complete the resection. Reconstruction starts with pancreatic anastomosis. Pancreatic duct-jejunal anastomosis is performed in all cases with interrupted stitches. Then, hepaticojejunostomy is performed at 8–15 cm from the pancreatic anastomosis. Finally, end to side gastrojejunostomy or duodenojejunostomy is performed.

Distal Pancreatectomy

The operation begins with the sectioning of the splenic artery at its origin, sectioning of the neck of the pancreas and mobilization of the surgical specimen from right to left. The pancreas is transected using a scalpel and the stump sutured with interrupted stitches after elective ligation of the Wirsung's duct. No firm data support splenectomy in all cases. A valid alternative is the 'Warshaw technique' which, with resection of splenic vessels but preservation of the spleen, can achieve lymph node retrieval comparable to distal pancreatectomy with en bloc splenectomy [12].

Total Pancreatectomy

Total pancreatectomy is needed in the presence of multifocal disease or completion when the resection margin is involved by the tumor. The procedure for total pancreatectomy begins as a cephalic pancreaticoduodenectomy when this indication is considered from the onset, and the lack of vascular infiltration to contraindicate resection is confirmed. The splenic artery is tied at its origin, and the adjacent spleen and pancreas are mobilized from left to right. Finally, the retroportal lamina is sectioned.

Atypical Resection

Middle Pancreatectomy

Whereas neoplastic lesions located in the pancreatic head or body tail are usually resected by pancreaticoduodenectomy or distal pancreatectomy, tumors in the neck can be removed through middle pancreatectomy [20]. In these cases, standard or extended pancreatectomies performed for benign or borderline cases can determine the loss of a great amount of glandular tissue, significantly increasing the risk of diabetes, impaired exocrine function and splenic loss. During middle pancreatectomy the gastrocolic ligament is opened, preserving the gastroepiploic vessels, and the pancreatic gland is exposed. The posterior peritoneum along the superior and inferior margin of the pancreas is incised. The superior mesenteric vein and the portal vein must be identified and their surfaces cleared below the gland. The splenic artery and vein are dissected free and separated from the gland. Next, the posterior surface of the pancreatic neck is isolated from the portomesenteric axis. The segment of the pancreas with the tumor is subsequently transected through a knife to the left and to the right of the lesion. The cephalic stump is sutured with interrupted stitches after elective ligation of the Wirsung's duct. Then, the pancreaticojejunostomy is performed on the tail stump. The surgeon must be sure to achieve tumor-free proximal and distal resection margins after performing middle segment pancreatectomy and, for this reason, a frozen section examination is mandatory. There is the possibility of leaks from both the closed cut edge of the head and the pancreaticojejunostomy considering that in most patients we are dealing with a normal soft pancreatic texture with a small Wirsung's duct.

Enucleation

Enucleation is an adequate alternative for small, benign and low-grade malignant tumors, such as endocrine and cystic neoplasms of the pancreas. Unfortunately, this conservative procedure cannot always be used. When the neoplastic lesion measures up to 2 cm or more, or it is encased within the pancreatic gland, enucleation is associated with a high risk of Wirsung's duct damage. Moreover, in the case of tumors with uncertain biological behavior this approach should be avoided because of the risk of tumor recurrence [5].

The enucleation consists of a resection of a localized pancreatic lesion. It is feasible in a limited number of circumstances (small, benign neoplasms or low aggressiveness, especially if the diameter is <2 cm). A pancreatic enucleoresection can be performed safely if the lesion is superficial and far away from the main pancreatic duct. If these conditions are not met, the risk of injury to a minor pancreatic duct or the main pancreatic duct is high. It is recommended to study the relationship between the tumor and the main pancreatic duct preoperatively with magnetic resonance cholangiopancreatography at a minimum safety distance of 3–4 mm. The distance between the tumor and the product can be confirmed by intraoperative ultrasound, which is also performed at the end of surgery to confirm the integrity of the product itself.

Middle-Preserving Pancreatectomy

Total pancreatectomy is the treatment of choice for multicentric diseases involving the pancreas, especially for pathologies with frank malignancy. In recent years, there has been an increased use of pancreatic resection for benign or low-grade malignant lesions, especially in young patients with a long life expectancy. When the lesions involve both the head and tail of the pancreas only, the body of the gland may be spared by means of a middle-preserving pancreatectomy, preventing the consequences of the complete loss of the pancreatic parenchyma [21].

After a midline incision, the peritoneal cavity is carefully explored and the pancreas is exposed. Intraoperative ultrasound is used to confirm the lesions in the head and tail of the pancreas. A standard pylorus-preserving pancreaticoduodenectomy is performed followed by a spleen-preserving distal pancreatectomy with careful dissection of the splenic vessels. Both resection lines must be negative at the frozen section and the distal pancreatic stump is sutured. The remaining body of the pancreas is anastomosed end-to-end to a Roux-en-Y jejunal loop. An end-to-end duodenojejunostomy and an end-to-side hepaticojejunostomy are also performed.

Open or Laparoscopic Approach?

Laparoscopic procedures play an important role in the treatment of pNETs. It has been demonstrated that laparoscopic distal pancreatectomy and enucleation are safe and feasible in patients with pancreatic endocrine tumors [22]. Insulinomas in non-MEN1 patients are increasingly being treated by a laparoscopic approach. In 85% of patients they are single tumors, almost always intrapancreatic, and, if they can be localized preoperatively, they can be cured in 70–100% of cases using a laparoscopic approach [23].

The laparoscopic approach for insulinomas is adequate, while the role of laparoscopic surgery for gastrinomas appears to be limited. The laparoscopic procedure needs to be integrated with the use of intraoperative ultrasonography to correctly define the area of pancreatic transection during distal pancreatectomy. The advantages of minimally invasive surgery are lower postoperative pain, better cosmetic outcomes, a shorter length of hospital stay and a faster return to normal activity with a rate of pancreatic fistula comparable to that observed after open surgery.

References

1 Metz DC, Jensen RT: Gastrointestinal neuroendocrine tumors: pancreatic endocrine tumors. Gastroenterology 2008;135:1469–1492.

2 Vagefi Razo O, Deshpande V, McGrath DJ, Lauwers GY, Thayer SP, Warshaw AL, Fernández-Del Castillo C: Evolving patterns in the detection and outcomes of pancreatic neuroendocrine neoplasms. Arch Surg 2007;142:347–354.

3 Büchler MW, Wagner M, Schmied BM, Uhl W, Friess H, Z'graggen K: Changes in morbidity after pancreatic resection: toward the end of completion pancreatectomy. Arch Surg 2003;138:1310–1314.

4 Partelli S, Gaujoux S, Boninsegna L, Cherif R, Crippa S, Couvelard A, Scarpa A, Ruszniewski P, Sauvanet A, Falconi M: Pattern and clinical predictor of lymph node involvement in nonfunctioning pancreatic neuroendocrine tumors (NF-PanNETs). JAMA Surg 2013;148:932–939.

5 Heeger K, Falconi M, Partelli S, Waldmann J, Crippa S, Fendrich V, Bartsch DK: Increased rate of clinically relevant pancreatic fistula after deep enucleation of small pancreatic tumors. Langenbecks Arch Surg 2014;399:315–321.

6 Crippa S, Zerbi A, Boninsegna L, Capitanio V, Partelli S, Balzano G, Pederzoli P, Di Carlo V, Falconi M: Surgical management of insulinomas: short- and long-term outcomes after enucleations and pancreatic resections. Arch Surg 2012;147:261–266.

7 Rindi G, Falconi M, Klersy C, Albarello L, Boninsegna L, Buchler MW, Capella C, Caplin M, Couvelard A, Doglioni C, Delle Fave G, Fischer L, Fusai G, de Herder WW, Jann H, Komminoth P, de Krijger RR, La Rosa S, Luong TV, Pape U, Perren A, Ruszniewski P, Scarpa A, Schmitt A, Solcia E, Wiedenmann B: TNM staging of neoplasms of the endocrine pancreas: results from a large international cohort study. J Natl Cancer Inst 2012;104:764–777.

8 Lopez CL, Falconi M, Waldmann J, Boninsegna L, Fendrich V, Goretzki PK, Langer P, Kann PH, Partelli S, Bartsch DK: Partial pancreaticoduodenectomy can provide cure for duodenal gastrinoma associated with multiple endocrine neoplasia type 1. Ann Surg 2013;257:308–314.

9 Bartsch DK, Waldmann J, Fendrich V, Boninsegna L, Lopez CL, Partelli S, Falconi M: Impact of lymphadenectomy on survival after surgery for sporadic gastrinoma. Br J Surg 2012;99:1234–1240.

10 Norton JA, Alexander HR, Fraker DL, Venzon DJ, Gibril F, Jensen RT: Possible primary lymph node gastrinoma: occurrence, natural history, and predictive factors: a prospective study. Ann Surg 2003;237:650–659.

11 Partelli S, Maurizi A, Tamburrino D, Baldoni A, Polenta V, Crippa S, Falconi M: GEP-NETs update: a review on surgery of gastro-entero-pancreatic neuroendocrine tumors. Eur J Endocrinol 2014;171:R153–R162.

12 NCCN: Clinical practice guidelines in oncology (NCCN guidelines) – neuroendocrine tumors, version 2.2014. 2013.

13 Crippa S, Partelli S, Zamboni G, Scarpa A, Tamburrino D, Bassi C, Pederzoli P, Falconi M: Incidental diagnosis as prognostic factor in different tumor stages of nonfunctioning pancreatic endocrine tumors. Surgery 2014;155:145–153.

14 Falconi M, Zerbi A, Crippa S, Balzano G, Boninsegna L, Capitanio V, Bassi C, Di Carlo V, Pederzoli P: Parenchyma-preserving resections for small non functioning pancreatic endocrine tumors. Ann Surg Oncol 2010;17:1621–1627.

15 Falconi M, Bartsch DK, Eriksson B, Klöppel G, Lopes JM, O'Connor JM, Salazar R, Taal BG, Vullierme MP, O'Toole D: ENETS consensus guidelines for the management of patients with digestive neuroendocrine neoplasms of the digestive system: well-differentiated pancreatic non-functioning tumors. Neuroendocrinology 2012;95:120–134.

16 Gaujoux S, Partelli S, Maire F, D'Onofrio M, Larroque B, Tamburrino D, Sauvanet A, Falconi M, Ruszniewski P: Observational study of natural history of small sporadic nonfunctioning pancreatic neuroendocrine tumors. J Clin Endocrinol Metab 2013;98:4784–4789.

17 Touzios JG, Kiely JM, Pitt SC, Rilling WS, Quebbeman EJ, Wilson SD, Pitt HA: Neuroendocrine hepatic metastases: does aggressive management improve survival? Ann Surg 2005;241:776–783.

18 Bettini R, Boninsegna L, Mantovani W, Capelli P, Bassi C, Pederzoli P, Delle Fave GF, Panzuto F, Scarpa A, Falconi M: Prognostic factors at diagnosis and value of WHO classification in a mono-institutional series of 180 non-functioning pancreatic endocrine tumours. Ann Oncol 2008;19:903–908.
19 Capurso G, Bettini R, Rinzivillo M, Boninsegna L, Delle Fave G, Falconi M: Role of resection of the primary pancreatic neuroendocrine tumor only in patients with unresectable metastatic liver disease: a systematic review. Neuroendocrinology 2011;93:223–229.
20 Crippa S, Bassi C, Warshaw AL, Falconi M, Partelli S, Thayer SP, Pederzoli P, Fernández-del Castillo C: Middle pancreatectomy: indications, short- and long-term operative outcomes. Ann Surg 2007;246:69–76.
21 Partelli S, Boninsegna L, Salvia R, Bassi C, Pederzoli P, Falconi M: Middle-preserving pancreatectomy for multicentric body-sparing lesions of the pancreas. Am J Surg 2009;198:49–53.
22 Fernández-Cruz L, Blanco L, Cosa R, Rendón H: Is laparoscopic resection adequate in patients with neuroendocrine pancreatic tumors? World J Surg 2008;32:904–917.
23 Kulke MH, Anthony LB, Bushnell DL, de Herder WW, Goldsmith SJ, Klimstra DS, Marx SJ, Pasieka JL, Pommier RF, Yao JC, Jensen RT: NANETS treatment guidelines: well-differentiated neuroendocrine tumors of the stomach and pancreas. Pancreas 2010;39:735–752.

Massimo Falconi
Ospedale San Raffaele
via Olgettina 60
IT–20132 Milan (Italy)
E-Mail falconi.massimo@hsr.it

Papotti M, de Herder WW (eds): Neuroendocrine Tumors: A Multidisciplinary Approach.
Front Horm Res. Basel, Karger, 2015, vol 44, pp 149–163 (DOI: 10.1159/000382144)

Gastrointestinal Surgery of Neuroendocrine Neoplasms

Carsten Palnæs Hansen[a] · Ingrid Holst Olsen[a, b] · Ulrich Knigge[a, b]

Departments of [a]Surgical Gastroenterology and [b]Endocrinology, Neuroendocrine Tumor Centre of Excellence, Rigshospitalet, Copenhagen University Hospital, Faculty of Health Sciences, University of Copenhagen, Copenhagen, Denmark

Abstract

Surgery is the only treatment that may cure the patient with gastroenteropancreatic (GEP) neuroendocrine neoplasms (NENs) and should always be considered as the first-line treatment if radical resection can be achieved. Even in cases where radical surgery is not possible, palliative resection may be performed to reduce local or hormone-induced symptoms and to improve quality of life. The surgical procedures for GEP-NENs are accordingly described below. In most patients life-long follow-up is required, even following radical surgery, as recurrence may occur several years later.

Surgery of gastroenteropancreatic (GEP) neuroendocrine neoplasms (NENs) should always be considered as the first-line treatment, since surgery is the only treatment able to cure the patient. This also includes patients with resectable metastases as well as patients in whom a reduction of the tumor burden (debulking surgery) may relieve discomfort from the size of the tumor or endocrine symptoms. Furthermore, if tumor burden is reduced by other treatments in patients not considered for surgery as first-line therapy due to extensive or disseminated disease, surgical intervention should always be reconsidered. Several guidelines for the surgical management of GEP-NENs have been published in recent years [1–12]. However, prospective studies on surgery in NENs are missing. There is no evidence for adjuvant or neoadjuvant chemotherapy in NENs, although many patients with radically resected neuroendocrine carcinomas (NECs) receive adjuvant chemotherapy.

Esophageal Neuroendocrine Neoplasms

NENs of the esophagus and the cardiac region are rare, but the incidence is increasing as pathologists have become more aware of NENs in this area. Most tumors are NECs with a very high Ki-67 proliferation index and metastases at diagnosis [13, 116]. Patients should be offered surgery if radical resection, including lymph node dissection, can be obtained.

Gastric Neuroendocrine Neoplasms

NENs of the stomach are classified into four types [6]. In the type 1 category, more than 98% of neoplasms are less than 1 cm in size and have a benign behavior. Endoscopic surveillance with or without endoscopic ultrasonography should be performed every 6–12 months. Tumors greater than 1 cm should be endoscopically resected either by snare or by endoscopic mucosal resection. Resection of the gastrin-producing antral G cells by an antrectomy is an option to reduce the stimulatory effect of gastrin on the enterochromaffin-like cells, but when to perform is not clarified. In the very few patients with multiple tumors greater than 1 cm or regional lymph node metastases, partial or total gastrectomy should be considered [14]. Type 2 tumors are rare and multiple, but have a benign behavior. They occur in patients with gastrinomas associated with multiple endocrine neoplasia type 1 (MEN1). Tumors should be treated as type 1 tumors and pancreaticoduodenal gastrinomas should be resected. Type 3 tumors are solitary, malignant and without relation to hypergastrinemia. The tumors should be treated with partial or total gastrectomy, including lymph node dissection and removal of resectable liver metastases. Type 4 tumors (NECs) are diagnosed with an increasing incidence [116]. Surgery is rarely an option due to dissemination at the time of diagnosis. Resectable tumors should be treated as type 3 tumors.

Duodenal Neuroendocrine Neoplasms

Duodenal NENs account for less than 3% of duodenal tumors and less than 3% of all GEP-NENs [3, 15]. Gastrinomas are most frequent (up to 50%), mainly found in the first and second part of the duodenum and giving rise to the Zollinger-Ellison syndrome. The tumors are often multiple and often associated to MEN1. Less frequently are somatostatinomas in the periampullary area and other NENs. Metastases to regional lymph nodes and the liver are seen in 40–60 and <10% of cases, respectively. Endoscopic ultrasonography should be performed to evaluate invasion before resection. Tumors less than 1 cm located to the mucosa or submucosa may be resected endoscopically. Tumors between 1 and 2 cm without local lymph node metastases may be removed endoscopically or by surgical resection. Tumors invading muscularis mucosa, tumors greater than 2 cm and all tumors with lymph node metastases require a duodenal resection, duodenectomy or a pancreaticoduodenectomy, including regional lymph node dissection [16–18]. Duodenotomy with bidigital palpation of the duodenal wall is the best way to detect duodenal NENs and should be performed in cases of local resection to ensure radicality [17]. Intraoperative endoscopy is another option to identify small tumors. In localized NECs, a pancreaticoduodenectomy with extensive lymph adenectomy, including the para-aortic glands, should be performed. For ampullary NENs, a pancreaticoduodenectomy is generally recommended as even small tumors may have a higher propensity of metastatic disease [19–21].

Pancreatic Neuroendocrine Neoplasms

Pancreatic NENs (pNENs) account for 2–4% of pancreatic neoplasms. Around 70% are nonfunctioning and 30% are functioning with endocrine symptoms. Apart from insulinomas, the majority of pNENs have a malignant potential and more than 70% have metastases at the time of diagnosis. Because of the lack of hormonal symptoms, nonfunctioning tumors are often disseminated at the time of diagnosis [22, 23].

Nonfunctioning pNENs

There is no agreement about the size of the tumor for which surgery is indicated. Only 6% of pNENs less than 2 cm have been found to be malignant when detected incidentally [24]. At present, there is no evidence that surgical treatment of tumors less than 2 cm may improve overall survival. Therefore, it has been suggested that histologically proven pNENs smaller than 2 cm that have been found incidentally and do not tend to increase in size should be monitored closely with follow-up every 3 months for the first year and then every 6 months for at least 3 years with CT or MRI [5, 25–27]. However, before a surveillance approach is decided on, a low Ki-67 proliferation index should be verified. Tumors larger than 2 cm or tumors that increase in size during follow-up should always be considered for resection.

The survival benefit of resection of pNENs has been demonstrated in patients with localized, regional and distant metastases. A median survival of 7 and 10 years has been reported in patients that undergo resection for locoregional disease compared to a survival of 2 years in unresectable patients [28–30]. Patients with distant metastases have an expected shorter survival while the presence of regional node metastases has no impact on survival [31]. Invasion into nearby organs or invasion or encroachment upon the portomesenteric vessels is not a contraindication for surgery. Resection of the superior mesenteric vein or the portal vein is not associated with an increased morbidity or mortality compared with nonvascular surgery in high-volume centers [32–34].

Tumors of the pancreatic head are treated with a pancreaticoduodenectomy and lesions of the body and tail with a pancreatic resection to the left of the superior mesenteric vessels. Splenic preservation should only be attempted in benign tumors [35]. Large infiltrating tumors or multiple lesions may need a total pancreatectomy.

Laparoscopic left pancreatectomy is possible for tumors in the body and tail, while laparoscopic or laparoscopically assisted pancreaticoduodenectomy is only performed in selected patients. Radicality and complications after laparoscopic resection should be comparable with open surgery, but open surgery is advocated in patients with malignant tumors and regional metastases [36, 37].

Enucleation by open or laparoscopic surgery is an option in small pNENs with an expected benign behavior. The major advantage is avoidance of exocrine and endocrine insufficiency and a fast recovery. Enucleation should be undertaken under guidance of intraoperative ultrasonography in order to locate the tumor and its relation to the major pancreatic duct. The procedure is not advisable if the tumor is close to the major pancreatic duct (<3 mm) due to the risk of duct leakage with the development of pancreatic fistula (30%) [38–40].

In the case of liver metastases, resection of the primary and metastases should be undertaken if R0/R1 resection can be achieved. However, there is no evidence of a survival benefit from debulking of locally advanced tumors (R2 resection), although this may have a palliative effect in some patients [41], nor has resection of the primary tumor in the presence of nonresectable metastases shown increased survival [42, 43].

Functioning pNENs

Insulinomas and gastrinomas are most frequent and have a longer 5-year survival than other functioning and nonfunctioning pNENs. Resection should always be considered in order to relieve the patient from endocrine symptoms and to avoid dissemination of a potential malignant tumor. Patients with liver metastases may be eligible for surgery if an R0/R1 resection is possible.

Insulinomas

More than 90% of insulinomas are benign, encapsulated and equally distributed in the gland. Due to their small size (<1–2 cm) preoperative localization may be a challenge. CT, MRI and endoscopic ultrasonography are the preferred imaging modalities as somatostatin receptor imaging is usually negative. At operation mobilization with palpation and intraoperative ultrasonography of the gland is mandatory for the localization of one or more tumors and tumor relation to the major pancreatic duct. Small benign insulinomas may be enucleated if appropriate distance to the main pancreatic duct is achieved. Otherwise pancreatic resection independent of localization should be performed. Malignant insulinomas are usually disseminated at diagnosis and rarely curatively resectable, although palliative resection may reduce severe symptoms [44, 45].

Gastrinomas
Most gastrinomas are located in the duodenum (>60%) or the pancreas (<40%) [2]. More than 60% are malignant or have a malignant potential. At diagnosis, pancreatic gastrinomas have metastasized to the liver in about 50% of patients compared to 10% of their duodenal counterparts.

Resection of sporadic gastrinomas is the mainstay in patients without liver metastases as it is the only possibility for cure, although endocrine symptoms may be relieved by proton pump inhibitors. In addition, resection of the primary tumor decreases the risk of development of liver metastases, which is the most important prognostic factor for long-term survival [46]. Although small pancreatic gastrinomas may be enucleated, a more radical approach with pancreaticoduodenal resection and regional lymph node dissection should be considered, as it may increase radicality and prevent recurrence [47]. Depending on the tumor location, a pancreaticoduodenectomy or a distal pancreatectomy is performed. As liver metastases are the main predictor for survival, resectable liver metastases should always be considered for resection [46, 48, 49].

Rare Functioning Tumors
Rare functioning pNENs include glucagonomas, somatostatinomas, VIPomas and other even rarer hormone-releasing tumors. Most are malignant, with lymph node or liver metastases at diagnosis. The surgical procedures follow those of nonfunctioning pNENs and also palliative resections should be considered to relieve the patient from severe endocrine symptoms [2].

Multiple Endocrine Neoplasia Type 1
Pancreaticoduodenal NENs are associated with MEN1 in 10–20% of cases [50, 51]. These tumors may run a more benign course compared with their sporadic counterparts, but disease progression varies individually and pancreatic malignancies are the major cause of death in patients with MEN1 [2, 51, 52]. However, there is no consensus about the type of surgery. The conservation of the endocrine and exocrine function of the gland and the rate of complications must be weighed against the aim of achievement of radical surgery.

Insulinomas in relation to MEN1 should always be considered for pancreatic resection due to severe and uncontrollable attacks of hypoglycemia despite medical treatment [51]. Patients with gastrinomas and the Zollinger-Ellison syndrome normally have multiple duodenal and pancreatic tumors and regional lymph node metastases at the time of diagnosis. A pancreaticoduodenectomy is the recommended surgical procedure [2]. However, patients with tumors less than 2 cm usually have a good prognosis even in the presence of local lymph node metastases [53, 54]. Therefore, operation should mostly be reserved for patients with tumors greater than 2 cm.

Nonfunctioning tumors are usually multifocal and distributed throughout the whole gland, often together with functioning tumors. Tumors larger than 2 cm or any tumor that increases in size should be considered for resection [55]. The procedure depends on the location of the lesions.

Small Intestinal Neuroendocrine Neoplasms

Data from the SEER database indicate that at diagnosis 30% of patients with small intestinal NENs have localized disease, whereas 40 and 30% of the patients have regional or distant metastases, respectively [15]. However, in other series the percentage of regional or distant metastases has been found to be much higher [56–58].

Patients with localized tumors with or without mesenteric lymph node metastases should always be considered for curative surgery [7, 59–62]. Resection of the small intestine and/or right-sided hemicolectomy (RSH) with meticulous mesenteric lymph node dissection, including the central nodes, is advocated to obtain radical resection.

If feasible, the intestinal resection may be performed by a laparoscopic approach as long as the central lymph node metastases can be securely resected. Comparison of laparoscopic and open resections revealed that similar radicality, progression-free and overall survivals were recorded [63].

Extensive small bowel resection should be avoided as patients may develop short bowel syndrome. Furthermore, intestinal bypass operations with residual mesenteric tumor masses should be avoided as it may cause difficulties for later operations with curative intent.

In patients with lymph node and liver metastases, surgery should be considered if radical resection of the primary as well as regional and distant metastases can be achieved [7, 62]. Even in patients where radical resection of distant metastases is not possible, resection of the primary and regional mesenteric metastases should be considered to prevent imminent or later bowel obstruction or vascular encasement as well as further progression of disease [7, 12, 56, 64–67].

Patients who had resection of the primary, even though distant metastases were not resectable, may have a longer survival than nonoperated patients [56, 60, 61, 68]. In a recent review, it was calculated that overall survival ranged from 75 to 139 months in resected patients, compared to 50 to 88 months in nonresected patients [65]. However, the results are controversial and have not been confirmed in other studies [69, 70]. All studies were retrospective and should be considered with caution due to selection bias as patients with huge tumor burden, widespread metastatic disease, poor condition, severe comorbidity and old age may not have been considered as candidates for surgery [65].

Patients with metastatic disease but with unknown primary should also be considered for surgery as the primary, most frequently localized to the ileum, is found intraoperatively in around 90% of the patients [71]. To avoid carcinoid crises caused by excess release of serotonin and other vasoactive substances in relation to surgery, liver embolization and anesthesia, patients with small intestinal NENs and with metastatic disease from unknown primary should be treated with octreotide perioperatively, either as constant intravenous infusion or as subcutaneous injections preoperatively, followed by intravenous injections in case of imminent carcinoid crisis.

Prophylactic cholecystectomy in neuroendocrine tumor (NET) patients has been advocated in those treated with somatostatin analogs in order to avoid the development of bile stones and in patients before liver embolization in order to avoid accidental necrosis of the gallbladder [72–74]. However, most bile stones are asymptomatic and liver embolization techniques have been significantly improved. Thus, the indication for prophylactic cholecystectomy remains doubtful, also considering the not negligible complication rate to cholecystectomy [7].

Appendiceal Neuroendocrine Neoplasms

NENs of the appendix occur with an incidence of around 0.5/100,000/year [75, 76]. The tumors are divided into serotonin-producing carcinoids, glucagon-producing tubular carcinoids and goblet cell carcinoids (GCCs) [77, 78]. The first two types have a benign and indolent growth pattern, while GCCs may have a more aggressive behavior [117].

More than 70% of the tumors are located in the tip of the appendix, while GCCs are frequently found in the mid-appendix. Most tumors are incidental findings at the pathological examination of the surgical specimen after appendectomy [7].

More than 80% of the tumors are less than 1 cm in diameter without invasion to the mesoappendix or regional metastases. In these cases, simple appendectomy is a sufficient treatment [7, 64]. In tumors greater than 2 cm in diameter, a supplementary RSH is recommended as regional metastases may be seen in 20–30% of patients [7, 64, 77]. For tumors 1–2 cm in diameter, RSH is advocated in the case of tumor localization at the appendix base, uncertain resection margins, invasion into the mesoappendix (extended for more than 3 mm), angioinvasion and regional lymph node metastases [7, 64, 77]. In a recent study of 28 patients with appendiceal NENs who underwent subsequent RSH, residual disease was found in 5 out of 13 patients with a tumor size between 1 and 2 cm. It was suggested that RSH should be performed in all patients with appendiceal NENs larger than 1 cm [79]. The Ki-67 proliferation index has never been sufficiently applied for appendiceal NENs [7] although a high Ki-67 index has been shown to correlate with decreased survival [80].

GCCs are more aggressive than classical appendiceal NENs [117]. Therefore, it is generally recommended that patients with GCCs, regardless of tumor size, have an RSH performed after the initial appendectomy [7, 12, 61, 67, 82]. It has been suggested that female patients with localized GCCs have a prophylactic bilateral salpingo-oophorectomy performed to prevent ovarian metastases [83]. Considering that the median age of females with localized and disseminated disease is identical at around 59 years [117], this approach cannot be advocated.

Women with carcinomatosis and ovarian metastases should be offered peritonectomy, hysterectomy and bilateral salpingo-oophorectomy, RSH and required additional intestinal resections. Additional hyperthermic intraperitoneal chemotherapy (HIPEC) has been advocated but the effect on survival is uncertain. Remarkable disseminated disease is rarely found in men [117].

Colonic Neuroendocrine Neoplasms

The majority of NENs in the cecum and ascending colon are G1 or G2 NETs originating from enterochromaffin cells and should be treated with an RHS with mesenterial and retroperitoneal lymph node dissection. Likewise, G1 and G2 NETs in other parts of the colon should have bowel resections as recommended for adenocarcinomas [4]. Open surgery is generally recommended in order to achieve sufficient lymph node dissection, but laparoscopic resections have been more common. Endoscopic resection of small tumors cannot be recommended due to the risk of insufficient resection margins or bowel perforation. In cases of lymph node and liver metastases, these should be resected if radicality can be obtained. If metastatic disease is not radically resectable a resection of the primary may be required to prevent bowel obstruction.

For colonic G3 NECs resection should only be performed if a radical resection of the primary and metastatic disease can be achieved [116]. However, this is rarely possible as most NECs have unresectable metastatic disease at the time of diagnosis. As surgery may delay the start of chemotherapy, bowel resection should only be performed if bowel obstruction is pending.

Rectal Neuroendocrine Neoplasms

The surgical approach to rectal NENs depends on the tumor size, TNM stage and grade. Most rectal NENs are found incidentally and are less than 1 cm and without muscular invasion. In patients with G1 NETs less than 2 cm and G2 NETs less than 1 cm without muscular invasion (T1/T2) endoscopic resection may be a sufficient treatment. In cases of G2 NETs of 1–2 cm without mucosal invasion, transanal endoscopic microsurgery or endoscopic submucosal dissection is recommended if regional lymph node metastases are excluded by rectal ultrasonography and/or MRI. Patients with G3 NECs, all NETs greater than 2 cm, T3/T4 stage or regional lymph node metastases should be offered low anterior resection or abdominoperineal resection as up to 80% have a risk of metastatic disease [4, 84, 116]. In patients with distant metastases, resection of the primary should only be undertaken if radical resection of the primary and regional and distant metastases is possible. If not possible, resection of the primary should only be offered if bowel obstruction is imminent [4, 85–88].

Neuroendocrine Carcinomas

NECs are defined as small or large cell NECs with a Ki-67 index >20% according to the WHO 2010 classification [89, 116]. Most carcinomas have a Ki-67 index above 70%. The primary is most frequently found in the pancreas, colon-rectum, esophagus and stomach, but unknown primary with metastases is seen in approximately one third of patients [13]. Curative surgery is rarely possible because most patients have metastatic disease at the time of diagnosis [13, 90, 91, 116]. Therefore, surgery should only be offered if radical resection can be obtained. There is no consensus for adjuvant chemotherapy but it should generally be offered.

Mixed Adenocarcinomas and Neuroendocrine Carcinomas

Mixed adenocarcinomas and NECs are carcinomas with >30% of each component [89]. They are most frequently found in the esophagus, stomach and colon-rectum, and their incidence is increasing, probably due to the increasing awareness of pathologists. The surgical treatment is the same as for adenocarcinomas if radical surgery can be obtained. However, this is rarely possible due to disseminated disease of both tumor components at the time of diagnosis. Adjuvant chemotherapy is directed toward the largest component, but no consensus exists. Whether neoadjuvant chemotherapy should be offered is unknown.

Neuroendocrine Liver Metastases

Liver metastases are found in 25–90% of patients with GEP-NENs at the time of diagnosis [15, 61, 92, 93]. Patients with untreated liver metastases have a 5-year survival <40% [94–97]. The benefit of surgical treatment of liver metastases has been demonstrated both in terms of greater than 90% symptom control, quality of life and survival, but is seldom curative since recurrence of hepatic metastases has been reported in most studies, with a rate up to 98%. Overall survival after hepatic resection has a wide range, from 46 to 86% at 5 years to 35 to 79% at 10 years [97–101]. At preoperative staging, liver metastases may be divided into: type I, a single metastasis of any size in one lobe; type II, large metastatic bulk with smaller metastases in both lobes, and type III, disseminated metastases in all liver segments [100]. Only patients with type 1 and selected patients with type II are eligible for radical liver surgery. The number of patients that are candidates for radical (R0) liver resection varies between 15 and 60% depending on patient selection at individual centers and local expertise. In all cases of liver surgery, intraoperative ultrasonography is mandatory to detect all and even small lesions.

Debulking is an option in patients with severe local or endocrine symptoms that cannot be relieved by medical treatment or liver embolization. It was suggested that at least

90% of the metastatic burden should be resected [98]. However, this value is arbitrary and resection of less may be indicated in case of uncontrollable endocrine symptoms.

In a noncirrhotic liver, resection of up to 80% of the liver volume is generally tolerated. The risk is minor if the resected specimen has been replaced by an extensive tumor mass as compensated hypertrophy of the unaffected liver has already occurred. If lobar resection is necessary but the remaining liver is too small, ligation of the portal vein of the affected lobe will lead to hypertrophy of the contralateral lobe in an otherwise healthy liver within 4–6 weeks, thereby allowing hemihepatectomy. Resection of liver metastases and of the primary during a one-stage operation is possible, but in case of large-scale liver surgery with hemihepatectomy or multiple bilateral segmentectomies, resection of the primary should be postponed to reduce the surgical risk [102].

Nonanatomical 'cherry picking' surgery in patients with multifocal bilobar metastases has recently been suggested to preserve normal liver tissue and avoid major resections, which may cause liver insufficiency [103].

In patients with right-sided heart disease due to carcinoid syndrome, valvular replacement should be performed at least 3 months before liver surgery to reduce central venous pressure and the risk of severe bleeding during the operation. In patients with liver metastases from small intestinal NETs or unknown primary tumor, perioperative treatment with octreotide should always be administrated to avoid carcinoid crisis.

Radiofrequency ablation (RFA) is the preferred ablative procedure performed either percutaneously or intraoperatively under ultrasonographic guidance in functioning and nonfunctioning NETs. RFA is an option when liver surgery is unfavorable or in combination with liver resection to obtain complete tumor removal and preserve as much normal liver tissue as possible [104–106]. However, RFA is still a supplement or a secondary treatment to liver resection. Metastases should not exceed 5 cm in diameter in order to achieve radical ablation, and less than 8–10 in number to avoid complications. The effect of RFA is reduced when metastases are close to the major intrahepatic vessels due to heat loss. Microwave ablation may be an option in these cases. RFA reduces local and hormone-related symptoms in 70–80% of patients for a period of 1 year [105, 107].

Liver Transplantation

The indication for liver transplantation in NEN patients has been controversial, since all patients have recurrence of intra- or extrahepatic metastases. A retrospective study with a total of 213 patients showed a 5-year survival and a disease-free survival of 50 and 30%, respectively [108]. A prospective study in 36 patients using strict selection criteria, including low-grade tumors, stable disease for at least 6 months before transplantation and age <55 years showed a 5-year survival of 85% and a disease-free survival of 34% [109]. Predictors of poor outcome were enlargement of the explanted liver by more than 25%, age >45 years and resection of the primary tumor concomitant to transplantation [108, 110, 111]. Transplantation may be offered to young patients with unresectable well-differentiated, low-grade metastases confined to the liver, without extrahepatic disease and refractory to other treatments [8, 108, 110–113].

Peritoneal Metastases

Peritoneal metastases are seen in 17% of patients with NENs and the frequency increases with the presence of liver metastases and extensive disease [56, 114]. A French retrospective study evaluated surgical treatment with and without HIPEC. There was no difference in the overall 5- and 10-year survival, which was 69 and 52%, respectively, but patients in the HIPEC group had a longer disease-free survival. Sixty-six percent of the patients received concomitant hepatic surgery for liver metastases [115]. Due to the lack of randomized studies, it is difficult to draw conclusions.

Follow-Up

Most patients with radical or nonradical surgery for NENs should have follow-up. For patients with residual tumor, the follow-up must be lifelong. Radically resected patients should be followed for at least 10 years, although no definite consensus exists. However, it has to be taken into consideration that patients with small intestinal NETs may have recurrence up to 15–20 years later. Patients with small radically resected insulinomas, appendiceal or rectal NETs may have one or two follow-ups with measurement of relevant hormones and tumor markers.

Conclusion

The treatment of NENs is a multidisciplinary task. As surgery is presently the only treatment able to cure the patient, the multidisciplinary team should include surgeons with expert skills and knowledge concerning gastrointestinal, pancreatic and hepatic surgery in NENs.

References

1 Salazar R, Wiedenmann B, Rindi G, Ruszniewski P: ENETS 2011 consensus guidelines for the management of patients with digestive neuroendocrine tumors: an update. Neuroendocrinology 2012;95:71–73.

2 Jensen RT, Cadiot G, Brandi ML, et al: ENETS consensus guidelines for the management of patients with digestive neuroendocrine neoplasms: functional pancreatic endocrine tumor syndromes. Neuroendocrinology 2012;95:98–119.

3 Lawrence B, Gustafsson BI, Chan A, et al: The epidemiology of gastroenteropancreatic neuroendocrine tumors. Endocrinol Metab Clin North Am 2011;40:1–18.

4 Caplin M, Sundin A, Nillson O, et al: ENETS consensus guidelines for the management of patients with digestive neuroendocrine neoplasms: colorectal neuroendocrine neoplasms. Neuroendocrinology 2012;95:88–97.

5 Falconi M, Bartsch DK, Eriksson B, et al: ENETS consensus guidelines for the management of patients with digestive neuroendocrine neoplasms of the digestive system: well-differentiated pancreatic nonfunctioning tumors. Neuroendocrinology 2012;95:120–134.

6 Delle Fave G, Kwekkeboom DJ, van Cutsem E, et al: ENETS consensus guidelines for the management of patients with gastroduodenal neoplasms. Neuroendocrinology 2012;95:74–87.

7 Pape U-F, Perren A, Niederle B, et al: ENETS consensus guidelines for the management of patients with neuroendocrine neoplasms from the jejuno-ileum and the appendix including goblet cell carcinomas. Neuroendocrinology 2012;95:135–156.
8 Pavel M, Baudin E, Couvelard A, et al: ENETS consensus guidelines for the management of patients with liver and other distant metastases from neuroendocrine neoplasms of foregut, midgut, hindgut, and unknown primary. Neuroendocrinology 2012; 95:157–176.
9 Kulke MH, Anthony LB, Bushnell DL, et al: NANETS treatment guidelines: well-differentiated neuroendocrine tumors of the stomach and pancreas. Pancreas 2010;39:735–752.
10 Strosberg JR, Coppola D, Klimstra DS, et al: The NANETS consensus guidelines for the diagnosis and management of poorly differentiated (high-grade) extrapulmonary neuroendocrine carcinomas. Pancreas 2010;39:799–800.
11 Ramage JK, Ahmed A, Ardill J, et al: Guidelines for the management of gastroenteropancreatic neuroendocrine (including carcinoid) tumours (NETs). Gut 2012;61:6–32.
12 Janson ET, Sorbye H, Welin S, et al: Nordic Guidelines 2010 for diagnosis and treatment of gastroenteropancreatic neuroendocrine tumours. Acta Oncol 2010;49:740–756.
13 Sorbye H, Welin S, Langer SW, et al: Predictive and prognostic factors for treatment and survival in 305 patients with advanced gastrointestinal neuroendocrine carcinoma (WHO G3): The NORDIC NEC study. Ann Oncol 2013;24:152–160.
14 Merola E, Sbrozzi-Vanni A, Panzuto F, et al: Type I gastric carcinoids: a prospective study on endoscopic management and recurrence rate. Neuroendocrinology 2011;95:207–213.
15 Yao JC: One hundred years after 'carcinoid': epidemiology of and prognostic factors for neuroendocrine tumors in 35,825 cases in the United States. J Clin Oncol 2008;26:3063–3072.
16 Zyromski NJ, Kendrick ML, Nagorney DM, et al: Duodenal carcinoid tumors: how aggressive should we be? J Gastrointest Surg 2001;5:588–593.
17 Norton JA, Jensen RT: Resolved and unresolved controversies in the surgical management of patients with Zollinger-Ellison syndrome. Ann Surg 2004; 240:757–773.
18 Mullen JT, Wang HM, Yao JC, et al: Carcinoid tumors of the duodenum. Surgery 2005;138:971–977.
19 Clements W: Ampullary carcinoid tumors: rationale for an aggressive surgical approach. J Gastrointest Surg 2003;7:773–776.
20 Hartel M, Wente MN, Sido B, et al: Carcinoid of the ampulla of Vater. J Gastroenterol Hepatol 2005;20: 676–681.
21 Albores-Saavedra J, Hart A, Chablé-Montero F, Henson DE: Carcinoids and high-grade neuroendocrine carcinomas of the ampulla of Vater: a comparative analysis of 139 cases from the surveillance, epidemiology, and end results program – a population based study. Arch Pathol Lab Med 2010;134:1692–1696.
22 Zerbi A, Capitanio V, Boninsegna L, Pasquali C: Surgical treatment of pancreatic endocrine tumours in Italy: results of a prospective multicentre study of 262 cases. Langenbecks Arch Surg 2011;296:2757–2764.
23 Fernandez-Cruz L, Molina V, Vallejos R, et al: Outcome after laparoscopic enucleation for non-functional neuroendocrine pancreatic tumours. HPB (Oxford) 2012;14:171–176.
24 Bettini R, Partelli S, Boninsegna L, et al: Tumor size correlates with malignancy in nonfunctioning pancreatic endocrine tumor. Surgery 2011;150:75–82.
25 Figueiredo FAF, Giovannini M, Monges G, et al: EUS-FNA predicts 5-year survival in pancreatic endocrine tumors. Gastrointest Endosc 2009;70:907–914.
26 Chatzipantelis P, Konstantinou P, Kaklamanos M, et al: The role of cytomorphology and proliferative activity in predicting biologic behavior of pancreatic neuroendocrine tumors: a study by endoscopic ultrasound-guided fine-needle aspiration cytology. Cancer 2009;117:211–216.
27 Gaujoux S, Partelli S, Maire F, et al: Observational study of natural history of small sporadic nonfunctioning pancreatic neuroendocrine tumors. J Clin Endocrinol Metab 2013;98:4784–4789.
28 Schurr PG, Strate T, Rese K, et al: Aggressive surgery improves long-term survival in neuroendocrine pancreatic tumors – an institutional experience. Ann Surg 2007;245:273–281.
29 Hill JS, McPhee JT, McDade TP, et al: Pancreatic neuroendocrine tumors. Cancer 2009;115:741–751.
30 Watzka FM, Laumen C, Fottner C, et al: Resection strategies for neuroendocrine pancreatic neoplasms. Langenbecks Arch Surg 2013;398:431–440.
31 Franko J, Feng W, Yip L, et al: Non-functional neuroendocrine carcinoma of the pancreas: incidence, tumor biology, and outcomes in 2,158 patients. J Gastrointest Surg 2010;14:541–548.
32 Kelly KJ, Winslow E, Kooby D, et al: Vein involvement during pancreaticoduodenectomy: is there a need for redefinition of 'borderline resectable disease?' J Gastrointest Surg 2013;17:1209–1217.
33 Haugvik S-P, Labori KJ, Waage A, et al: Pancreatic surgery with vascular reconstruction in patients with locally advanced pancreatic neuroendocrine tumors. J Gastrointest Surg 2013;17:1224–1232.

34 Storkholm JH, Hansen CP: Mesenterico-portal vein resection in patients with pancreatico-duodenal cancer is safe and may increase survival. Dan Med J 2014;61:A4757.
35 Kimura WW, Yano MM, Sugawara SS, et al: Spleen-preserving distal pancreatectomy with conservation of the splenic artery and vein: techniques and its significance. J Hepatobiliary Pancreat Sci 2010;17:813–823.
36 Iacobone M, Citton M, Nitti D: Laparoscopic distal pancreatectomy: up-to-date and literature review. World J Gastroenterol 2012;18:5329–5337.
37 Asbun HJ, Stauffer JA: Laparoscopic vs open pancreaticoduodenectomy: overall outcomes and severity of complications using the Accordion Severity Grading System. J Am Coll Surg 2012;215:810–819.
38 Pitt SC, Pitt HA, Baker MS, et al: Small pancreatic and periampullary neuroendocrine tumors: resect or enucleate? J Gastrointest Surg 2009;13:1692–1698.
39 Casadei R, Ricci C, Rega D, et al: Pancreatic endocrine tumors less than 4 cm in diameter: resect or enucleate? A single-center experience. Pancreas 2010;39:825–828.
40 Falconi M, Zerbi A, Crippa S, et al: Parenchyma-preserving resections for small nonfunctioning pancreatic endocrine tumors. Ann Surg Oncol 2010;17:1621–1627.
41 Bloomston M, Muscarella P, Shah MH, et al: Cytoreduction results in high perioperative mortality and decreased survival in patients undergoing pancreatectomy for neuroendocrine tumors of the pancreas. J Gastrointest Surg 2005;10:1361–1370.
42 Bettini R, Mantovani W, Boninsegna L, et al: Primary tumour resection in metastatic nonfunctioning pancreatic endocrine carcinomas. Dig Liver Dis 2008;41:49–55.
43 Capurso G, Bettini R, Rinzivillo M, et al: Role of resection of the primary pancreatic neuroendocrine tumour only in patients with unresectable metastatic liver disease: a systematic review. Neuroendocrinology 2010;93:223–229.
44 Crippa S, Zerbi A, Boninsegna L, et al: Surgical management of insulinomas: short- and long-term outcomes after enucleations and pancreatic resections. Arch Surg 2012;147:261–266.
45 Su A-P, Ke N-W, Zhang Y, et al: Is laparoscopic approach for pancreatic insulinomas safe? Results of a systematic review and meta-analysis. J Surg Res 2014;186:126–134.
46 Norton JA, Fraker DL, Alexander HR, et al: Surgery increases survival in patients with gastrinoma. Ann Surg 2006;244:410–419.
47 Bartsch DK, Waldmann J, Fendrich V, et al: Impact of lymphadenectomy on survival after surgery for sporadic gastrinoma. Br J Surg 2012;99:1234–1240.
48 Norton JA: Surgical treatment and prognosis of gastrinoma. Best Pract Res Clin Gastroenterol 2005;19:799–805.
49 Norton JA: Endocrine tumours of the gastrointestinal tract: surgical treatment of neuroendocrine metastases. Best Pract Res Clin Gastroenterol 2005;19:577–583.
50 Metz DC, Jensen RT: Gastrointestinal neuroendocrine tumors: pancreatic endocrine tumors. Gastroenterology 2007;135:1469–1492.
51 Jensen RI, Berna MJ, Bingham DB, Norton JA: Inherited pancreatic endocrine tumor syndromes: advances in molecular pathogenesis, diagnosis, management, and controversies. Cancer 2008;113:1807–1843.
52 Kouvaraki MA, Shapiro SE, Cote GJ, et al: Management of pancreatic endocrine tumors in multiple endocrine neoplasia type 1. World J Surg 2006;30:643–653.
53 Norton JA, Fang TD, Jensen RT: Surgery for gastrinoma and insulinoma in multiple endocrine neoplasia type 1. J Natl Compr Canc Netw 2006;4:148–153.
54 Morrow EH, Norton JA: Surgical management of Zollinger-Ellison syndrome: state of the art. Surg Clin North Am 2009;89:1091–1103.
55 Triponez F, Goudet P, Dosseh D, et al: Is surgery beneficial for MEN1 patients with small (≤2 cm), nonfunctioning pancreaticoduodenal endocrine tumor? An analysis of 65 patients from the GTE. World J Surg 2006;30:654–662.
56 Norlén OO, Stålberg PP, Oberg KK, et al: Long-term results of surgery for small intestinal neuroendocrine tumors at a tertiary referral center. World J Surg 2012;36:1419–1431.
57 Landerholm KK, Zar NN, Andersson RER, et al: Survival and prognostic factors in patients with small bowel carcinoid tumour. Br J Surg 2011;98:1617–1624.
58 Chambers AJ, Pasieka JL, Dixon E, Rorstad O: Role of imaging in the preoperative staging of small bowel neuroendocrine tumors. J Am Coll Surg 2010;211:620–627.
59 Fendrich V, Bartsch DK: Surgical treatment of gastrointestinal neuroendocrine tumors. Langenbecks Arch Surg 2011;396:299–311.
60 Hellman P, Lundström T, Ohrvall U, et al: Effect of surgery on the outcome of midgut carcinoid disease with lymph node and liver metastases. World J Surg 2002;26:991–997.
61 Ahmed A, Turner G, King B, et al: Midgut neuroendocrine tumours with liver metastases: results of the UKINETS study. Endocr Relat Cancer 2009;16:885–894.
62 Sutton R, Doran HE, Williams E, et al: Surgery for midgut carcinoid. Endocr Relat Cancer 2003;10:469–481.
63 Figueiredo MN, Maggiori L, Gaujoux S, et al: Surgery for small-bowel neuroendocrine tumors: is there any benefit of the laparoscopic approach? Surg Endosc 2014;28:1720–1726.

64 Knigge U, Hansen CP: Surgery for GEP-NETs. Best Pract Res Clin Gastroenterol 2012;26:819–831.
65 Capurso G, Rinzivillo M, Bettini R, et al: Systematic review of resection of primary midgut carcinoid tumour in patients with unresectable liver metastases. Br J Surg 2012;99:1480–1486.
66 Akerstrom G, Hellman P, Hessman O, Osmak L: Management of midgut carcinoids. J Surg Oncol 2005;89:161–169.
67 Boudreaux JP, Klimstra DS, Hassan MM, et al: The NANETS consensus guideline for the diagnosis and management of neuroendocrine tumors: well-differentiated neuroendocrine tumors of the jejunum, ileum, appendix, and cecum. Pancreas 2010;39:753–766.
68 Givi B, Pommier SJ, Thompson AK, et al: Operative resection of primary carcinoid neoplasms in patients with liver metastases yields significantly better survival. Surgery 2006;140:891–897.
69 van der Horst-Schrivers ANA, Post WJ, Kema IP, et al: Persistent low urinary excretion of 5-HIAA is a marker for favourable survival during follow-up in patients with disseminated midgut carcinoid tumours. Eur J Cancer 2007;43:2651–2657.
70 Strosberg J, Gardner N, Kvols L: Survival and prognostic factor analysis of 146 metastatic neuroendocrine tumors of the mid-gut. Neuroendocrinology 2009;89:471–476.
71 Bartlett EK, Roses RE, Gupta M, et al: Surgery for metastatic neuroendocrine tumors with occult primaries. J Surg Res 2013;184:221–227.
72 Attanasio R, Mainolfi A, Grimaldi F, et al: Somatostatin analogs and gallstones: a retrospective survey on a large series of acromegalic patients. J Endocrinol Invest 2008;31:704–710.
73 Norlén O, Hessman O, Stalberg P, et al: Prophylactic cholecystectomy in midgut carcinoid patients. World J Surg 2010;34:1361–1367.
74 Drougas JG, Anthony LB, Blair TK, et al: Hepatic artery chemoembolization for management of patients with advanced metastatic carcinoid tumors. Am J Surg 1998;175:408–412.
75 Hof KHI, van der Wal HC, Kazemier G, Lange JF: Carcinoid tumour of the appendix: an analysis of 1,485 consecutive emergency appendectomies. J Gastrointest Surg 2008;12:1436–1438.
76 Goede AC, Caplin ME, Winslet MC: Carcinoid tumour of the appendix. Br J Surg 2003;90:1317–1322.
77 Misdraji J: Neuroendocrine tumours of the appendix. Curr Diagn Pathol 2005;11:180–193.
78 Tang LH, Shia J, Soslow RA, et al: Pathologic classification and clinical behavior of the spectrum of goblet cell carcinoid tumors of the appendix. Am J Surg Pathol 2008;32:1429–1443.
79 Grozinsky-Glasberg S, Alexandraki KI, Barak D, et al: Current size criteria for the management of neuroendocrine tumors of the appendix – are they valid? Clinical experience and review of the literature. Neuroendocrinology 2013;98:31–37.
80 Liu E, Telem DA, Warner RR, et al: The role of ki-67 in predicting biological behavior of globlet cell carcinoid tumor in appendix. Am J Surg 2011;202:400–403.
81 Hsu C, Rashid A, Xing Y, et al: Varying malignant potential of appendiceal neuroendocrine tumors: importance of histologic subtype. J Surg Oncol 2012;107:136–143.
82 Roy PP, Chetty RR: Goblet cell carcinoid tumors of the appendix: an overview. World J Gastrointest Oncol 2010;2:251–258.
83 Plöckinger U, Couvelard A, Falconi M, et al: Consensus guidelines for the management of patients with digestive neuroendocrine tumours: well-differentiated tumour/carcinoma of the appendix and goblet cell carcinoma. Neuroendocrinology 2007;87:20–30.
84 Shields CJ, Tiret E, Winter DC, Group IRCS: Carcinoid tumors of the rectum: a multi-institutional international collaboration. Ann Surg 2010;252:750–755.
85 Ishii N, Horiki N, Itoh T, et al: Endoscopic submucosal dissection and preoperative assessment with endoscopic ultrasonography for the treatment of rectal carcinoid tumors. Surg Endosc 2010;24:1413–1419.
86 Kinoshita T, Kanehira E, Omura K, et al: Transanal endoscopic microsurgery in the treatment of rectal carcinoid tumor. Surg Endosc 2007;21:970–974.
87 Wang AY, Ahmad NA: Rectal carcinoids. Curr Opin Gastroenterol 2006;22:529–535.
88 Kwaan MR, Goldberg JE, Bleday R: Rectal carcinoid tumors: review of results after endoscopic and surgical therapy. Arch Surg 2008;143:471–475.
89 Bosman FT, Carneiro F, Hruban RH, Theise NT (eds): WHO Classification of Tumours of the Digestive System. Lyon, IARC, 2010.
90 Garcia-Carbonero R, Capdevila J, Crespo-Herrero G, et al: Incidence, patterns of care and prognostic factors for outcome of gastroenteropancreatic neuroendocrine tumors (GEP-NETs): results from the National Cancer Registry of Spain (RGETNE). Ann Oncol 2010;21:1794–1803.
91 Kang H, O'Connell JB, Leonardi MJ, et al: Rare tumors of the colon and rectum: a national review. Int J Colorectal Dis 2007;22:183–189.
92 Modlin IM, Lye KD, Kidd M: A 5-decade analysis of 13,715 carcinoid tumors. Cancer 2003;97:934–959.
93 Ekeblad SS, Sundin AA, Janson ETE, et al: Temozolomide as monotherapy is effective in treatment of advanced malignant neuroendocrine tumors. Clin Cancer Res 2007;13:2986–2991.

94 Chen H, Hardacre JM, Uzar A, et al: Isolated liver metastases from neuroendocrine tumors: does resection prolong survival? J Am Coll Surg 1998;187:88–92.
95 Chamberlain RS, Canes D, Brown KT, et al: Hepatic neuroendocrine metastases: does intervention alter outcomes? J Am Coll Surg 2000;190:432–445.
96 House MG, Cameron JL, Lillemoe KD, et al: Differences in survival for patients with resectable versus unresectable metastases from pancreatic islet cell cancer. J Gastrointest Surg 2005;10:138–145.
97 Glazer ES, Tseng JF, Al-Refaie W, et al: Long-term survival after surgical management of neuroendocrine hepatic metastases. HPB (Oxford) 2010;12:427–433.
98 Sarmiento JM, Heywood G, Rubin J, et al: Surgical treatment of neuroendocrine metastases to the liver: a plea for resection to increase survival. J Am Coll Surg 2002;197:29–37.
99 Mayo SC, de Jong MC, Bloomston M, et al: Surgery versus intra-arterial therapy for neuroendocrine liver metastasis: a multicenter international analysis. Ann Surg Oncol 2011;18:3657–3665.
100 Frilling A, Sotiropoulos GC, Li J, et al: Multimodal management of neuroendocrine liver metastases. HPB (Oxford) 2010;12:361–379.
101 Frilling A, Modlin IM, Kidd M, et al: Recommendations for management of patients with neuroendocrine liver metastases. Lancet Oncol 2014;15:E8–E21.
102 Steinmueller T, Kianmanesh R, Falconi M, et al: Consensus guidelines for the management of patients with liver metastases from digestive (neuro) endocrine tumors: foregut, midgut, hindgut, and unknown primary. Neuroendocrinology 2008;87:47–62.
103 Krausch M, Raffel A, Anlauf M, et al: 'Cherry picking,' a multiple non-anatomic liver resection technique, as a promising option for diffuse liver metastases in patients with neuroendocrine tumours. World J Surg 2014;38:392–401.
104 Berber E, Flesher N, Siperstein AE: Laparoscopic radiofrequency ablation of neuroendocrine liver metastases. World J Surg 2002;26:985–990.
105 Mazzaglia PJ, Berber E, Milas M, Siperstein AE: Laparoscopic radiofrequency ablation of neuroendocrine liver metastases: a 10-year experience evaluating predictors of survival. Surgery 2007;142:10–19.
106 Evrard S, Becouarn Y, Fonck M, et al: Surgical treatment of liver metastases by radiofrequency ablation, resection, or in combination. Eur J Surg Oncol 2003;30:399–406.
107 Akyildiz HY, Mitchell J, Milas M, et al: Laparoscopic radiofrequency thermal ablation of neuroendocrine hepatic metastases: long-term follow-up. Surgery 2010;148:1288–1293.
108 Le Treut YP, Gregoire E, Klempnauer J, et al: Liver transplantation for neuroendocrine tumors in Europe – results and trends in patient selection: a 213-case European liver transplant registry study. Ann Surg 2013;257:807–815.
109 Mazzaferro V, Pulvirenti A, Coppa J: Neuroendocrine tumors metastatic to the liver: how to select patients for liver transplantation? J Hepatol 2007;47:460–466.
110 Gedaly RR, Daily MFM, Davenport DD, et al: Liver transplantation for the treatment of liver metastases from neuroendocrine tumors: an analysis of the UNOS database. Arch Surg 2011;146:953–958.
111 Nguyen NTT, Harring TR, Goss JA, O'Mahony CA: Neuroendocrine liver metastases and orthotopic liver transplantation: the US experience. Int J Hepatol 2011;2011:742890.
112 Pascher A, Klupp J, Neuhaus P: Endocrine tumours of the gastrointestinal tract: transplantation in the management of metastatic endocrine tumours. Best Pract Res Clin Gastroenterol 2005;19:637–648.
113 Gregoire E, Le Treut YP: Liver transplantation for primary or secondary endocrine tumors. Transpl Int 2010;23:704–711.
114 Mitry E, Rougier P: Treatment strategy for pancreatic endocrine tumours (in French). Gastroenterol Clin Biol 2003;27(3 suppl):S31–S36.
115 Elias D, David A, Sourrouille I, et al: Neuroendocrine carcinomas: optimal surgery of peritoneal metastases (and associated intra-abdominal metastases). Surgery 2014;155:5–12.
116 Ilett E, Langer SW, Olsen IH, Federspiel B, Kjær A, Knigge U: Neuroendocrine carcinomas of the gastroenteropancreatic system: a comprehensive review. Diagnostics 2015;5:119–176.
117 Olsen IH, Holt N, Langer SW, Hasselby JP, Grønbæk H, Hillingsø J, Mahmoud M, Ladekarl M, Iversen LH, Kjær A, Federspiel B, Knigge U: Goblet cell carcinoids: characteristics of a Danish cohort of 85 patients. PLoS One 2015;10:e0117627.

Ulrich Knigge
Department of Surgical Gastroenterology C, 2122
Neuroendocrine Tumor Centre of Excellence, Rigshospitalet, Copenhagen University Hospital
Blegdamsvej 9, DK–2100 Copenhagen Ø (Denmark)
E-Mail ulrich.peter.knigge@regionh.dk; uknigge@sund.ku.dk

Papotti M, de Herder WW (eds): Neuroendocrine Tumors: A Multidisciplinary Approach.
Front Horm Res. Basel, Karger, 2015, vol 44, pp 164–176 (DOI: 10.1159/000382145)

Transplantation and Debulking Procedures for Neuroendocrine Tumors

A. Frilling[a] • A. Al-Nahhas[b] • A.K. Clift[c]

Departments of [a]Surgery and Cancer and [b]Imaging (Nuclear Medicine) and [c]School of Medicine, Imperial College London, London, UK

Abstract

An array of treatment modalities is currently available in the management of patients with neuroendocrine tumors (NETs). Complete resection of the primary tumor and all metastatic lesions represents the only approach possessing intent to cure. However, due to patients' disease frequently being at an advanced stage on initial diagnosis only a minority of individuals are candidates for radical procedures. Cytoreductive surgery (debulking) may potentially confer improvements in quality of life and prolong overall survival. In light of the recent introduction of effective nonsurgical treatment options, the indication for cytoreductive surgery needs to be carefully assessed. The presence of nonresectable liver metastases is not a contraindication for resection of the primary tumor including locoregional disease in small bowel NETs. Resection of primary pancreatic NETs in the setting of unresectable metastatic liver disease may have a beneficial effect on the prognosis of selected patients with a tumor requiring less aggressive local surgery. Liver transplantation presents a generally accepted approach in meticulously selected patients with unresectable liver metastases. Stringent and validated selection criteria are not available. While overall survival is satisfactory, high recurrence rates hinder outcomes and call for the development and implementation of neoadjuvant and adjuvant concepts. Advances in intestinal transplantation over time may justify consideration of an individual with advanced neuroendocrine tumor disease unresponsive to standard medical or surgical treatment.

Historically referred to as carcinoids and more recently termed neuroendocrine neoplasms, neuroendocrine tumors (NETs) are a collective of heterogeneous neoplasms arising from the diffuse neuroendocrine system, most commonly originating in the gastroenteropancreatic and bronchopulmonary systems. Over the last 3 decades a steady increase in their incidence alongside changes in anatomic distribution have been observed. In a UK population-based cancer registry, the overall incidence increased from 0.27 to 1.32 for men and from 0.35 to 1.33 for women per 100,000 individuals per year [1]. Most NETs, especially those not secreting hormones, are considered as malignant or of indeterminate behavior. The disposition to metastasize depends strongly upon the anatomic tumor localization and the grade of tumor differentiation. While metastases are very rarely seen in low-grade (G1) gastric, rectal or appendiceal NETs, about 30–85% of G1 or intermediate grade (G2) pancreatic NETs and up to 90% of small intestinal NETs are metastatic at initial diagnosis [2]. High-grade (G3) NETs are almost always diagnosed at an advanced stage with extensive metastatic spread. Tumor differentiation and the presence of liver metastases (LM) represent the most powerful prognostic determinants irrespective of the primary tumor site. Based on morphologic growth patterns, three types of neuroendocrine LM have been observed; these are crucial for informing treatment strategies and bear prognostic relevance [3].

Complete resection of the primary tumor, locoregional lymph node metastases and liver deposits represent the mainstay of treatment for patients with advanced G1 and G2 NETs by offering curative intent and instantaneous symptomatic relief. Accurate preoperative staging including somatostatin receptor-based imaging is crucial for treatment decision making and surgical planning [4, 5]. In small bowel NETs, radical surgery of the primary tumor and mesenteric lymph node metastases is feasible in about 72% of patients [6]. For pancreatic NETs, complete locoregional resectability in up to 65% of patients, in some cases with concomitant vascular reconstruction, has been reported [7]. Due to their predominantly bilobar and multifocal growth, less than 30% of neuroendocrine LM are amenable to complete resection. In selected cases, implementation of advanced surgical technology has the potential to achieve complete elimination of LM initially deemed unresectable [8, 9]. For patients with advanced disease who are not candidates for radical resection, an armamentarium of palliative treatment options exists, including cytoreductive resection (debulking), percutaneous liver-directed ablation, angiographic liver-directed ablation, peptide receptor radionuclide therapy, molecularly targeted drugs and chemotherapy. Highly selected patients with nonresectable disease may be considered for isolated liver or intestinal transplantation [10]. In this chapter, we review the data regarding cytoreductive surgical procedures for NETs and analyze the experience pertaining to abdominal visceral transplantation in this clinical setting.

Debulking

Cytoreductive or debulking surgery reduces the tumor load with an aim to ameliorate symptoms of hormonal excess or local effects of tumor bulk and may prolong survival. Although this benchmark has never been accurately validated, debulking is generally recommended only for patients in whom at least 70–90% of the tumor burden can be eliminated.

Table 1. Results from hepatic resection in patients with neuroendocrine LM – selected studies published since 2000

First author	Year	Total patients, n	R0/R1 resection			R2 resection		
			n	OS	PFS	n	OS	PFS
Saxena [38]	2011	74	48	median 98 months	median 48 months	26	median 27 months	median 24 months
Scigliano [39]	2009	41	37	88% R0 82% R1	31% R0 9% R1	4	50%	0%
Frilling [3]	2009	119	23	100%	96%	4		
Gomez [40]	2007	18	15	86%	90%	3		25%
Elias [41]	2003	47	37	74% R0 70% R1	66% R0 46% R1	10	47%	30%
Sarmiento [42]	2003	170	75		24%	95		9%
Norton [43]	2003	16	16	82%		0		
Nave [44]	2001	31	10	86%		21	26%	
Coppa [45]	2001	29	20	67%	29%	0		
Yao [46]	2001	36	16	70%		0		
Chamberlain [47]	2000	85	15	85%		19	63%	
Pascher [48]	2000	41	16	median 70 months		10	median 50 months	

OS = 5-year overall survival; PFS = 5-year progression-free survival.

Debulking of LM

Although NETs are heterogeneous with regards to prognosis and predilection to liver metastasis, hepatic spread is a major negative prognosticator for patients with NETs irrespective of primary location. For example, patients with gastrinoma without LM can expect a 95% 20-year survival, whereas with diffuse bilobar hepatic involvement this diminishes to 15% survival at 10 years [11]. Classification of neuroendocrine LM according to their morphologic growth as type I (single metastasis), type II (isolated metastatic bulk with accompanying smaller deposits) or type III (disseminated metastatic spread) influences therapeutic decisions [3].

Surgical resection remains the gold standard treatment option for neuroendocrine LM, yielding an overall survival of 67–100% at 5 years and 35–79% at 10 years (table 1) [10]. A recent systematic review of 29 case series demonstrated median 5- and 10-year overall survival of 70.5% (range 31–100) and 42% (range 0–100), respectively [12]. The median progression-free survival was 21 months (range 13–46) with median 1-, 3-, 5- and 10-year progression-free survival of 63% (range 50–80), 32% (range 24–69), 29% (range 6–66) and 1% (range 0–11), respectively. The median rate of resection with macroscopic clear margins (R0/R1) was 71% (range 6–100), whereas that of debulking (R2) was 18% (range 0–36). Poor tumor differentiation, extrahepatic disease and incomplete resection were identified as independent factors indicating dismal prognosis.

In an international multi-institutional analysis, Mayo et al. [13] reported the outcomes of 339 patients with neuroendocrine LM undergoing surgical treatment. Sixty-five patients had R2 margin status following the first surgical procedure. Overall survival for the entire cohort at 1, 5 and 10 years was 92, 74 and 51%, respectively, whilst 1-, 3- and 5-year progression-free/disease-free survival was 56.9, 24.2 and 5.9%, respectively. Almost all (99%) patients' disease had recurred at 10 years. R2 resection status was not significantly associated with increased risk of recurrence, but did adversely affect survival overall – palliative surgery led to an average survival of 77.5 versus 156.9 months for surgery with curative intent. Furthermore, R0/R1 resection was associated with superior survival in patients with LM from functional NETs, yet resection margin status had no effect on survival in those with nonfunctioning tumors. In conjunction with the demonstration from meticulous pathological examination of resection specimens that preoperative imaging grossly underestimates the actual burden of disease [14], the authors posited that their results infer that R0, R1 and R2 all in fact represent cytoreductive approaches of varying fervor as opposed to any being strictly curative. In line with this hypothesis, Glazer et al. [15] showed in their series of 172 patients with neuroendocrine LM who underwent various types of hepatic surgery that positive resection margins (R1 or R2) were not associated with significantly worse overall and recurrence/progression-free survival.

It appears that although the efficacies of curative and palliative approaches are both attenuated by the shared hindrance of recurrence, debulking is associated with poorer overall survival outcomes generally. A recent study from the Mayo clinic retrospectively analyzed outcomes of 72 patients with LM from nonfunctioning pancreatic NETs treated between 1987 and 2008 [16]. Thirty-nine patients received curative resection, 32 received palliative resections of LM with removal of ≥90% tumor bulk, and 1 had <90% tumor removal. Interestingly, 1-, 5- and 10-year overall survival of patients receiving R0 resection and ≥90% debulking were 100, 69.6 and 54.2% versus 93.8, 48.1 and 32.1%, and were not statistically different in a univariate model. Such differences were, however, significant using a multiple variable model ($p = 0.02$). Disease recurrence at 1 and 5 years in R0 patients was roughly comparable with 1- and 5-year progression-free survival in a ≥90% debulking group: 53.7 and 10.7% versus 58.1 and 3.5%. By combining surgical debulking with intraoperative and in some cases repeated postoperative percutaneous radiofrequency ablation, Taner et al. [17] achieved a 5- and 10-year overall survival of 80 and 59%, respectively, and a symptom-free survival of 34 and 16% at 3 and 5 years, respectively, in a cohort of patients with neuroendocrine LM in whom curative resection was not feasible.

With numerous options for unresectable LM within the NET armamentarium, some reports have assessed outcomes of palliative resection compared with other

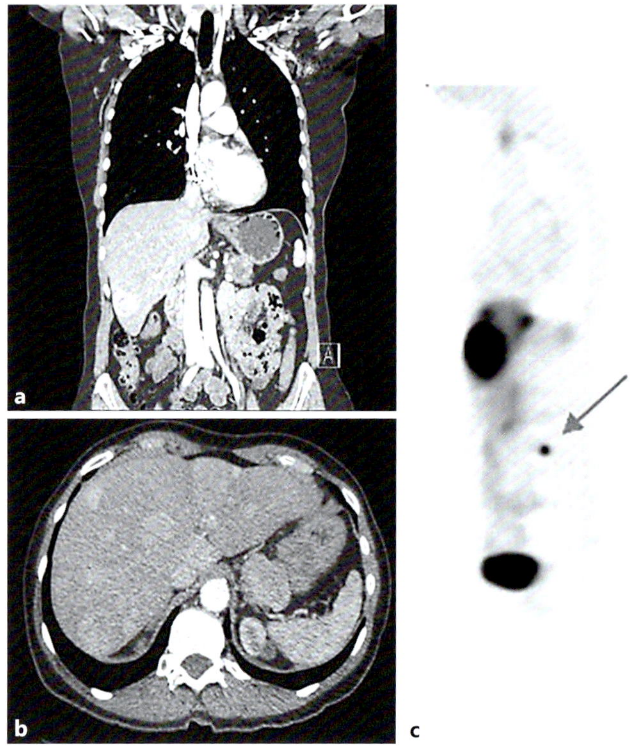

Fig. 1. a, **b** CT scan of a 52-year-old patient with a G1 NET of the pancreatic tail and bilobar nonresectable liver metastases. **c** A single-bone metastasis not detectable on standard imaging was seen on ^{68}Ga-DOTATOC PET/CT (arrow). The patient was offered first-line chemotherapy (streptozotocin and 5-FU) for pancreatic NETs. In cases of good response within the liver and skeletal system, primary tumor resection will be considered.

modalities. In their study of 120 patients with symptomatic neuroendocrine LM (38 of which underwent palliative resection whilst 59 underwent embolisation), Osborne et al. [18] demonstrated a significantly favorable outcome with debulking over transarterial embolisation, with a mean survival of 32 ± 18.9 and 24 ± 15.8 months, respectively. All these reports are of a retrospective nature and are burdened by a bias of patient selection. Indeed, a Cochrane review on interventions for neuroendocrine LM found a lack of evidence regarding patient benefit from hepatic lesion debulking when compared to nonsurgical treatment options [19].

Resection of the Primary Tumor in the Presence of Unresectable LM

There is little sound evidence that resection of the primary tumor will positively impact on the prognosis of patients with unresectable neuroendocrine LM (fig. 1). While some groups argue that resection of a pancreatic primary decelerates the progression of LM [20] and contributes to a better quality of life by avoidance of symptoms associated with hormonal production and local mass effect, including vascular and biliary obstruction [21], others have shown that overall survival did not differ between resected and nonresected patient groups [22]. In a series of Solorzano et al. [23], 9% of patients with pancreatic NETs experienced complications, including bleeding from isolated gastric varices secondary to splenic vein occlusion caused by the nonresected primary tumor. A systematic review of a few cohort studies related to this topic suggested a possible benefit of resecting the primary tumor in terms of survival provided that surgical morbidity is low, although a bias toward offering surgery to patients possessing good functional capacity and tumor localization within the pancreatic body or tail requiring less extensive resections was presumed [24]. More recently, younger age, low Ki-67% of the primary tumor and <25% liver involvement have been identified as helpful selection criteria for those patients who may benefit from primary tumor resection [22]. For patients with small intestinal NETs and unresectable LM, a median overall survival of 75–139 months was extrapolated from six studies for those who underwent primary tumor resection, compared to 50–88 months when the primary tumor remained in situ [25]. In the largest of these series comprising 314 patients, cumulative survival was 67% at 5 years if the primary and the mesenteric lymph nodes were resected, and only 42% if no resection was performed [26]. Irrespective of the primary tumor site, the 'liver first' approach in terms of upfront treatment of hepatic metastases followed by resection of the primary tumor might be an appealing strategy for this clinical scenario. A multimodal strategy would allow identification of those patients with LM refractory to treatment who consequentially would not benefit from removal of the primary tumor.

Transplantation

Liver Transplantation

Predicated by their relatively less aggressive behavior as compared to other secondary malignancies, neuroendocrine LM are accepted indications for liver transplantation. Following initial reports of the use of orthotopic liver transplantation (OLT), including patients with neuroendocrine LM in the 1980s, experience with approximately 700 cases has been reported worldwide in a number of single- and multicenter series (table 2). Although there appears to be consensus regarding exclusion criteria for OLT in neuroendocrine LM, such as higher tumor grade, nonportal tumor drainage, extrahepatic metastases (fig. 2) with the exception of resectable perihilar lymph node metastases and advanced carcinoid heart disease, other selection criteria vary between centers. The Milan criteria for liver transplantation in neuroendocrine LM as defined by Mazzaferro et al. [27] require low-grade NETs (with or without clinical syndrome), drainage of the primary tumor by the portal venous system, complete resection of the primary tumor alongside any extrahepatic disease prior to liver transplantation, ≤50% hepatic involvement, response or stable disease for 6 months prior to transplantation, and patient age ≤55 years.

In contrast, Olausson et al. [28] reported favorable outcomes from a series of patients in which they allowed older age (up to 64 years), >50% tumor volume (in 12 of 15 patients) and Ki-67 index of up to 10% for OLT (n = 10) and multivisceral transplantation (MVT; n = 5). The Gothenburg group attained 5-year overall survivals of

Table 2. Selected single-center studies reporting survival outcomes from liver transplantation for neuroendocrine LM (published since 2000)

First author	Year	Patients, n	Overall survival, %					Disease-free survival, %			
			1 year	2 years	3 years	5 years	10 years	1 year	3 years	5 years	10 years
Bonaccorsi-Riani [29]	2010	9	88		77	33[c]		67	33	11	
Olausson [28]	2007	15[a]				90			70	20	
Marin [49]	2007	10	86		57				38		
Mazzaferro [27]	2007	24				90				77	
van Vilsteren [50]	2006	19	88					80			
Frilling [51]	2006	15[b]	78.3			67.2		69.4		48.3	
Florman [52]	2004	11	73			36					
Cahlin [53]	2003	7		80							
Rosenau [54]	2002	19	89			80	50	56		21	21
Coppa [45]	2001	9				70				53	

[a] Includes 5 patients undergoing multivisceral transplantation.
[b] Includes 1 patient undergoing multivisceral transplantation.
[c] Includes 4 patients transplanted prior to 1990.

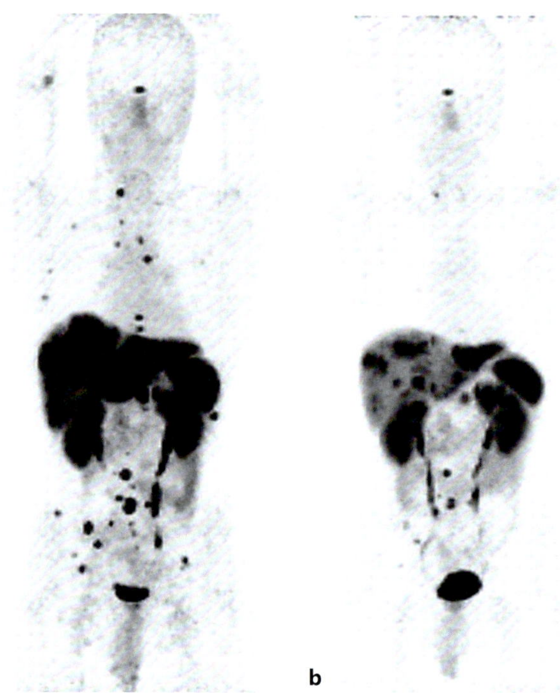

Fig. 2. ^{68}Ga-DOTATOC PET/CT of a 36-year-old patient with a malignant insulinoma evaluated for liver transplantation for nonresectable liver metastases. **a** Multiple extrahepatic metastases were considered as contraindication for transplantation. The patient underwent five cycles of ^{117}Lu peptide receptor radionuclide therapy. **b** A posttreatment ^{68}Ga-DOTATOC PET/CT confirmed very good response to treatment.

90 and 70% for OLT and the entire cohort, respectively, with a 1-year recurrence-free survival of 70% for all patients. Furthermore, they reported that neither age, tumor burden >50% nor Ki-67 index exerted significant prognostic influence on recurrence in their case series. Another divergence from the Milan group was the use of a highly aggressive surgical approach in some patients; those with tumors localized within the pancreatic head underwent resection and transplantation of the stomach, liver, duodenum and pancreas alongside resection of the primary tumor, lymph nodes and LM within the same procedure.

Five year overall and disease-free survival of 33–90 and 11–77%, respectively, have been reported in single-center series (table 2). This wide range of outcomes may reflect the different biological behaviors of primary tumors (e.g. pancreatic NETs vs. intestinal NETs) included in these series, inconsistency of selection criteria in the early time eras, and the lack of uniform standardized follow-up protocols. In a series from Belgium, for example, 1-, 3- and 5-year overall and disease-free survivals were 10, 75 and 25 and 75, 0 and 0%, respectively, in the patients undergoing transplantation in the period between 1987 and 1989, compared to 80, 80 and 60 and 80, 40 and 20%, respectively, for those who underwent the procedure between 2000 and 2003 [29]. A multicenter analysis of the UNOS database examined the outcomes of 150 patients undergoing liver transplantation either as a single procedure (n = 137) or as part of MVT (n = 13) in the USA between 1988 and 2008 [30]. The overall 1-, 3- and 5-year survival for isolated OLT and for all patients was 81, 65 and 49%, respectively, versus 80, 64 and 48%, respectively. These were comparable to the survival of patients undergoing transplantation for hepatocellular carcinoma in the same time period. There was no significant distinction in survival outcomes between carcinoid and noncarcinoid tumors. The authors identified that patients receiving transplantation after the median waiting time of 67 days had significantly better outcomes irrespective of age for those transplanted before this time, with 63 and 36% 5-year survival, respectively, suggesting potential benefits from disease stabilization prior to transplantation.

A more recent analysis of the UNOS database by Nguyen et al. [31] considered 184 patients with neuroendocrine LM transplanted from 1988 to 2011 (0.17% of all transplants) with an emphasis on the effect of MELD (model for end-stage liver disease) score criteria on survival outcomes. When considering the entire timespan, patients with neuroendocrine LM showed significantly lower overall survival compared to patients with hepatocellular carcinoma, with 1-, 3- and 5-year overall survival of 79.5, 61.4 and 49.2 versus 85.8, 71.1 and 60.6, respectively, and those transplanted for nonmalignant conditions with a 1-, 3- and 5-year overall of 85.2, 78.3 and 73.0%, respectively. Lack of recording of recurrence rates and disease-free survival has been noted as an important shortcoming of this database. After the implementation of MELD in 2002, 1-, 3- and 5-year overall survival for neuroendocrine LM patients increased to 84.7, 65 and 57.8%, respectively, and was comparable to the outcomes observed in patients with hepatocellular carcinoma transplanted in the MELD era, but was still marginally lower than in patients who received liver allografts for benign indications.

Analyses of potentially prognostic clinical parameters showed that in those transplanted for neuroendocrine LM after implementation of MELD, higher recipient total bilirubin, lower recipient albumin and higher donor creatinine at the time of transplantation were adverse factors for patient survival, whilst allograft survival was likewise affected by the necessity of retransplantation, higher recipient total bilirubin and higher donor creatinine. Notably, these parameters serve as surrogates for outcome irrespective of the indication for transplantation.

A similar retrospective analysis by Le Treut et al. [32] reviewed 213 European patients and reported 1-, 2-, 3-, 4- and 5-year overall survival and disease-free survival of 81, 73, 65, 55 and 52%, respectively, versus 65, 49, 40, 33 and 30%, respectively. Three-month postoperative mortality was 10%. Univariate analyses did not identify age as a prognostic factor (at any threshold), but did demonstrate the significance of concomitant major resection, poor tumor differentiation and hepatomegaly as independent unfavorable prognosticators. It remained unclear if the morbidity of a major resection in addition to liver transplantation rather than tumor biology contributed to a dismal outcome. After identifying an improved 5-year overall survival of 59% in patients transplanted after 2000, the authors executed a multivariate analysis on this subcohort which found hepatomegaly, age >45 years and additional resection as predictors of poor prognosis. The authors designed a 4-point scale (0–3) to score patients on the basis of their possessing adverse prognostic factors. A score of 0 or 1 was associated with 79% 5-year overall survival and 57% 5-year disease-free survival compared to 35 and 19%, respectively, in patients who reached 2 or 3 points on the scale. In a previous French multicentric study including 85 patients transplanted in the period 1989–2005, 5-year overall and disease-free survival amounted to 47 and 20%, respectively, and the 3-month mortality was 14% [33]. The improved outcomes noted in patients transplanted for neuroendocrine LM in the current era documented in a single-center series and in the three large multicenter reports may be attributed to the application of more stringent selection criteria, refinement of surgical techniques, introduction of novel immunosuppressive agents with antiproliferative side effects, and overall improvement in the management of transplanted patients.

Several issues related to liver transplantation in patients with neuroendocrine LM remain controversial. The data generated from recent publications suggest that 5-year overall and disease-free survival is around 50 and 30%, respectively, implying that liver transplantation should be considered as a palliative rather than a curative treatment option. A high recurrence rate is a matter of concern and calls for neoadjuvant and adjuvant treatment strategies utilizing concepts followed for patients transplanted for other malignancies and newly introduced, targeted drugs. A 6-month waiting policy aiming to identify patients with stable disease, as favored by some centers, bears robust evidence. With regards to the optimal timing of liver transplantation during the course of the disease, some advocate this approach as a last-resort modality after standard therapy options have been exhausted, whereas others prefer its consideration at an earlier stage, an approach which most likely contributes to better outcome. There is urgent need for novel patient- and tumor-specific biomarkers which would facilitate more accurate patient selection and monitoring during the treatment journey.

Intestinal Transplantation

Simultaneous transplantation of the stomach, duodenum, pancreas and small bowel with (MVT) or without the liver (modified MVT) [34] has only been offered to a few patients with nonresectable NETs worldwide. The incidence and severity of rejections, which were considered in the initial era to be the Achilles' heel of the procedure, decremented markedly following the introduction of tacrolimus-based immunosuppressive regimens and antilymphocyte globulins. In a series of 100 multivisceral transplants in 98 patients performed at the University of Miami from 1994 to 2005, there were 2 patients with NETs, a carcinoid and a VIPoma, respectively [35]. At the Indiana University, 4 of 95 patients had NETs (insulinoma, gastrinoma, VIPoma, carcinoid) and diffuse LM and underwent MVT during a 7-year period [36]. Two of 4 patients had disease recurrence during the study period. The patient with the carcinoid tumor developed recurrence at 10 months after transplant and died. In the gastrinoma patient who was alive at 40 months, the disease had recurred at 23 months. Of the 5 patients with pancreatic NET who underwent MVT at the Sahlgrenska University Hospital in Gothenburg, 2 died at 2 and 4 months, respectively, due to transplant-related morbidity, 1 died of disease recurrence at 27 months (recurrence diagnosed at 25 months), and 2 were alive at 12 and 66 months, respectively; the last had developed disease recurrence at 48 months [28]. A review of the outcomes of 15 adult patients from Sweden and Norway referred for intestinal transplantation disclosed a 2-year overall survival of 67% for a cohort of 6 patients with NETs (all of pancreatic origin) which was identical to the outcome of patients transplanted for intestinal failure [37]. Ultimately, all patients with NETs experienced disease recurrence, with 2 patients consequently dying at 2 and 8 years posttransplantation, respectively. There is some evidence from the UNOS database suggesting that outcomes in NET patients who had MVT are comparable to OLT, demonstrating almost indistinguishable outcomes when MVT was included within survival analyses [30].

References

1 Ellis L, Shale MJ, Coleman MP: Carcinoid tumors of the gastrointestinal tract: trends in incidence in England since 1971. Am J Gastroenterol 2010;105: 2563–2569.

2 Miller HC, Drymousis P, Flora R, Goldin R, Spalding D, Frilling A: Role of Ki-67 Proliferation Index in the Assessment of Patients with Neuroendocrine Neoplasias Regarding the Stage of Disease. World J Surg 2014;38:1353–1361.

3 Frilling A, Li J, Malamutmann E, Schmid K-W, Bockisch A, Broelsch CE: Treatment of liver metastases from neuroendocrine tumours in relation to the extent of hepatic disease. Br J Surg 2009;96:175–184.

4 Frilling A, Sotiropoulos GC, Radtke A, Malago M, Bockisch A, Kuehl H, et al: The impact of ^{68}Ga-DOTATOC positron emission tomography/computed tomography on the multimodal management of patients with neuroendocrine tumors. Ann Surg 2010;252:850–856.
5 Ruf J, Heuck F, Schiefer J, Denecke T, Elgeti F, Pascher A, et al: Impact of multiphase ^{68}Ga-DOTATOC-PET/CT on therapy management in patients with neuroendocrine tumors. Neuroendocrinology 2010;91:101–109.
6 Norlén O, Stålberg P, Öberg K, Eriksson J, Hedberg J, Hessman O, et al: Long-term results of surgery for small intestinal neuroendocrine tumors at a tertiary referral center. World J Surg 2012;36:1419–1431.
7 Norton JA, Harris EJ, Chen Y, Visser BC, Poultsides GA, Kunz PC, et al: Pancreatic endocrine tumors with major vascular abutment, involvement, or encasement and indication for resection. Arch Surg 2011;146:724–732.
8 Kianmanesh R, Sauvanet A, Hentic O, Couvelard A, Lévy P, Vilgrain V, et al: Two-step surgery for synchronous bilobar liver metastases from digestive endocrine tumors: a safe approach for radical resection. Ann Surg 2008;247:659–665.
9 Schadde E, Ardiles V, Slankamenac K, Tschuor C, Sergeant G, Amacker N, et al: ALPPS offers a better chance of complete resection in patients with primarily unresectable liver tumors compared with conventional-staged hepatectomies: results of a multicenter analysis. World J Surg 2014;38:1510–1519.
10 Frilling A, Modlin IM, Kidd M, Russell C, Breitenstein S, Salem R, et al: Recommendations for management of patients with neuroendocrine liver metastases. Lancet Oncol 2014;15:e8–e21.
11 Norton JA, Jensen RT: Resolved and unresolved controversies in the surgical management of patients with Zollinger-Ellison syndrome. Ann Surg 2004;240:757–773.
12 Saxena A, Chua TC, Perera M, Chu F, Morris DL: Surgical resection of hepatic metastases from neuroendocrine neoplasms: a systematic review. Surg Oncol 2012;21:e131–e141.
13 Mayo SC, de Jong MC, Pulitano C, Clary BM, Reddy SK, Gamblin TC, et al: Surgical management of hepatic neuroendocrine tumor metastasis: results from an international multi-institutional analysis. Ann Surg Oncol 2010;17:3129–3136.
14 Elias D, Lefevre JH, Duvillard P, Goéré D, Dromain C, Dumont F, et al: Hepatic metastases from neuroendocrine tumors with a 'thin slice' pathological examination: they are many more than you think. Ann Surg 2010;251:307–310.
15 Glazer ES, Tseng JF, Al-Refaie W, Solorzano CC, Liu P, Willborn KA, et al: Long-term survival after surgical management of neuroendocrine hepatic metastases. HPB (Oxford) 2010;12:427–433.
16 Cusati D, Zhang L, Harmsen WS, Hu A, Farnell MB, Nagorney DM, et al: Metastatic nonfunctioning pancreatic neuroendocrine carcinoma to liver: surgical treatment and outcomes. J Am Coll Surg 2012;215:117–124, discussion 124–125.
17 Taner T, Atwell TD, Zhang L, Oberg TN, Harmsen WS, Slettedahl SW, et al: Adjunctive radiofrequency ablation of metastatic neuroendocrine cancer to the liver complements surgical resection. HPB (Oxford) 2013;15:190–195.
18 Osborne DA, Zervos EE, Strosberg J, Strosberg J, Boe BA, Malafa M, et al: Improved outcome with cytoreduction versus embolization for symptomatic hepatic metastases of carcinoid and neuroendocrine tumors. Ann Surg Oncol 2006;13:572–581.
19 Gurusamy KS, Pamecha V, Sharma D, Davidson BR: Palliative cytoreductive surgery versus other palliative treatments in patients with unresectable liver metastases from gastro-entero-pancreatic neuroendocrine tumours. Cochrane Database Syst Rev 2009:CD007118.
20 Bruzoni M, Parikh P, Celis R, Are C, Ly QP, Meza JL, et al: Management of the primary tumor in patients with metastatic pancreatic neuroendocrine tumor: a contemporary single-institution review. Am J Surg 2009;197:376–381.
21 Hung J-S, Chang M-C, Lee P-H, Tien Y-W: Is surgery indicated for patients with symptomatic nonfunctioning pancreatic neuroendocrine tumor and unresectable hepatic metastases? World J Surg 2007;31:2392–2397.
22 Bettini R, Mantovani W, Boninsegna L, Crippa S, Capelli P, Bassi C, et al: Primary tumour resection in metastatic nonfunctioning pancreatic endocrine carcinomas. Dig Liver Dis 2009;41:49–55.
23 Solorzano CC, Lee JE, Pisters PW, Vauthey JN, Ayers GD, Jean ME, et al: Nonfunctioning islet cell carcinoma of the pancreas: survival results in a contemporary series of 163 patients. Surgery 2001;130:1078–1085.
24 Capurso G, Bettini R, Rinzivillo M, Boninsegna L, Delle Fave G, Falconi M: Role of resection of the primary pancreatic neuroendocrine tumour only in patients with unresectable metastatic liver disease: a systematic review. Neuroendocrinology 2011;93:223–229.
25 Capurso G, Rinzivillo M, Bettini R, Boninsegna L, Delle Fave G, Falconi M: Systematic review of resection of primary midgut carcinoid tumour in patients with unresectable liver metastases. Br J Surg 2012;99:1480–1486.
26 Hellman P, Lundström T, Ohrvall U, Eriksson B, Skogseid B, Oberg K, et al: Effect of surgery on the outcome of midgut carcinoid disease with lymph node and liver metastases. World J Surg 2002;26:991–997.

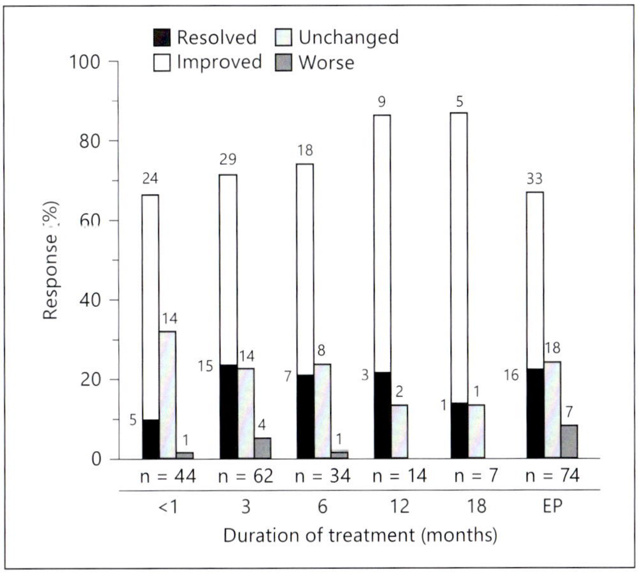

Fig. 1. Carcinoid diarrhea response to octreotide: categorical rating versus baseline of octreotide therapy in symptomatic carcinoid subjects. The numbers at the top of each column represent the number of patients responding. The scale and rating are described in the text. EP = End-point evaluation. Reproduced with permission from Dunne et al. [12].

marker reduction by 10% or greater; 3 = no change; 4 = symptom worsening or increase in biomarkers by 10% or greater; 5 = new symptoms. This scale was necessary because of considerable clinical heterogeneity, the relative paucity of the eligible subjects with this rare cancer [13], and the varied background and clinical research experience of the 78 investigators from 13 countries, including the USA. Therefore, at the outset, case-report forms for internal use were established wherein the severity of presenting clinical and biochemical features were converted to standardized nomenclatures [12].

Carcinoid Tumors Subjects

A total of 85 subjects were included (47 US, of which 26 were treated at the Mayo Clinic and, although included in this database, were published separately [13], and 38 non-US). Dosages ranged between 100 and 1,500 μg per day in the subjects reported. The duration of treatment ranged from as few as 2 weeks (lack of efficacy) to 24 months. The mean daily dose in the Mayo Clinic subjects was 479 μg after 1 month [13].

Results in 74 subjects with carcinoid diarrhea demonstrated control within 14 days (fig. 1). Individual responses during those first 14 days showed that 29 of 44 subjects (66%) either improved or had complete resolution, and 5 of 44 (11%) were without a response. At 6 months 74% had improvement or reduction, and at 12 months 86% demonstrated improvement or complete resolution. Nine percent experienced worsening of diarrhea. While this could have reflected the severity of progressive carcinoid disease, 25% of normal volunteers studied in parallel had documented subclinical fat

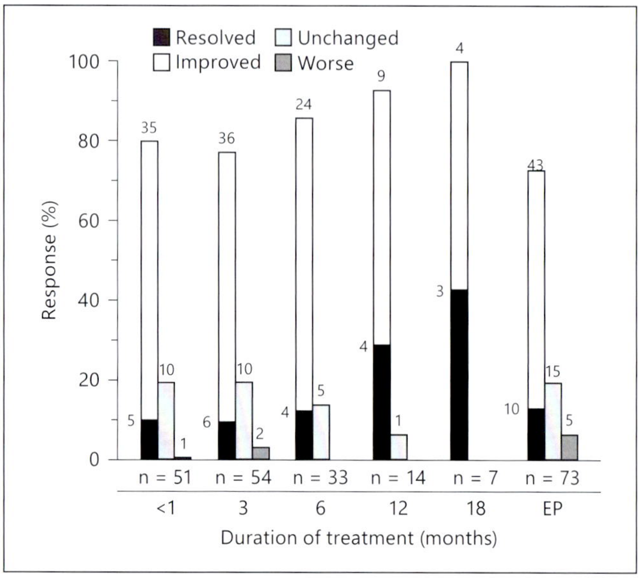

Fig. 2. Carcinoid flushing response to octreotide: categorical rating versus baseline of octreotide therapy in symptomatic carcinoid subjects. The numbers at the top of each column represent the number of patients responding. EP = End-point evaluation. Reproduced with permission from Dunne et al. [12].

absorption. This may have been, in retrospect, steatorrhea from octreotide-induced meal-stimulated pancreatic enzyme inhibition in the symptomatic carcinoid group. The regular use of pancreatic enzyme replacement may have improved those 7% with worsening diarrhea [12, 14]. Empiric use of pancreatic enzyme replacement was not done on the original volunteer subjects or the affected patients. Also noted in figure 1, at the end point, 66% of the 74 subjects studied had durable resolution or improvement of their diarrhea.

The results of the combined US and non-US registration patients and their flushing response to octreotide are shown in figure 2. In the FDA registration, 73 patients experienced flushing as part of their syndrome preoctreotide acetate treatment. Within 14 days, flushing had improved in 40 of 51 patients (78%), and resolved completely in 5 of 51 (10%). At 6 months 85% (28 of 33) had improvement or resolution and by 12 months, 13 of 14 accessible (93%) had improvement or resolution of flushing. Five patients had worsening of facial flushing [12]. At the end point, flushing was improved or resolved in 73% of the studied subjects (53 of a total of 73).

Figure 3 shows the 5-HIAA biomarker responses to octreotide acetate in the registry carcinoid subjects. Circulating serotonin is the predominant biomarker secreted by metastatic (mid-gut) carcinoid tumors (hepatic metastasis), with degradation to its metabolic product, 5-HIAA. This had been (and continues to be) measured as a 24-hour urine collection. A commercial plasma 5-HIAA measurement is now available in the USA and Europe which correlates very well with 24-hour urine 5-HIAA and is more convenient [15]. In the FDA registration data, a trial of 60 patients had elevated urinary 5-HIAA excretion levels prior to beginning octreotide acetate. There was a 58% reduction (35 of 60 subjects) with 3 obtaining complete normalization with

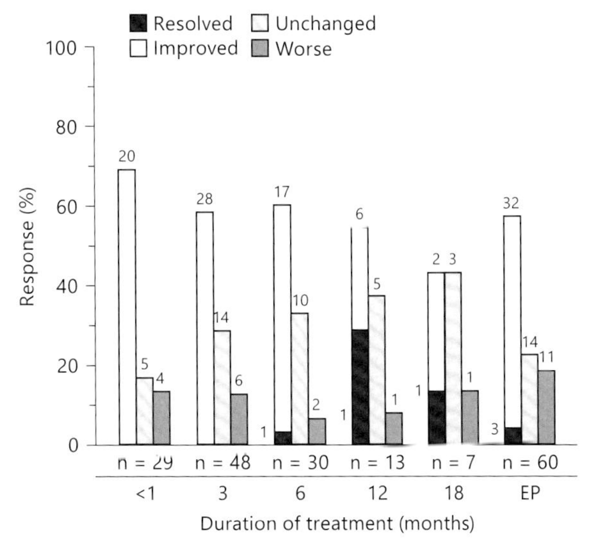

Fig. 3. Carcinoid biomarker response to octreotide: categorical rating versus baseline of octreotide therapy in symptomatic carcinoid subjects. The numbers at the top of each column represent the number of patients responding. EP = End-point evaluation. Reproduced with permission from Dunne et al. [12].

octreotide acetate during the study. In 23% (14 of 60) there were no changes, and in 22%, there was a paradoxical increase from pretreatment levels. The 5-HIAA reductions associated with octreotide clearly allude to what we have learned; namely, when somatostatin subtype 2 receptors are expressed in GEP-NETs, octreotide (and lanreotide) can decrease amino acid and neuropeptide hormone release.

Although radiographic responses were not an objective in the FDA registration, no predictable antitumor action or effect on tumor size, growth or progression of metastasis could be discerned from this initial study. Two European patients did, however, demonstrate tumor shrinkage. It should be recalled that all of these patients in the FDA registry study were on varying doses of subcutaneous (SQ) octreotide. Higher sustained octreotide levels were not achieved until 1999, 10 years after SQ octreotide acetate registration, wherein the effects of sustained elevated octreotide levels could be more consistently observed [16]. Phase I octreotide and lanreotide trials were performed after octreotide approval and radiographic responses were observed at higher doses [17].

The most significant single institution work leading and supporting the FDA registration of octreotide use in carcinoid syndrome patients was the study by Kvols et al. [13] at Mayo Clinic in 1986. As noted above, 27 of the 85 evaluable patients with malignant carcinoid syndrome that were in the initial FDA registration submission to the FDA were reported separately. The overall rating responses used in the FDA subjects were similarly applied in the Mayo article [12]. The Mayo article also evaluated categories of response – diarrhea, flushing and changes of 5-HIAA levels treated with octreotide acetate.

According to the Kvols et al. [13] report, of the 25 patients with active carcinoid syndrome diarrhea, 19 (76%) had a greater than 50% decrease in the number and volume of bowel movements. This effect was durable for a median time of 12 months. Furthermore, of the 24 patients with daily flushing, octreotide acetate resulted in a 79% reduction in the number and intensity of the daily episodes with a median durable response of 12 months. Finally, in 25 patients with elevated 24-hour urine 5-HIAA levels (range 14–1,079 mg/24 h, average 265 mg) 18 subjects (72%) had a greater than 50% urinary 5-HIAA reduction with a median durable response of 12 months.

Pancreatic Neuroendocrine Tumor Subjects

The second FDA indication and approval of octreotide acetate was for the watery diarrhea of vasoactive intestinal peptide (VIP)-secreting tumors [12]. This very rare functional pancreatic NET made up 17% (25 of 173) of the total GEP-NETs treated with octreotide acetate and submitted to the FDA in both the USA and Europe (table 1) [12].

From a total of 25 valuable subjects, 19 of 20 subjects showed improvement in the secretory area within 1 month with a mean rating of 1.8 (1.5–2.4, being classified as 'improved'). Individual responses were equally impressive. Eighteen of 21 (86%) improved or had complete resolution of their diarrhea. The effect was durable as 13 of 13 had improved or complete resolution at 6 and 12 months. Most importantly, in the effectively treated VIPoma patients suffering the consequences of secreting diarrhea, (hypokalemia, metabolic acidosis, dehydration), parenteral support was completely stopped in 13 of 15 patients responding to octreotide acetate [12].

Overall, no predictable antitumor action or effect on tumor size was observed. However, shrinkage of metastatic VIPoma tumors using various radiologic testing was reported in 4 non-US patients during their treatment.

A similar supporting case report was observed in a patient with VIPoma watery diarrhea syndrome in the USA. The case was reported in early 1985 [18]. The patient was a 65-year-old woman who had had a VIP secreting tumor and episodic 'pancreatic cholera' syndrome since 1973 (age 53 years). She had temporary/no improvement with trials of lithium, glucocorticoid, phenothiazines, indomethacin and combination of doxorubicin, 5-fluorouracil, streptozocin or dacarbazine and chlorozotocin. For 6 days prior to the trial of octreotide acetate (SMS 201-995), the patient averaged 10-bowel movements per day, both day and night. Her average fecal loss was 5,816 g per day with daily sodium, potassium, chloride and bicarbonate repletion requirements. She also required 3 liters daily of fluid and electrolyte replacement (especially high doses of potassium). SQ octreotide was given at only 100 μg twice daily.

Figure 4 demonstrates the dramatic diminution of stool weight output and the decreased requirement of high potassium replacement within 24 h of initiating SQ octreotide acetate (SMS 201-995). Also shown are the dramatic decreases in several elevated neuropeptides with the initiation of octreotide acetate in this VIPoma subject

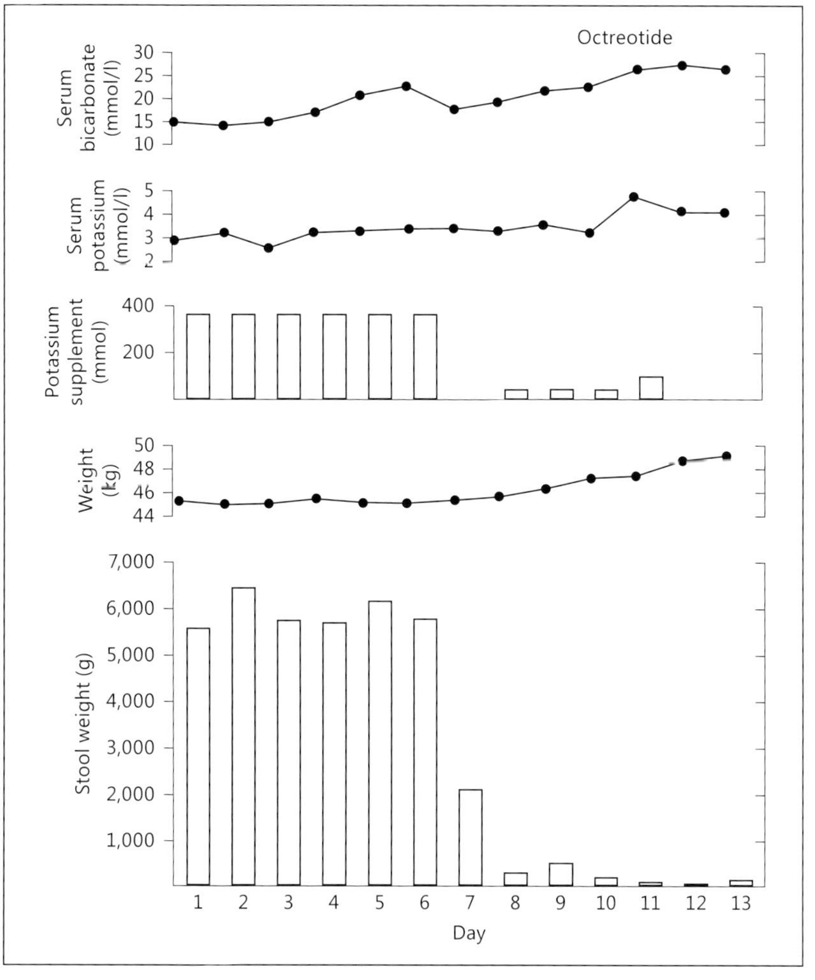

Fig. 4. Clinical and laboratory parameters of the first VIPoma patient in the USA: effect of somatostatin on serum bicarbonate and potassium concentrations, required potassium supplementation, stool weight and body weight. Reproduced with permission from Maton et al. [18].

(fig. 5) [18]. Dramatic reductions of high circulating neuropeptides were observed in the first 7 days following the initiation of octreotide. Octreotide acetate continued to control the diarrhea for 3 months, after which time acute respiratory failure developed with gastrointestinal bleeding and fungal septicemia, followed by death.

Although FDA-indicated approval did not include symptomatic glucagon syndrome patients, 16 patients (9 from the USA and 7 non-US) were evaluated for efficacy in the initial FDA application (table 1). All were malignant glucagonoma subjects with symptoms of necrolytic migratory erythema, diarrhea, diabetes mellitus and the elevated biomarker glucagon [12, 14]. Overall, responses were observed in 16 evaluable subjects and 11 were evaluable over 3 months taking octreotide acetate 200–300 μg

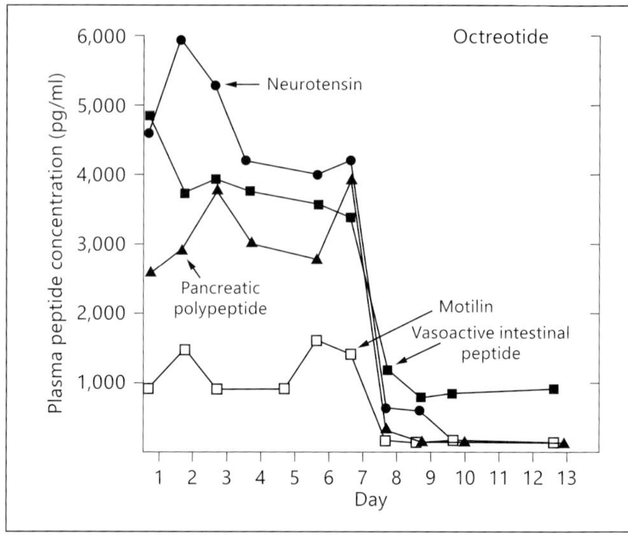

Fig. 5. Biochemical markers of the first VIPoma patient in the USA: effect of somatostatin on plasma concentrations of neurotensin, pancreatic polypeptide, VIP and motilin. Reproduced with permission from Maton et al. [18].

daily. After the first 2 weeks, 6 of 11 (55%) improved with resolution of their rash. Those that reportedly improved initially continued to improve at 6 and 12 months. Relapse was observed beyond the observation period of 12 months in 19% of these patients. Of the 6 subjects with the diarrhea aspect of the syndrome, 6 patients resolved their diarrhea completely over 6 months of therapy. In the 16 subjects with diabetes mellitus, little effect on improving the elevated glucose levels was observed [12].

Plasma glucagon levels, which were elevated in 6 subjects prior to initiation of octreotide acetate, did not improve their levels with the octreotide acetate doses used in the study; yet the rash did improve, suggesting an independent mechanism for the classic glucagonoma rash. Gastrinoma was also evaluated in 26 patients (14 US and 12 non-US) and were included in the 171 patients submitted for FDA registration (table 1) [12]. The mean dosage was lower than for other functioning pancreatic NETs in the FDA application, and ranged from 170 to 250 μg/daily for 6 months. Inadequate dosing probably affected the overall response of the 26 patients studied. Sixteen subjects discontinued drug use due to ineffectiveness. Of 7 evaluable patients with intact stomachs and diarrhea, within the first 3 months diarrhea (acid excess mediated) resolved in 3 patients and improved (50% or more acid diarrhea reduction) in 2, with 2 unchanged. Of 12 subjects with abdominal pain, 50% experienced improvement or resolution. Plasma gastrin was suppressed in 15 patients, unchanged in 3 and elevated above the baseline in 7 subsequent to octreotide acetate therapy. No consistent response between clinically treated octreotide and pretreatment circulating gastrin levels were observed. However, the patients with the best clinical response were those with marked suppression of plasma gastrin by octreotide.

Also included in the original FDA registration demonstrating the effects of octreotide acetate were data from 15 patients with insulinoma (7 benign and 8 with malignant and metastatic tumors). We now know that in benign insulinoma the predominant somatostatin subtype receptor is somatostatin receptor subtype 5 [11, 19]. Somatostatin receptor subtype 2 appears to be present, however, when insulinoma metastasizes to the liver [11]. Utilizing the marker of hypoglycemia, the overall effectiveness of the 15 patients was mixed, with glucose improvement in 50% of the patients in first 3 months of therapy. Four of the initial 7 responders were worse at the end point. Insulin levels were also uneven; these findings imply that octreotide may act more on insulin at its target tissues (e.g. meal-stimulated insulin hepatic glycogen storage) than on the insulin tumor itself. When it is effective, octreotide doses used for insulinoma patients range from 220 to 675 μg, with 1 metastatic insulinoma patient who responded for a year with a higher dose of 990 μg daily, suggesting that higher doses of octreotide for malignant insulinoma may have a more potent effect on somatostatin receptor subtype 5 agonism [11, 12].

Four GRFomas[m1] with clinical symptoms associated with excessive secondary growth hormone secretion were also evaluated over 18 months in the original FDA registration application. The range of octreotide dose was for 200–600 μg/daily. Symptomatic improvement was achieved in 3 of 4 patients with a tendency to increase daily octreotide doses to 12 months of therapy [12].

As noted above, although FDA US and European approvals of octreotide acetate in 1988 and 1989, respectively, were specifically for diarrhea in carcinoid syndrome and the secretory diarrhea of VIP syndrome, GEP-NETs, both functional and nonfunctional, were subsequently treated widely and reported for the next several years [14]. It is felt that this was due in large part to the very low side effect profile and safety of octreotide acetate [14].

Somatostatin Congener Depot Formulations

In 1999, a longer-acting octreotide acetate preparation (octreotide long-acting repeatable; LAR) registrational trial was published by Rubin et al. [16]. The long-acting formulation involving octreotide acetate contained mostly inside microspheres that release slowly into the circulation affected by cleavage of the polymer ester linkage through tissue fluid hydrolysis. The pharmacokinetics of octreotide-LAR are similar to that of SQ octreotide with a combined peak of 15–30 min, plateau of 30–60 min, and half-life of 60–120 min [20]. However, a portion of the mixed precipitate octreotide acetate is around the microspheres causing a rapid ‘spike' of octreotide during the first 12 h following intramuscular injection. Lanreotide Depot is not in a microsphere formulation. As a result, lanreotide gives more of a ‘square wave' distribution with very little peak-trough kinetic. It is given deep SQ versus octreotide-LAR that is given intramuscularly [20].

The Rubin et al. [16] paper led to FDA approval of the octreotide-LAR preparation in 1999. It was a randomized trial comparing LAR at 10, 20 and 30 mg every 4 weeks

Table 2. AEs in GEP tumors: comparing FDA octreotide acetate submission and lanreotide Depot publication

AE	Octreotide GEP tumors	Lanreotide GEP tumors
Total AEs studied	(n = 193)	(n = 101)
Diarrhea	12% (n = 6)	26% (n = 26)
Nausea	17% (n = 9)	7% (n = 7)
Flatulence	1% (n = 0.5)	8% (n = 8)
Fatty stools/loose stools	13% (n = 9)	–[a]
Emesis	6% (n = 3)	12% (n = 12)
Cholelithiasis	Documented[b]	10% (n = 10)
Hyperglycemia	Documented	5% (n = 5)
Hypothyroidism	Suggested	Not mentioned
Vitamin D insufficiency	Not mentioned	Not mentioned

Data was modified to include similar descriptions and percent occurrence in each AE for each somatostatin congener-affected population.
[a] No AE category for lanreotide Depot; possibly included in the diarrhea percentage.
[b] Documented but not quantified (see text).

with open label use of SQ octreotide every 8 h. This included 'rescue' with SQ octreotide in the octreotide-LAR group. The criteria for efficacy was rather strictly defined by SQ octreotide effectiveness in achieving two or fewer flushing episodes per day, and three or fewer bowel movements per day with an SQ octreotide dose that ranged between 300 and 900 μg daily in divided doses. Ninety-three patients were enrolled and randomized to receive octreotide-LAR 10 (n = 22), 20 (n = 20) or 30 mg (n = 25), or continuous SQ acetate octreotide every 8 h (n = 26). Seventy-nine patients were efficacy accessible for at least the 20-week visit/evaluations. Compared to SQ steady state levels, steady state intramuscular octreotide LAR was at least as effective in controlling and reducing the average number of daily bowel movements in all three groups. The 10-mg LAR dose was least effective in controlling the daily flushing episodes as compared to either the SQ octreotide group or the 20- and 30-mg LAR groups. The starting LAR dose was recommended to be 20 mg monthly [16]. Of interest, because of the overlapping of mean octreotide LAR blood levels in the 10-mg versus 20-mg groups, the eventual pricing after FDA approval of these two LAR preparations was similar in the USA.

While the antiproliferative action of both octreotide-LAR [21] and lanreotide Depot [22] will be discussed later, more common adverse events (AEs) relating to both octreotide SQ LAR and lanreotide Depot will now be discussed. Table 2 compares more common AEs submitted to the FDA for 1989 approval of octreotide acetate (which also used a group of volunteers) [12] with AEs for lanreotide Depot [22]. The AEs reported in the octreotide LAR paper were lower, namely 5 months [16], due in part (in our opinion) to the relatively short duration of study. Therefore, these AEs

[16] are not included since few were noted and they were similar to both AEs of the original octreotide acetate SQ submission as well as the AEs from the lanreotide Depot paper.

Although the criteria and interpretation of AEs were not designed to be identical, the major GEP-NET tumors had similar AE responses noted in the carcinoid tumor groups, which comprised 49% of the FDA GEP-NET study group [12]. Forty-four percent of the GEP-NET patients were carcinoid syndrome patients in the lanreotide Depot paper [22]. Of interest, both studies alluded to higher AE tolerability in the affected carcinoid patients due to the effectiveness of controlling the carcinoid complex/syndrome. The lanreotide Depot study documented cholelithiasis in 10% of the treated GEP-NET population. The SQ octreotide data submitted to the FDA noted that 'gall bladder paresis were documented' but did not list the percentage of occurrence of cholelithiasis in this group of patients [12].

Also, and possibly due to the relative brevity of the two trials (24 months), the metabolic consequences of steady high levels of the two somatostatin congeners, octreotide acetate and lanreotide Depot, were not well quantified or documented or mentioned, except for the 5% hypothyroid AE in the lanreotide Depot trial. Clearly, the short-term duration of both somatostatin congeners can be predicted/determined from the extensive body of work on native somatostatin 1–14 that began almost immediately following its description in 1973 by Brazeau et al. [3]. Reviews since 1973 of both somatostatin 1–14 and its congeners (octreotide and lanreotide) have shown the seamless transition and interrelationships between the native form of somatostatin1–14 and its congeners octreotide and lanreotide [5, 6, 23].

The following clinical observations and long-term side effects, observed over several years of use of octreotide acetate, particularly, have been derived from an almost 60-year combined GEP-NET octreotide experience of the authors. The authors also have a combined 40-year experience in managing and monitoring GEP-NET patients on a regular 4-, 6- and 12-month basis. The long-term effects of sustained chronic dosing of octreotide acetate in both SQ and LAR forms reflect persistent elevated levels and supraphysiological hormone (endocrine) action and effects. This is especially true in our experience, with both octreotide LAR and lanreotide Depot. The AE of subclinical fat malabsorption is a persistent issue, especially in mid-gut serotonin-driven diarrheal states. This appears to be both an issue of serotonin-induced hypermotility with subsequent insufficient pancreatic enzyme residence time to allow fat absorption. Inhibition of prandial exocrine functions, experienced at higher somatostatin congener doses, is an expected adverse event. The prandial inhibition of enzyme release with subsequent fat malabsorption appears to be persistent and may occur during the actual improvement of the serotonin-induced (hypermotility) diarrhea, confounding the effectiveness of either congener in improving the serotonin-mediated postprandial diarrhea. The most reproducible symptoms of both congeners in terms of subclinical fat malabsorption are stools 1–3 h after a meal, which are foul smelling, foamy, floaty, observed to have a greasy oily appearance, and are difficult to flush. Loose bowel movements usually occur in the early morning, with a more solid stool followed by gradual semi-soft and then liquid stools comprising 3–5 bowel movements before 1 p.m. in the afternoon. Over time, vitamin D (fat soluble vitamin) absorption becomes impaired and vitamin D_{25} levels will decrease and remain low. For this constellation of symptoms (most often associated with either octreotide LAR or lanreotide Depot) we have found that a trial of SQ octreotide 'rescue' 30 min before eating may help to slow the serotonin-induced fat malabsorptive hypermotile type of bowel movement. Empiric use of pancreas-lipase (e.g. Creon/ZENPEP), or vegetable pancreatic enzymes (e.g. DIGEST GOLD, a kosher enzyme replacement) or fruit pancreatic enzymes (e.g. papaya/chewable tablets-t or papaya-pineapple/chewable tablets – the latter two over the counter) will often improve the enzyme-deficient diarrhea, flatulence, abdominal cramps, nausea symptoms which were parceled out in the individual AEs of either the octreotide SQ and lanreotide-LAR study (table 2) [12, 22].

Some of our patients will restrict their meal fat enough to have manageable loose stools and would only take the pancreatic enzyme replacements for a higher fat meal (i.e. supper). Regular SQ octreotide 30 min before a meal with pancreatic enzymes with vitamin D at least once daily may slowly improve vitamin D_{25} blood levels over time. However, on occasion vitamin $D_{1,\,25}$ (intravenous or oral) with oral 1,200–1,800 mg of calcium citrate twice weekly may be required. The intravenous vitamin $D_{1,\,25}$ is usually twice weekly. Chronic management and monitoring is important to try and maintain mineral density over long periods of time, especially in affected women.

In this regard SQ octreotide acetate is effective in symptomatic carcinoid patients who exercise avidly or appreciate an alcoholic beverage before supper. In these cases, a simple SQ injection of 100 μg 30 min before the exercise (or stressful event) or ingestion of an alcoholic beverage will protect and prevent the serotonin surges induced by exercise, excitability or ethanol ingestion. Procedures or intercurrent illnesses may provoke symptom exacerbation despite the use of octreotide LAR. Prophylactic use or 'breakthrough' use of octreotide 100–500 μg SQ every 6–12 h may provide effective symptom control. The week prior to octreotide LAR injection is associated with worsening symptoms and the potential for rescue SQ octreotide.

Chronic sustained elevation of either octreotide acetate or lanreotide plasma levels invariably result in gall bladder sludge/cholelithiasis. The long-term treatment with octreotide acetate of 'greater than one injection per month' is associated with cholesterol gallstones in 20–30% of patients [23]. This author further notes that 'in most cases, the gallstones remain asymptomatic; only approximately 1% of patients will have symptoms per year of treatment'. Our combined experience of over 2,500 GEP-NET patients followed over a combined 30 patient-year experience suggests that virtually all patients on chronic octreotide LAR (and probably lanreotide Depot) develop sludge/gall stones, probably supporting tonic cholecystokinin suppression with subsequent paresis of food-stimulated gall bladder contraction [24]. While we have not systematically examined symptomatic gall stone disease, we have observed an increased risk of morbidity in carcinoid patients with full-blown carcinoid syndrome when an acute bladder attack presents itself. Therefore, we support the recommendation of Akerström and Hellman [25] to remove the gall bladder as prophylaxis when exploratory laparotomy is contemplated for the removal of primary GEP-NETs or debulking procedures.

Regarding hyperglycemia, our long-term experience suggests that, over a long-term period of chronic octreotide usage, average blood glucose levels (measured by serial HgA1c, with normal being <6%) invariably rise between 6.1 and 6.4% and remain in that range throughout the usage of octreotide LAR or daily 3× injections of SQ octreotide. If patients are not prone to type 2 (noninsulin dependent) diabetes mellitus, HgA1c will rarely rise in the diabetes mellitus range of greater than 6.5%. Once again, dose-dependent physiologic mechanisms, wherein somatostatin preferentially inhibits glucagon (vs. insulin), may be in play as the congeners achieve pharmacologic blood levels. This would have a tendency toward hypoglycemia. However, hypomotile actions that affect both gastric emptying and small intestine motility are also relevant, which might be predicted to allow more nutrients such as glucose to be absorbed, with a contributing component of hyperglycemia [6, 23]. Overall, it appears that blood sugars are higher with chronic congener usage and do not appear to completely autoregulate to normal glycemia over time. Treatment of these modest persistent blood sugar elevations is usually not necessary.

Chronic elevated octreotide-lanreotide blood levels will be associated many times with functional hypothyroidism. Measuring the biologically active thyroid hormone free T3 most often makes the diagnosis. Thyroid-stimulating hormone (TSH) is normally in the low/normal range and free T4 is often in the normal range. Low free T3 may well be due to the inhibition of TSH from the pituitary with a subsequent decrease of peripheral T4 to T3 conversion by TSH. Initial lower dosages of levothyroxine (e.g. 0.05 μg) with TSH, free T4, free T3 and testing every 12–16 weeks with subsequent adjustment is recommended. This may well contribute, in part, to the chronic fatigue carcinoid GEP-NET patients suffer.

Two studies, one with octreotide LAR [21] and one with lanreotide Depot [22], and both placebo controlled have introduced somatostatin congeners for not only symptomatic control, but as antiproliferative therapeutic agents. Table 3 compares and contrasts these two seminal studies on the clinical antiproliferative action of these two somatostatin congeners.

Together, these two placebo-controlled randomized studies strengthen, support and demonstrate the therapeutic antiproliferative action previously suggested from uncontrolled clinical studies [26]. Although strict comparison between these placebo-controlled studies is difficult, similar reported hazard ratios of the two studies – 0.34 (95% CI, octreotide) and 0.47 (95% CI, lanreotide) – argue forcefully that either somatostatin congeners exert an antiproliferative action. Furthermore, the CLARINET study includes both WHO grade 1 and 2 GEP-NET subjects compared to PROMID,

Table 3. Comparison and contrast between PROMID [21] and CLARINET [22] placebo-controlled studies of therapeutic action in GEP-NETs

	PROMID	CLARINET
Type and drug	Placebo-controlled double-blind Randomized: OCT-LAR	Placebo-controlled double-blind Randomized: LAN Depot
Study centers	19 (Germany)	48 (14 countries)
Tumor types	Mostly nonfunctional GEP	Nonfunctional GEP
Proliferation index (ki-67)	95% (<2%)	100% (<10%)
Patient distribution	42 OCT; 43 placebo; noncrossover	101 LAN; 103 placebo; crossover
Primary endpoint	TTP	PFD
Outcome	Median TTP 14.3 (vs. 6 months placebo) when primary tumor resected/liver metastasis <10%, TTP 29 months	Median TTP not reached vs. 18 months placebo

OCT = Octreotide; LAN = lanreotide; TTP = time to progression; PFD = progression-free disease.

which included mostly WHO grade 1 patients. Together, these two studies support the use of octreotide LAR/lanreotide Depot in grade 1 (and mid-grade 2) subjects, especially for symptomatic GEP-NETs or subjects that have CT criteria of regional or distant metastasis either at presentation or documented over time as antiproliferative agents.

Future Considerations

Imaging GEP-NET patients includes scintigraphy, classically with ^{111}In-pentetreotide [27]. PET technology with ^{68}Ga-DOTANOC, DOTATOC, or DOTATATE provides improved patient convenience and clinical decision making [28]. Theranostics incorporates somatostatin receptor expression with the potential of using therapeutic injectable radioisotopes. ^{177}Lu and ^{90}Y somatostatin congeners offer improved tumor and symptom control [29, 30].

Clinical decision making in GEP-NET patients includes correlating symptoms with hyperhormonal excess, identifying the tumor grade and location while developing a continuum care plan that incorporates hormonal and (depending upon the grade) cytotoxic agents. As therapeutic options have increased over the last decade, survival outcomes have increased as well depending upon the primary site and grade. Patients survive now for many years with metastatic disease, which was not the case before the somatostatin era.

References

1 Bauer W, Briner U, Doepfner W, Haller R, Huguenin R, Marbach P, Petcher TJ, Pless J: Sms 201–995: A very potent and selective octapeptide analogue of somatostatin with prolonged action. Life Sci 1982;31:1133–1140.

2 Liebow C, Reilly C, Serrano M, Schally AV: Somatostatin analogues inhibit growth of pancreatic cancer by stimulating tyrosine phosphatase. Proc Natl Acad Sci U S A 1989;86:2003–2007.

3 Brazeau P, Vale W, Burgus R, Ling N, Butcher M, Rivier J, Guillemin R: Hypothalamic polypeptide that inhibits the secretion of immunoreactive pituitary growth hormone. Science 1973;179:77–79.

4 Arimura A, Fishback JB: Somatostatin: Regulation of secretion. Neuroendocrinology 1981;33:246–256.

5 Reichlin S: Somatostatin. N Engl J Med 1983;309: 1495–1501.

6 O'Dorisio T, Redfern S: Somatostatin and somatostatin-like peptides: clinical research and clinical applications; in Mazzaferri EL, et al. (eds): Advances in Endocrinology and Metabolism. St. Louis, Mosley, 1990, vol 1, pp 175–230.

7 Reichlin S: Neuroendocrine-immune interactions. N Engl J Med 1993;329:1246–1253.

8 Sheppard M, Shapiro B, Pimstone B, Kronheim S, Berelowitz M, Gregory M: Metabolic clearance and plasma half-disappearance time of exogenous somatostatin in man. J Clin Endocrinol Metab 1979;48: 50–53.

9 Patel YC, Srikant CB: Subtype selectivity of peptide analogs for all five cloned human somatostatin receptors (hsstr 1–5). Endocrinology 1994;135:2814–2817.

10 Bruns C, Weckbecker G, Raulf F, Kaupmann K, Schoeffter P, Hoyer D, Lubbert H: Molecular pharmacology of somatostatin-receptor subtypes. Ann NY Acad Sci 1994;733:138–146.

11 Reubi JC, Maurer R, von Werder K, Torhorst J, Klijn JG, Lamberts SW: Somatostatin receptors in human endocrine tumors. Cancer Res 1987;47:551–558.

12 Dunne MJ, Elton R, Fletcher T, Hopkes P, Shui J: Sandostatin and gastroenteropancreatic endocrine tumors-therapeutic characteristics; in O'Dorisio TM (ed): Sandostatin in the Treatment of GEP Endocrine Tumors. Berlin, Springer, 1987, pp 93–117.

13 Kvols LK, Moertel CG, O'Connell MJ, Schutt AJ, Rubin J, Hahn RG: Treatment of the malignant carcinoid syndrome: evaluation of a long-acting somatostatin analogue. N Engl J Med 1986;315:663–666.

14 Harris AG: Octreotide in the treatment of disorders of the gastrointestinal tract. Drug Invest 1993;4:1–54.

15 Tellez MR, Mamikunian G, O'Dorisio TM, Vinik AI, Woltering EA: A single fasting plasma 5-HIAA value correlates with 24-hour urinary 5-HIAA values and other biomarkers in midgut neuroendocrine tumors (NETs). Pancreas 2013;42:405–410.

16 Rubin J, Ajani J, Schirmer W, Venook AP, Bukowski R, Pommier R, Saltz L, Dandona P, Anthony L: Octreotide acetate long-acting formulation versus open-label subcutaneous octreotide acetate in malignant carcinoid syndrome. J Clin Oncol 1999;17:600–606.

17 Anthony L, Johnson D, Hande K, Shaff M, Winn S, Krozely M, Oates J: Somatostatin analogue phase I trials in neuroendocrine neoplasms. Acta Oncol 1993;32:217–223.

18 Maton PN, O'Dorisio TM, Howe BA, McArthur KE, Howard JM, Cherner JA, Malarkey WB, Collen MJ, Gardner JD, Jensen RT: Effect of a long-acting somatostatin analogue (SMS 201-995) in a patient with pancreatic cholera. N Engl J Med 1985;312:17–21.

19 Rossowski WJ, Coy DH: Specific inhibition of rat pancreatic insulin or glucagon release by receptor-selective somatostatin analogs. Biochem Biophys Res Commun 1994;205:341–346.

20 Lancranjan I, Bruns C, Grass P, Jaquet P, Jervell J, Kendall-Taylor P, Lamberts SW, Marbach P, Orskov H, Pagani G, Sheppard M, Simionescu L: Sandostatin LAR: a promising therapeutic tool in the management of acromegalic patients. Metabolism 1996;45:67–71.

21 Rinke A, Muller HH, Schade-Brittinger C, et al: Placebo-controlled, double-blind, prospective, randomized study on the effect of octreotide LAR in the control of tumor growth in patients with metastatic neuroendocrine midgut tumors: a report from the PROMID Study Group. J Clin Oncol 2009;27:4656–4663.

22 Caplin ME, Pavel M, Cwikla JB, et al: Lanreotide in metastatic enteropancreatic neuroendocrine tumors. N Engl J Med 2014;371:224–233.

23 Lamberts SW, van der Lely AJ, de Herder WW, Hofland LJ: Octreotide. N Engl J Med 1996;334:246–254.

24 Dowling RH, Hussaini SH, Murphy GM, Besser GM, Wass JA: Gallstones during octreotide therapy. Metabolism 1992;41:22–33.

25 Akerström G, Hellman P: Surgery on neuroendocrine tumours. Best Pract Res Clin Endocrinol Metab 2007;21:87–109.

26 Toumpanakis C, Caplin ME: Update on the role of somatostatin analogs for the treatment of patients with gastroenteropancreatic neuroendocrine tumors. Semin Oncol 2013;40:56–68.

27 Krenning EP, Kwekkeboom DJ, Bakker WH, Breeman WA, Kooij PP, Oei HY, van Hagen M, Postema PT, de Jong M, Reubi JC, et al: Somatostatin receptor scintigraphy with [111in-Dtpa-D-Phe1]- and [123i-Tyr3]-octreotide: the Rotterdam experience with more than 1000 patients. Eur J Nucl Med 1993;20:716–731.

28 Herrmann K, Czernin J, Wolin EM, Gupta P, Barrio M, Gutierrez A, Schiepers C, Mosessian S, Phelps ME, Allen-Auerbach MS: Impact of ^{68}Ga-DOTATATE PET/CT on the management of neuroendocrine tumors: the referring physician's perspective. J Nucl Med 2015;56:70–75.

29 van Vliet EI, Teunissen JJ, Kam BL, de Jong M, Krenning EP, Kwekkeboom DJ: Treatment of gastroenteropancreatic neuroendocrine tumors with peptide receptor radionuclide therapy. Neuroendocrinology 2013;97:74–85.

30 Bushnell DL Jr, O'Dorisio TM, O'Dorisio MS, Menda Y, Hicks RJ, van Cutsem E, Baulieu JL, Borson-Chazot F, Anthony L, Benson AB, Oberg K, Grossman AB, Connolly M, Bouterfa H, Li Y, Kacena KA, LaFrance N, Pauwels SA: ^{90}Y-edotreotide for metastatic carcinoid refractory to octreotide. J Clin Oncol 2010;28:1652–1659.

Lowell B. Anthony, MD
Department of Internal Medicine, Division of Medical Oncology
Markey NCI Designated Comprehensive Cancer Center
University of Kentucky, Lexington, KY 40536 (USA)
E-Mail lowell.anthony@uky.edu

Papotti M, de Herder WW (eds): Neuroendocrine Tumors: A Multidisciplinary Approach.
Front Horm Res. Basel, Karger, 2015, vol 44, pp 193–197 (DOI: 10.1159/000402752)

Medical Therapy of Pulmonary Neuroendocrine Neoplasms: Targeted, Symptomatic and Chemotherapy

Piero Ferolla

Multidisciplinary Group for Diagnosis and Therapy of Neuroendocrine Tumors, ENETS Center of Excellence, Umbria Regional Cancer Network, Perugia, Italy

Abstract

Whenever feasible, surgery represents the treatment of choice for pulmonary neuroendocrine neoplasms (NENs). In patients with hypersecreting tumors, wide metastatic spread or those not candidates for a surgical treatment, medical therapies may assure a control of the secretory pattern and slow the rate of tumor growth. No specific trials have been designed so far for pulmonary NENs and the first randomized trial entirely dedicated to thoracic NENs (the LUNA trial) is ongoing. International scientific society guidelines (ESMO and NANETS) and recommendations (ENETS) are therefore necessarily based on expert experience, on the subgroup analysis of large multicenter trials not focused on pulmonary NENs, and on the analysis of small retrospective series. Somatostatin analogs represent the therapy of choice in the presence of associated carcinoid syndrome and ectopic acromegaly and a reasonable first-line in slow-progressing tumors. Due to the low rate of proliferation, platinum-based chemotherapy is generally reserved to rapidly progressing tumors. Temozolomide alone or in association has shown activity in small retrospective series or monocentric trials – larger multicenter trials will better define its efficacy. Everolimus alone or in combination with somatostatin analogs has shown activity in the subgroup analysis of a large multicenter trial (RADIANT II). Many other drugs have shown activity in the preclinical models but, at the moment, no prospective and randomized data are available.

Control of Associated (Neuro) Endocrine Hypersecretions

Thoracic neuroendocrine tumors (NETs) are associated with clinically evident endocrine hypersecretions in a percentage of cases inferior to the gastroenteropancreatic (GEP) counterpart [1–5]. Somatostatin analogs represent the drug of choice in the control of most of the associated hypersecretions, including typical and atypical carcinoid syndrome. The percentage of response to these drugs in thoracic NETs is similar to GEP-NETs; however, the results have been reported in only small series. H1 and H2 blockers and loperamide may be associated with somatostatin analogs to control some of the symptoms, and steroids may be required in patients with atypical carcinoid syndrome while β-blockers are contraindicated whenever bronchostenosis is present. Telotristat etiprate, an inhibitor of tryptophan hydroxylase, is currently under investigation in the course of phase II and III trials to increase the percentage of control of carcinoid syndrome in patients not completely controlled by somatostatin analogs [6].

The other more frequently associated hypersecretions are ectopic adrenocorticotrophin hypersecretion, hypersecretion of growth hormone-releasing hormone and the syndrome of inappropriate secretion of antidiuretic hormone. The treatment of these hypersecretions does not differ in a relevant manner from those indicated when other causes are recognized. The use of debulking strategies to reduce the mass of secreting cells, including surgery, locoregional treatments and peptide receptor radiotherapy, may be evaluated in the multidisciplinary tumor board. The addition of α-interferon has been reported to have some efficacy.

Control of Tumor Growth in the Metastatic Setting or in Patients Not Candidates for Surgery

At the time of writing, the first multicenter randomized prospective trial entirely dedicated to thoracic NETs (LUNA trial, ClinicalTrials.gov ID: NCT01563354) is ongoing. No other prospective trials focused on bronchial NETs have been published, therefore the only available results come from small retrospective series and from the subgroup analysis of a few larger multicenter studies that allowed the inclusion of thoracic NETs.

Since they originate from the same cells of the neuroendocrine diffuse system, sharing most of the biological features, it is reasonable to speculate that some of the results obtained in other neuroendocrine cells, such as in the ileal carcinoid, may also be applicable in the bronchial carcinoid.

Somatostatin Analogs

Two large phase III studies focused on small intestine NETs have clearly demonstrated an impact in terms of progression-free survival (PFS) of the long-acting somatostatin analogs octreotide (PROMID study) [7] and lanreotide (CLARINET study) [8]. Based on these data and the lack of any other larger studies with any type of drugs, somatostatin analogs appear the preferable first step in the treatment of inoperable (including multicentric forms) or metastatic well-differentiated bronchial NETs (typical and atypical carcinoids according to the WHO classification).

The proliferation indexes (mitotic count and ki-67), the grade of uptake at somatostatin receptor scintigraphy and the rate of radiological progression may be evaluated case by case in a multidisciplinary tumor board to better define the need for additional therapies in the clinical management of advanced disease.

The role of somatostatin analogs in the treatment of multicentric forms and precursor lesions such as diffuse idiopathic pulmonary neuroendocrine cell hyperplasia appear reasonable, but need to be evaluated in specific studies. The same consideration should be reserved to their possible role in the adjuvant setting in patients at high risk of recurrences, such as atypical carcinoids stage N1 or N2, for which a clinical trial is urgently needed.

When progressive disease occurs in the course of therapy with somatostatin analogs, no standard therapies are available. When available, a clinical trial should always be preferred. The first international randomized trial specifically dedicated to thoracic neuroendocrine neoplasms (NENs), the LUNA trial, will clarify the efficacy and safety of everolimus and pasireotide, while a multicenter Italian trial assessing the safety and efficacy of the association between lanreotide and temozolomide will start within a year.

Target Therapies

Everolimus alone or in combination with somatostatin analogs has shown activity in the subgroup analyses of a large multicenter trial (RADIANT II) [9]. The subgroup comprised 44 patients and the trend of impact on PFS was superior than 8 months, although an imbalance in the subdivision between the two arms of the study does not allow a correct statistical analysis [10]. However, it should be remembered that in both phase II studies and expanded access programs, the impact of everolimus on PFS seems more relevant for carcinoid tumors when compared to pancreatic NETs.

Prospective phase III trials are ongoing in other similar NETs (ileal carcinoids) with peptide receptor radiotherapy and locoregional therapies. Despite the lack of large trials, the analysis of a small subgroup of metastatic thoracic NETs revealed a rate of response similar to that obtained in GEP-NETs [11]. A large phase III study (RADIANT IV) also including nonsecreting lung NETs has completed recruitment and is currently ongoing. It will explore the efficacy of everolimus as a single agent when compared to placebo in patients with progressive disease. The LUNA trial entirely dedicated to thoracic NETs will assess the efficacy and safety of everolimus as a single agent compared to the association with pasireotide or pasireotide alone in patients with progressive disease. Many other target agents are theoretically active or seem promising in the preclinical models, single patients or subgroups included in other small phase II trials, but these preliminary results need further investigation.

Chemotherapy

The use of mono- or polychemotherapy in thoracic well-differentiated NETs has been associated with poor results in recent decades. Results reported in the literature generally derive from small series, and the study methods include several biases. Among these are the criteria of inclusion that often comprise tumors with different grades of differentiation, the lack of information regarding the progression of disease before the start of therapy and the criteria of evaluation of response. The percentage of G3–4 toxicity was generally relatively high. The cisplatin-etoposide scheme, which represents the standard first-line treatment for poorly differentiated tumors, should be reserved, in well-differentiated tumors, to patients that became rapidly progressive or when a rapid control of the associated endocrine syndrome is clinically needed (in association with the drugs reported in the previous paragraph).

Temozolomide alone or in association constitutes an exception, although the results are reported in small retrospective series [12, 13]. The first prospective multicenter trial entirely dedicated to thoracic NENs will start this year. It will assess the efficacy and safety of temozolomide in association with lanreotide ('EUDRACT 2014-005579-10'). The activity of the enzyme O^6-alkylguanine DNA alkyltransferase (MGMT) appears crucial for the efficacy of this drug; however, the three methods of evaluation of this activity present different limitations and not all the reports were concordant in the correlation of enzymatic expression levels with the response to the drugs. Based on these considerations, it is probably not ethical at the moment to select patients on the basis of these methods, and in clinical trials an a posteriori analysis or the advent of new methods will better clarify the clinical indications for the selection of candidates for this therapy.

Conclusions

Based on the evidence resulting from small retrospective trials, and on the subgroup analysis of trials including pulmonary NENs, everolimus and temozolomide appear the probable best choice in progressive metastatic disease when progression occurs after somatostatin analogs, which may represent the first-line of treatment and the treatment of choice in secreting tumors. Temozolomide seems theoretically preferable when brain metastases are present and when concomitant radiotherapy is needed for bone metastases [14]. The toxicity profile of everolimus allows a long-term treatment, while the use of the alkylating agent temozolomide should be limited to a maximum of 24 months.

References

1 Daddi N, Ferolla P, Urbani M, Semeraro A, Avenia N, Ribacchi R, Puma F, Daddi G: Surgical treatment of neuroendocrine tumors of the lung. Eur J Cardiothorac Surg 2004;26:813–817.

2 Öberg K, Hellman P, Ferolla P, Papotti M, ESMO Guidelines Working Group: Neuroendocrine bronchial and thymic tumors: ESMO clinical practice guidelines for diagnosis, treatment and follow-up. Ann Oncol 2012;23(suppl 7):vii120–123.

3 Ferolla P, Daddi N, Urbani M, et al: Tumorlets, multicentric carcinoids, lymph-nodal metastases, and long-term behavior in bronchial carcinoids. J Thorac Oncol 2009;4:383–387.

4 Phan AT, Oberg K, Choi J, et al: NANETS consensus guideline for the diagnosis and management of neuroendocrine tumors: well-differentiated neuroendocrine tumors of the thorax (includes lung and thymus). Pancreas 2010;39:784–798.

5 Faggiano A, Ferolla P, Grimaldi F, Campana D, Manzoni M, Davì MV, Bianchi A, Valcavi R, Papini E, Giuffrida D, Ferone D, Fanciulli G, Arnaldi G, Franchi GM, Francia G, Fasola G, Crinò L, Pontecorvi A, Tomassetti P, Colao A: Natural history of gastro-entero-pancreatic and thoracic neuroendocrine tumors – data from a large prospective and retrospective Italian epidemiological study: the NET management study. J Endocrinol Invest 2012;35: 817–823.

6 O'Dorisio TM, Phan AT, Langdon RM, et al: Relief of bowel-related symptoms with telotristat etiprate in octreotide refractory carcinoid syndrome: preliminary results of a double-blind, placebo-controlled multicenter study (abstract). J Clin Oncol 2012; 30(suppl):4085.

7 Rinke A, Müller HH, Schade-Brittinger C, et al: Placebo-controlled, double-blind, prospective, randomized study on the effect of octreotide LAR in the control of tumor growth in patients with metastatic neuroendocrine midgut tumors: a report from the PROMID Study Group. J Clin Oncol 2009;27:4656–4663.

8 Caplin M, Ruszniewski P, Pavel M, et al: A randomized, double-blind, placebo-controlled study of lanreotide antiproliferative response in patients with gastroenteropancreatic neuroendocrine tumors (CLARINET). Paper presented at the European Cancer Congress, Amsterdam, September 27 to October 1, 2013.

9 Pavel ME, Hainsworth JD, Baudin E, et al: Everolimus plus octreotide long-acting repeatable for the treatment of advanced neuroendocrine tumours associated with carcinoid syndrome (RADIANT-2): a randomised, placebo-controlled, phase 3 study. Lancet 2011;378:2005–2012.

10 Fazio N, Granberg D, Grossman A, Saletan S, Klimovsky J, Panneerselvam A, Wolin EM: Everolimus plus octreotide long-acting repeatable in patients with advanced lung neuroendocrine tumors: analysis of the phase 3, randomized, placebo-controlled RADIANT-2 study. Chest 2013;143:955–962.

11 van Essen M, Krenning EP, Bakker WH, et al: Peptide receptor radionuclide therapy with ^{177}Lu-octreotate in patients with foregut carcinoid tumours of bronchial, gastric and thymic origin. Eur J Nucl Med Mol Imaging 2007;34:1219–1227.

12 Ekeblad S, Sundin A, Janson ET, Welin S, Granberg D, Kindmark H, Dunder K, Kozlovacki G, Orlefors H, Sigurd M, Oberg K, Eriksson B, Skogseid B: Temozolomide as monotherapy is effective in treatment of advanced malignant neuroendocrine tumors. Clin Cancer Res 2007;13:2986–2991.

13 Crona J, Fanola I, Lindholm DP, Antonodimitrakis P, Öberg K, Eriksson B, Granberg D: Effect of temozolomide in patients with metastatic bronchial carcinoids. Neuroendocrinology 2013;98:151–155.

14 Pavel M, Grossman A, Arnold R, et al: ENETS consensus guidelines for the management of brain, cardiac and ovarian metastases from neuroendocrine tumors. Neuroendocrinology 2010;91:326–332.

Piero Ferolla
Multidisciplinary Group for Diagnosis and Therapy of Neuroendocrine Tumors
ENETS Center of Excellence, Umbria Regional Cancer Network
via E. Dal Pozzo, IT–06126 Perugia (Italy)
E-Mail pferolla@alice.it

Papotti M, de Herder WW (eds): Neuroendocrine Tumors: A Multidisciplinary Approach.
Front Horm Res. Basel, Karger, 2015, vol 44, pp 198–215 (DOI: 10.1159/000402936)

Peptide Receptor Radionuclide Therapy of Neuroendocrine Tumors

Lisa Bodei[a] • Mark Kidd[b] • Vikas Prasad[c] • Irvin M. Modlin[b]

[a]Division of Nuclear Medicine, European Institute of Oncology, Milan, Italy; [b]Department of Gastroenterological Surgery, Yale School of Medicine, New Haven, Conn., USA; [c]Department of Nuclear Medicine, Campus Virchow-Klinikum, Charité University Hospital, Berlin, Germany

Abstract

Peptide receptor radionuclide therapy (PRRT) has been a well-accepted and effective therapeutic modality for inoperable or metastatic gastroenteropancreatic, bronchopulmonary and other neuroendocrine tumors for almost 2 decades. In general, PRRT is well tolerated with moderate toxicity in the majority of patients if the necessary precautions, appropriate dosage and coadministration of amino acids are undertaken. The two most commonly used radiopeptides, ^{90}Y-octreotide and ^{177}Lu-octreotate, produce significant objective response rates, with impact on progression-free survival and overall survival. In addition, biochemical and symptomatic responses are commonly observed. A key issue is the need to establish randomized controlled trials to standardize the treatment and facilitate comparison with other therapeutic strategies available.

Neuroendocrine tumors (NETs) are generally regarded as slow-growing tumors, but can exhibit highly aggressive behavior in some instances [1]. The majority of NETs are located in the gastroenteropancreatic (GEP) tract and in the bronchopulmonary system [2]. GEP-NETs were previously considered a rare disease, but it is now apparent that both their incidence (3.65/100,000/year) and prevalence (35/100,000) is increasing [3, 4]. The tumors may present either with symptoms related to excessive and often paroxysmal peptide and amine secretion or, if nonfunctional, with symptoms based upon local effects (mass, obstruction or bleeding) [2]. In many instances, the diagnosis is only established when the tumors have metastasized and curative treatments are no longer possible. Late diagnosis occurs even in functioning tumors since, despite the presence of a distinct clinical syndrome, symptoms are frequently misattributed to other prosaic diseases or afflictions (allergy, menopause, asthma, anxiety, psychological) [5]. Extension beyond the primary lesion usually involves mesenteric lymph nodes and local tissues, but distant metastasis to the liver is the most common site with advanced disease being evident in the bone and brain [6]. As a consequence, a large component of NET treatment involves the management of hepatic metastases [7].

Key issues involved in the development of an optimal management strategy include the precise type of tumor, the grade and stage of the lesion, and the overall condition of the patient. Ideally, removal of the primary tumor should be initially undertaken to preclude local invasion. Thereafter, appropriate strategies should be introduced for the management of residual disease depending upon location and extent. Surgery remains the only option with the potential to cure, but is rarely effective given that metastatic disease is often present at diagnosis and 'real' R0 resections are less common than previously thought [8, 9]. Since there exists a paucity of rigorous prospective randomized trials to support a clearly defined therapeutic strategy, in most cases management is usually determined by consensus discussion (tumor board), based on literature experience and subject to the local institution's particular bias. Although a variety of management guidelines have been developed based upon consensus conferences, they vary in detail and precise application from country to country [7]. In principle, however, the choice of therapy depends on the primary therapeutic aim for a particular individual, which may range from an attempt at complete surgical eradication of the disease to the amelioration of symptoms. For practical clinical purposes, most therapy is deployed with the objectives of diminishing the size of metastatic lesions, reducing metastatic growth, and ameliorating symptoms [10]. To achieve these goals, a diverse variety of therapeutic strategies have been developed (fig. 1). The surgical options include resection of the primary, hepatic metastasis resection, radiofrequency ablation and, in some cases, hepatic transplantation [11]. Interventional radiology techniques include embolization of hepatic metastases (with or without cytotoxic agents) or the use of radioactive microspheres. Medical therapy ranges from the deployment of bioactive agents, such as somatostatin analogs or interferon, to standard chemotherapy. More recently, a variety of novel molecular targeted agents, including everolimus, sunitinib and bevacizumab, have been used with marginal efficacy [12]. Of interest has been the development of targeted radiotherapy using a variety of different isotopes, including indium-111 (^{111}In), yttrium-90 (^{90}Y) and lutetium-177 (^{177}Lu) [13]. The latter therapeutic strategy, delivered by intravenous infusion, has been designated peptide receptor radionuclide therapy (PRRT).

PRRT has been utilized for almost 2 decades and is an established effective therapeutic modality in the treatment of inoperable or metastatic GEP, bronchopulmonary and other NETs. The two most commonly used radiopeptides, ^{90}Y-octreotide and ^{177}Lu-octreotate, produce objective response rates of 15–35% [13–18]. In addition to tumor shrinkage, biochemical and symptomatic responses are commonly observed [19]. Of particular relevance is the outcome in terms of both progression-free survival (PFS) and overall survival, which compare favorably with somatostatin analogs, chemotherapy and new, 'targeted', therapies such as everolimus and sunitinib [20, 21]. It

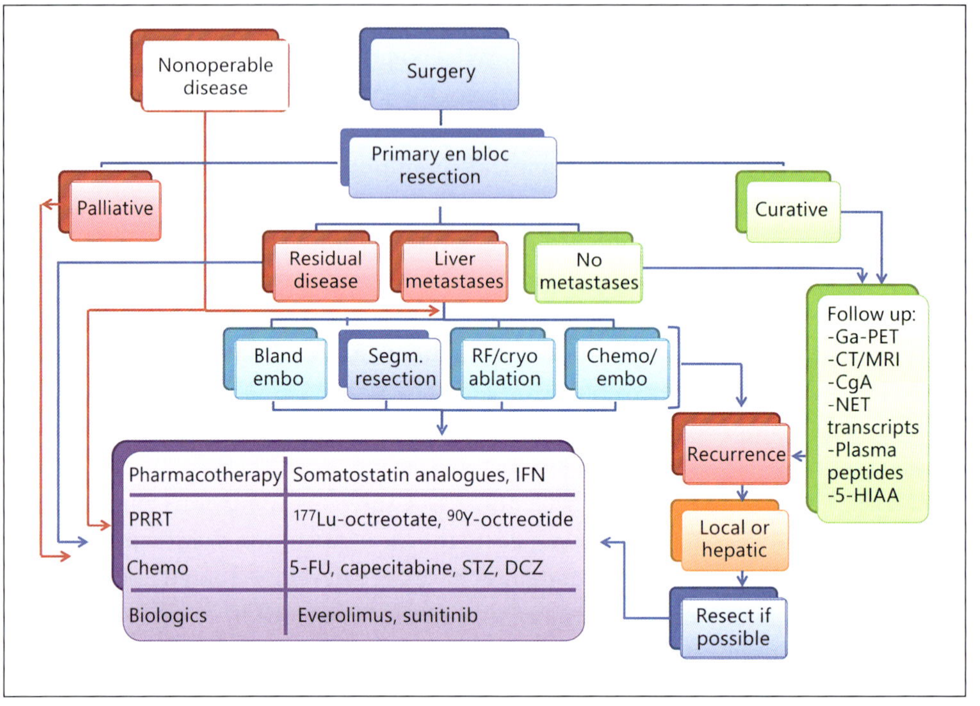

Fig. 1. Therapeutic algorithm for metastatic neuroendocrine neoplasms. CgA = Chromogranin A; chemo = chemotherapy; embo = embolization; Ga-PET = positron emission tomography with ^{68}Ga-peptides; RF = radiofrequency; STZ = streptozotocin; DCZ = dacarbazine.

is noteworthy that in the latter two novel therapies, the presence of the target in a particular tumor is not clinically identified prior to initiation of therapy [4]. Only radioisotope-based somatostatin receptor (SSTR) therapy (PRRT) implies the identification and quantification of the target (SSTR) prior to the administration of treatment [22].

In general, PRRT is well tolerated with only low to moderate toxicity in the majority of cases if the necessary precautions (e.g. coadministration of amino acids) are undertaken [13, 21]. The critical targets of long-term toxicity are the kidneys and bone marrow. There is a loss of renal function (grade 3–4 toxicity after ^{90}Y-peptides 3–9%, grade 4 toxicity after ^{177}Lu-peptides 0.4%). Reduced bone marrow reserve may occur and, very infrequently (1–2%), myelodysplastic syndrome (MDS) and occasionally leukemia have been sporadically reported [13, 14, 16, 21].

Historical Overview

PRRT was first used in 1994 and represented a logical step from the development of the isotopic diagnostic technique for in vivo localization of NETs. This technique used the radiolabeled SSA [^{111}In-DTPA^0-D-Phe^1]-octreotide or ^{111}In-pentetreotide. Using the same principle, but increasing the radionuclide activity (high-dose ^{111}In-pentetreotide), allowed transformation of a diagnostic strategy into a therapeutic modality. Partial remissions were, however, rare [13, 23]. As a consequence of these disappointing initial results, isotopes with higher energy and longer range, such as the pure β-emitter ^{90}Y, were evaluated. The β-particles emitted by ^{90}Y (maximum energy $E_{\beta max}$ 2.27 MeV, penetration range $R_{\beta max}$ 11 mm, half-life $T_{1/2}$ 64 h) allow for a simultaneous direct killing of somatostatin receptor-positive cells and a cross-fire effect that targeted adjacent receptor negative tumor cells. To further facilitate efficacy, a new analog, Tyr^3-octreotide, with a similar pattern of affinity for somatostatin receptors, was developed at the University of Basel. The advantages of this analog included its high hydrophilia, ease of labeling with ^{111}In and ^{90}Y, and tight binding to the bifunctional chelator DOTA (1,4,7,10-tetra-azacyclododecane-N,N',N",N"'-tetra-acetic acid) [24]. [^{90}Y-DOTA^0,Tyr^3]-octreotide, ^{90}Y-DOTATOC or ^{90}Y-octreotide was initially used in the treatment of metastatic NETs in 1996 [25]. The encouraging symptomatic and objective response following several cycles of ^{90}Y-octreotide therapy culminated in the establishment of further studies to examine the potential of PRRT in NET disease [16]. Based upon these positive clinical experiences, ^{90}Y-octreotide became the most widely used radiopeptide in the first decade of PRRT experience [17, 26, 27]. In 2000, the subsequent development of a new analog, octreotate (Tyr^3, Thr^8-octreotide), with 6- to 9-fold higher affinity for somatostatin receptor (SSR)2 engendered alterations in clinical practice. The chelated analog [DOTA]^0-Tyr^3-octreotate or DOTATATE was labeled with the β-γ-emitter ^{177}Lu ($E_{\beta max}$ 0.49 MeV, $R_{\beta max}$ 2 mm, $T_{1/2}$ 6.7 days) and investigated in several clinical phase I and II studies [15, 20, 28, 29]. Due to its enhanced efficacy and greater manageability, ^{177}Lu-octreotate has subsequently become one of the most frequently used radiopeptides for PRRT. ^{177}Lu-octreotate is currently being evaluated in a randomized phase III registration trial in small bowel NETs (www.netter-1.com).

Technique

The rationale for PRRT relies on amplified SSTR expression on the cell membrane of neuroendocrine tumor cells and the ability of a suitable radiolabeled peptide to bind predominantly to the SSTR2. The subsequent radiopeptide internalization, per normal receptor recycling dynamics, thereafter delivers the radioactivity directly into the tumor cell interior (fig. 2).

Systemic Administration

Standard clinical protocols of PRRT consist of the systemic administration of a radiolabeled SSA, fractionated in sequential cycles (usually 4–5), every 6–9 weeks, until the intended total amount of radioactivity has been delivered. The latter value depends on the limitations imposed by the level of renal, and to a lesser extent bone marrow

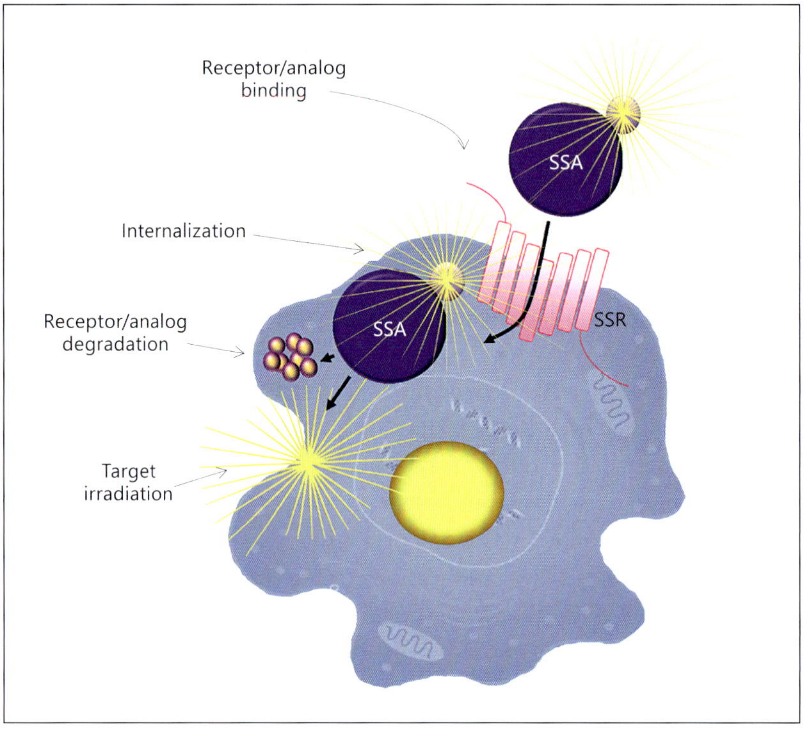

Fig. 2. Strategy and mechanism of action of PRRT. The somatostatin analog is linked to the isotope through a specific chelator. This radioanalog complex binds to the membrane somatostatin receptor and is internalized. Thus, radioactivity is transported into the intracellular receptor recycling compartment of the NET cell, where it exerts its action in proximity to the nucleus. SSA = Somatostatin analog.

irradiation. Coadministration of positively charged amino acids (lysine or arginine) is utilized to reduce the renal radioactivity dose through competitive inhibition of the proximal tubular reabsorption of the radiopeptide [14].

Intra-Arterial Administration

Since radiopeptides exhibit a high first-pass effect during intra-arterial administration and in many cases a higher uptake than with an intravenous route, PRRT with either ^{90}Y- or ^{177}Lu-DOTATOC has been tested intra-arterially in the management of hepatic metastases (G1/G2 GEP NETs not amenable to surgery). This strategy was noted to produce objective (partial + complete) responses in 60% [30, 31].

Peptide Receptor Radionuclide Therapy Results

The initial PRRT studies were undertaken in individuals with advanced disease in which all other treatment modalities had failed. Despite the severity of the disease, PRRT effectiveness led to confidence in its use in earlier phases of the disease. This

Table 1. Clinical GEP neuroendocrine neoplasm PRRT results derived from the different schedules utilized

Schedule	Reference	Patients, n	CR, %	PR, %	Progression at baseline, %	Response criteria	Outcome (PFS or TTP)
^{90}Y-octreotide							
7.4 GBq/m^2 in 4 cycles	[37]	36	4	20	100	WHO	n.a.
2.96–5.55 GBq/cycle ×2	[57]	21	0	28	n.a.	WHO	TTP 10 months
0.93–2.78 GB/m^2/cycle	[38]	58	0	9	81	SWOG	TTP 29 months
4.4 GBq/cycle ×3	[17]	90	0	4	100	SWOG	PFS 16 months
1–10 cycles (median 2), various activity	[16]	821	0.2	38	n.a.	RECIST	n.a.
^{177}Lu-octreotate							
27.8–29.6 GBq in 3–4 cycles	[20]	310	2	28	43	SWOG	PFS 33 months
3.7–29.2 GBq in 4–6 cycles of 3.7–7.4 GBq	[15]	39	3	31	76	RECIST	TTP 36 months

CR = Complete response; PR = partial response; TTP = time to progression; n.a. = not assessed.

reflected the recognition that radiopeptides exhibited a greater efficacy with decreased tumor burden. This observation was based upon a number of factors, including dosage to tumor volume ratio and the specific biological features of the neoplasm. Thus, it had become apparent that more advanced tumors were less responsive to treatment as a progression was associated with lower SSTR expression and increased genetic mutations, such as in the p53 gene [32]. In addition, studies have demonstrated that tumor load, especially in the liver, as well as grading and performance status, were relevant parameters for predicting the optimal PRRT outcome. Evaluation of such indices of prognosis and outcome concluded that treatment in a phase of 'early' progression rather than a 'wait and see' approach was advantageous [29]. Although it is apparent that PRRT treatment in advanced-stage disease is feasible, it is clear that it is substantially less effective. A further consideration is the type of disease being treated. Thus, pancreatic NETs are frequently more responsive to PRRT therapy compared to other types of NETs, although they tend to relapse rapidly [18] (table 1).

PRRT with ^{90}Y-Peptides

In the first decade of PRRT, ^{90}Y-octreotide was the most commonly used radiopeptide. The published results of the therapy were generated from individual phase I–II studies performed independently by a variety of centers. Current isotope administration protocols have developed administration schedules based upon the injection of standard radioactivities that were established using previous dose escalation studies, as well as 'individual' clinical experience. This resulted in substantial differences among individual protocols in respect of activities, which may be fixed or related to body weight or surface area, the number of cycles and time intervals between cycles. As a consequence, inclusion criteria and specific treatment schemes remain nonstandardized. A rigorous direct comparison between individual studies is, therefore, currently not feasible. Nevertheless, the aggregate of reported studies indicate that objective responses are apparent in up to 38% [13, 15, 16, 20, 33–36].

In a study carried out at Basel University, 39 NET patients (mostly of GEP origin) received four cycles of ^{90}Y-octreotide, with a cumulative activity of 7.4 GBq. Objective responses (WHO criteria) were identified in 23% (n = 9), with a complete remission in 2 patients, a partial response in 7 and a disease stabilization in 27. Pancreatic NETs (n = 13) exhibited a better objective response (38% partial + complete) than other tumors in other locations. Significant amelioration of related symptoms was noted in the majority (63%) of patients. In this series, 3 patients with progressive bronchial tumors were included. All demonstrated disease stabilization after PRRT [37].

In a multicenter phase I study carried out in Rotterdam, Louvain and Tampa, 60 patients with GEP-NETs were treated with four cycles of 0.9, 1.8, 2.8, 3.7, 4.6 and 5.5 GBq/m^2 of ^{90}Y-octreotide administered at 6- to 9-week intervals. The initial assessment of 32 evaluable patients indicated that objective responses (SWOG criteria) were evident. These constituted approximately 9% partial responses and 9% minor responses [27]. In a reanalysis of the 58 assessable patients (treated with cumulative activities of 1.7–32.8 GBq), a 57% clinical benefit, including stabilization and minor responses (SWOG criteria) was observed. Objective responses were described in 5%. The observed overall survival was 37 months (median) and PFS was 29 months. These results were considered to be comparable to the 12-month overall survival of a historical group treated with ^{111}In-pentetreotide [23]. Characteristically, patients stable at baseline had a better overall survival than those who were progressive at baseline. The extent of disease at baseline was also a predictive factor for survival [38].

The results of two phase I–II studies and a retrospective evaluation in 141 patients were published by the Milan group in 2004. Somatostatin receptor-positive tumors, mainly GEP- and bronchial tract NETs were treated with a cumulative activity of 7.4–26.4 GBq of ^{90}Y-octreotide, divided into 2–16 cycles, administered 4–6 weeks apart. The objective response rate was 26%, including partial and complete responses (SWOG criteria). Disease stabilization was observed in 55% and progression was noted in 18%. The mean duration of response ranged from 2 to 59 months (median 18). The majority who responded had GEP-NETs (3 gastric, 26 pancreatic, 27 small intestinal, 2 rectal). Pancreatic tumors showed higher responses. Individuals who were stable at baseline exhibited a better outcome (partial and complete responses in 32%) than individuals with progressive disease (partial and complete responses in 24%) [26].

In 2010, a multicenter study evaluated the role of ^{90}Y-octreotide in 90 patients with symptomatic, metastatic 'carcinoids' (small bowel NETs). The data identified stabilization of tumor response (SWOG criteria) in 74%, as well as a durable amelioration of symptoms related to the tumor mass and the hypersecretion of bioactive amines [17]. This trial reported a PFS of 16 months and an overall survival of 27 months.

More recently, the Basel group published the results of an open-label phase II trial in 1,109 patients treated with ^{90}Y-octreotide, divided into multiple cycles of 3.7 GBq/m^2 each. Objective morphologic responses (RECIST criteria) were observed in 378 (34.1%), biochemical responses in 172 (15.5%) and symptomatic responses in 329 (29.7%). In this series, the NET groups were 265 small bowel, 342 pancreatic tumors and 84 bronchial. The rates of objective response were 26.8, 47 and 28.6%, respectively. A longer survival was correlated with tumor and symptomatic response. The best predictor of survival was tumor uptake at baseline determined by OctreoScan [16].

Experience has also been obtained from studies with ^{90}Y-DOTATATE. Sixty patients with histologically proven GEP-NETs were treated with 4.1–16.2 GBq per patient (mean 3.7 GBq per therapy) in 1–3 cycles. Six months after PRRT completion, a partial response was evident in 13 patients (23%), while the remaining had stable disease (77%). The median PFS was 17 months and the median overall survival was 22 months. Hematological toxicity WHO grade 3 and 4 was noted during therapy in 10%, which persisted in 5%. After 24 months of follow-up, renal toxicity grade 2 was seen in 7 (11.6%) and the authors emphasized the need for careful renal monitoring [33].

PRRT with ^{177}Lu-Peptides

The radiopeptide DOTATATE labeled with ^{177}Lu, ^{177}Lu-DOTATATE or ^{177}Lu-octreotate has been widely used since its introduction in 2000. This reflects its higher affinity for SSR2, its easier manageability, a lower dosimetric burden in the kidney, and the possibility of obtaining scintigraphic images and dosimetric studies at the same time, given the gamma photon coemission of ^{177}Lu. Despite the absence of rigorous studies demonstrating a significant superiority over ^{90}Y-peptides, it is currently the most commonly used radiopeptide for PRRT (fig. 3, 4). The initial clinical trials were undertaken at Erasmus University, Rotterdam. Individual phase II studies, where the cumulative activity of 22.2–29.6 GBq of ^{177}Lu-octreotate was administered in four intended cycles of 7.4 Gbq each, culminated in the evaluation of a series of 504 patients, 310 of which were considered for efficacy. Complete and partial remissions occurred in 2 and 28%, with minor responses in 16% and stabilization in 35%, respectively (SWOG criteria). The median overall survival was >48 months and a median PFS of 33 months was calculated. A 'direct comparison' with data obtained from similar patients (published patient series) identified an 'estimated' 40- to 72-month survival benefit for PRRT-treated individuals. Although these data are not derived from robust/rigorous prospective randomized phase III trials, this survival difference likely reflects a real impact of PRRT as a therapeutic modality. It seems probable that such data can be viewed as favorable compared to other treatments, such as chemotherapy, both from the cost/benefit and the tolerability point of view [20]. Better responses were more frequent in individuals with a high uptake on baseline ^{111}In-pentetreotide scintigraphy and those with limited liver involvement. Conversely, progression was significantly more frequent in those with a low performance score and extensive

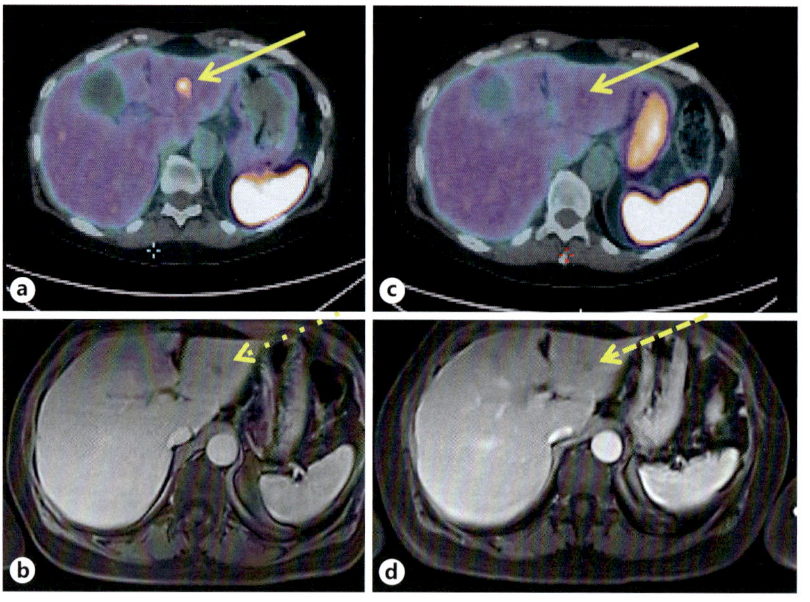

Fig. 3. The efficacy of ^{177}Lu-DOTATATE- PRRT in the treatment of a G2 ileal NET with liver metastases. **a** PET/CT with ^{68}Ga-DOTATOC, fused axial image (arrow). At baseline, the lesion in the II segment of the liver is evident at both functional and morphologic imaging. **b** T1 contrast-enhanced MRI, axial image (dotted arrow). **c** After completion of PRRT, the lesion is only very faintly visible on ^{68}Ga-DOTATOC (arrow). **d** A residual lesion is however still evident on MRI (dashed arrow).

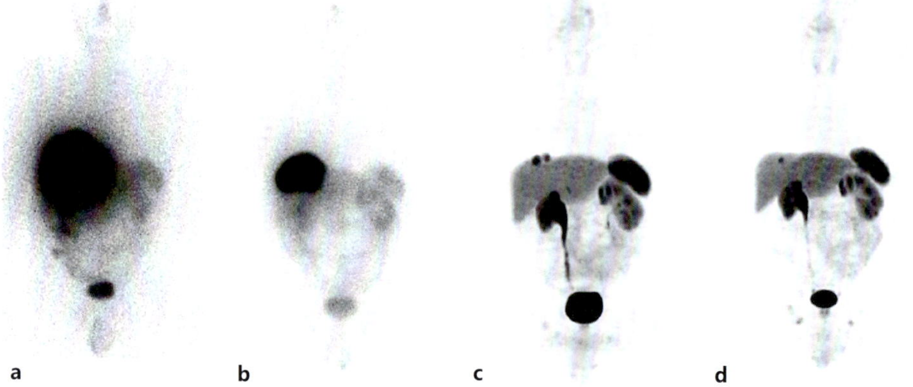

a b c d

Fig. 4. Response to ^{177}Lu-DOTATATE – PRRT in a rectal NET with a massive (21.5-cm diameter) inoperable right lobe liver metastasis. Previous therapy included recto-sigmoid resection and chemotherapy with capecitabine. **a** Anterior view, whole-body scan after the first ^{177}Lu-DOTATATE treatment. **b** Whole-body image, anterior view at the completion of 28.5 GBq of ^{177}Lu-DOTATATE. Post-therapy CT scan demonstrates tumor shrinkage (12.5-cm diameter). **c** ^{68}Ga-DOTATOC MIP image subsequent to 3 cycles of transarterial embolization. The post-treatment scan with ^{68}Ga-DOTATOC shows further response, corresponding to a diameter of 7.5-cm at CT. **d** MIP image after an additional course of PRRT with ^{177}Lu-DOTATATE (cumulative activity 43 GBq), tumor shrinkage to a diameter of 1.5 cm at CT occurred and hepatic resection of the residual was undertaken.

Table 2. Symptom control after PRRT

Patients, n	Symptom	Symptomatic response, n (%)	Median duration of response, weeks	Reference
^{90}Y-octreotide				
479	Carcinoid-related	143 (29.9)	–	[16]
47	Functional pancreatic NETs	7 (14.9)	–	
63	Flush	33 (51)	9.7	[17]
65	Diarrhea	38 (60)	13.8	
14	Flush	9 (64.3)	–	[37]
14	Diarrhea	6 (42.9)	–	
^{177}Lu-octreotate				
111	Diarrhea	74 (67)	–	[19]
10	Uncontrolled symptoms	7 (70)	–	[45]

disease at enrolment. Categorization of objective responses identified that pancreatic NETs tended to respond better than other GEP-NETs, and that functioning tumors, e.g. pancreatic gastrinomas, tended to relapse after a shorter interval (median time-to-progression 20 months vs. >36 in the remaining GEP-NETs) [18].

^{177}Lu-octreotate treatment, in addition, was also associated with a significant improvement in the global health/quality of life (QoL) on various symptom scales, particularly fatigue, insomnia and pain, as well as emotional and social functions. The effect was more frequent in individuals with tumor regression, but paradoxically was also evident in those with progressive disease [39]. Of note was the fact that there was no significant decrease in QoL in those who were asymptomatic prior to therapy (table 2) [19].

The results of a phase I–II escalation dose study aimed at defining the toxicity and efficacy of ^{177}Lu-octreotate were published in 2011 [15]. A cohort (n = 51) with unresectable/metastatic NETs, mainly of GEP origin, were divided into two dosage groups. One group received escalating activities, from 3.7–5.18 GBq and the second from 5.18–7.4 GBq, with dosimetry-based cumulative activities up to 29 GBq. Partial and complete responses were observed in 15 patients (32.6%). The median time-to-progression was 36 months, with an overall survival of 68% at 36 months. Nonresponders and patients with extensive tumor involvement had a lower survival [15]. A recent prospective phase II study used ^{177}Lu-octreotate and included a cohort (n = 52) with advanced well/moderately differentiated pancreatic NETs. Based on the existence of risk factors for renal toxicity, such as hypertension or diabetes (both of which reduce tolerance to the administered radiopeptides), patients were divided into two groups and treated with different levels of activity – full dose (21–28 GBq) compared to a reduced dose (11–20 GBq), respectively. Both regimens resulted in antitumor activity. However, PFS was not reached at the time of the analysis in the cohort treated with the full-dose regimen, while it was 20 months in those treated with reduced doses. This suggests the full-dose scheme should be recommended whenever possible [35]. A similar GEP-NETs study that differentiated the dosage according to risk factors for toxicity failed to identify significant differences in PFS among the two dosage groups [40].

A recent retrospective evaluation of a cohort with metastatic pancreatic NETs (n = 68, 52% at their first systemic treatment) treated with ^{177}Lu-octreotate (4 intended cycles, 8 GBq each, at 3-month intervals), 68% of whom were in progression at enrolment, showed partial responses in 60% with a median PFS of 34 months. Multivariate analysis indicated that G1 tumors were associated with a longer PFS, while reduced performance status (KPS ≤70), a high liver burden (≥25% of volume) and increased neuron-specific enolase (NSE; >15 ng/ml) were associated with a poorer prognosis [36]. To better define the predictors of long-term outcome, the same group performed a multivariate analysis in a cohort of metastatic GEP-NET patients (n = 74) who had previously undergone PRRT with ^{177}Lu-octreotate (4 cycles, 7.9 GBq each, at 3-month intervals). A Ki-67 index >10%, a Karnofsky performance status ≤70, a tumor burden in the liver ≥25% and a baseline NSE >15 ng/ml were independent predictors of shorter survival. However, even patients with Ki-67 >10% benefited from PRRT, with a median PFS of 19 months as opposed to 26 months for the entire cohort [29].

A phase II study has been performed in individuals with 'poorly responding' tumors, including bronchial and gastric NECs. Patients were treated with standard 22.2–29.6 GBq activities. Despite the limited numbers, the observed objective response (SWOG criteria) was comparable to GEP-NETs. The bronchopulmonary NET results were 5 partial responses, 1 minor response and 2 stabilizations in 9 patients. In the gastric tumor group there was 1 complete response, 1 minor response and 2 stabilizations (5 patients). The thymic tumor numbers were too small to draw any conclusions. The authors concluded that, contrary to previous findings, PRRT was as effective in bronchial and gastric NECs as in GEP-NETs [41].

Salvage Therapy

A recent study by the Rotterdam group described the use of a salvage protocol with ^{177}Lu-octreotate. Patients in progression were enrolled after an initial response to PRRT with ^{177}Lu-octreotate, administered using standard cumulative activities (22.2–29.6 GBq). In this series, 32 patients with bronchial or GEP-NETs received two additional cycles of ^{177}Lu-octreotate, with a cumulative activity of 15 GBq. Objective responses occurred in 8 patients (2 partial and 6 minor responses), while stabilization was identified in a further 8. The median time-to-progression was 17 months. Both the response rates and duration over time were lower than during the initial treatment. Nevertheless, 'salvage therapy' was well tolerated by the majority and has been proposed as a viable option for this category of patient [42].

Combination Therapy

In keeping with recent trends in oncology, PRRT experience has focused on combinations of therapy. In particular, the use of ^{177}Lu-octreotate, with the radio-sensitizer chemotherapy agent capecitabine, has been evaluated. An initial study in a small group (n = 7) of progressive GEP-NETs using four cycles of standard activity of ^{177}Lu-octreotate followed by capecitabine (1,650 mg/m^2) for 2 weeks was undertaken with encouraging results [43]. No severe toxicity, particularly hand-foot syndrome or hematological/renal-associated toxicity was evident. Objective responses were observed. A recent phase II study of progressive NETs (n = 35) treated with 4 cycles of 7.8 GBq of ^{177}Lu-octreotate followed by capecitabine, 1,650 mg/m^2 (2 weeks) produced a 24% objective response with 70% stable disease and 6% progression without adjunctive toxicity (RECIST criteria) [44].

A new version of the chemoradiotherapy protocol utilizing 5-fluorouracyl (5-FU) as opposed to its oral prodrug capecitabine has been investigated. A retrospective analysis of 68 patients with progressive disease or uncontrollable symptoms from NETs showed that the combination strategy (median cumulative activity of ^{177}Lu-octreotate 31 GBq and 200 mg/m^2/24 h 5-FU, from 4 days before to 3 weeks after PRRT cycle 2–4) resulted in a 70% benefit for at least 6 months for symptomatic patients and a 68% diseased control rate in progressive disease. Nonpancreatic primary site, dominant liver metastases, lesions <5 cm and the use of 5-FU were associated with an objective response [45].

Bone Metastases

The potential efficacy of PRRT in bone metastases has been demonstrated in a retrospective series (n = 68) treated with ^{177}Lu-octreotate (4 intended cycles, 8.1 GBq each, at 3-month intervals; followed up for a median of 48 months). The observed objective response rate was comparable to other studies of PRRT in GEP-NETs, with 2.9 and 33.8% of complete and partial responses, respectively. The median PFS was 35 months. Individuals with PRRT-responsive bone metastases exhibited longer overall survivals (median 56 vs. 39 months). In this patient group, high NSE values and Ki-67 >10% were associated with a shorter overall survival. Of note, however, was the conclusion that that Karnofsky performance status and multifocal of bone spread did not limit the efficacy of PRRT [46].

Combinations of ^{90}Y- and ^{177}Lu-Peptides

Protocols combining both ^{177}Lu- and ^{90}Y-peptides have been undertaken to take advantage of the different physical properties of each radionuclide. Theoretically, the combination of the two radioisotopes should allow simultaneous treatment of both large lesions (the higher energy and penetration range of the particles emitted by ^{90}Y) and small lesions (lower energy and penetration range of ^{177}Lu). Combination-isotope PRRT was performed in a Danish cohort of 69 patients treated in Basel. Complete responses were noted in 5 cases (7.4%), partial remissions in 11 (16.2%) and stabilization in 42 (61.8%). The median PFS was 29 months. Pancreatic NETs responded better than small bowel tumors [34]. This strategy, however, remains to be validated in a larger series. It should be noted that these studies included empirically designed ^{177}Lu and ^{90}Y treatment protocols rather than individualized dosimetric analyses [47, 48].

Table 3. Long-term PRRT toxicity in GEP neuroendocrine neoplasms

Patients, n	Follow-up, months	Renal toxicity	MDS	Leukemia	Reference
^{90}Y-octreotide					
40	19	10% grade 1	0	0	[57]
39	6	3% grade 2	0	0	[37]
58	18	3% grade 4	1	0	[38]
1,109	23	9.2% grade 3/4	1	1	[16]
^{177}Lu-octreotate					
504	19	0.4% grade 4	3	0	[20]
51	29	24% grade 1	0	0	[15]
74	21	1.3% grade 3/4	3	0	[49, 60]

PRRT Safety Profile

Renal

Two decades of follow-up have provided information that adverse events are mild-to-modest and it is accepted that both ^{90}Y- and ^{177}Lu-peptides are generally well tolerated. Acute side effects are usually mild and probably reflect the coadministration of amino acids (including nausea and, rarely, emesis), which have been used to offset renal damage. Other adverse events are directly related to the radiopeptide and include fatigue (common) and the exacerbation of an endocrine syndrome. Although the latter occurs infrequently, it may happen during the treatment of functional tumors. Chronic and permanent effects in the kidneys and the bone marrow are generally mild if the necessary precautions, such as dosage fractionation and attention to specific risk factors (e.g. hypertension or previous nephro- or myelotoxic chemotherapy regimens) are undertaken [14, 16, 34, 37, 49] (table 3). In this respect, appropriate dosimetry allows the delivery of elevated absorbed doses to the tumor, with relative sparing of healthy organs (kidneys, bone marrow).

Despite the very modest reported toxicity problems, concerns have been raised regarding PRRT given the general medical anxiety that is associated with the use of irradiation as a therapeutic modality. Renal irradiation is associated with reabsorption of the radiopeptides at the site of the proximal convoluted tubules, with a subsequent accumulation in the renal interstitium, where the radioactivity exerts its action. Studies with external radiotherapy indicate a threshold of tolerance in the range of 23–27 Gy. This dose range calculation will likely be superseded by the recently introduced bio-effective dose (BED) calculation. The latter is accurate for predicting toxicity, irrespective of the modality of delivery. This parameter identifies that the renal threshold for toxicity after PRRT is approximately 40 Gy [50, 51].

Renal toxicity is significantly decreased when positively charged amino acids, such as lysine or arginine, are coinfused with the radioisotope. These competitively inhibit radiopeptide reabsorption with a consequent 9–53% reduction in the renal radioactive dosage [52]. Overall, however, a mild loss of renal function does occur, with a median decline in creatinine clearance of 7.3% per year for ^{90}Y-octreotide and 3.8% per year for ^{177}Lu-octreotate [53]. Nevertheless, severe, end-stage renal damage remains rare (sporadic cases are reported in the literature) [13]. Early renal problems reported were mostly associated with the use of ^{90}Y-peptide PRRT, and reflected administration with very high activities in the absence of renal protection [54].

Long-term evaluation has rendered it evident that a higher and more persistent decline in creatinine clearance with the subsequent development of renal toxicity is more likely to occur in the presence of preexisting risk factors, for example long-standing hypertension and/or poorly controlled diabetes. Overall, PRRT with ^{90}Y-peptides is more frequently associated with a reduction of renal function; presumably reflecting the physical characteristics of the specific radioisotope, ^{90}Y. This observation was supported in a long-term evaluation of renal toxicity in a group (n = 28) undergoing PRRT with dosimetric analysis. Of the 23 treated with ^{90}Y-octreotide, a low (28 Gy BED) threshold was observed with risk factors (mainly hypertension and diabetes), in comparison to 40 Gy in the absence of such risk factors [55].

In a retrospective series (n = 1,109) treated with ^{90}Y-octreotide, 103 subjects (9.2%) experienced grade 4–5 permanent renal toxicity [16]. Multivariate regression revealed that the initial kidney uptake was predictive of severe renal toxicity. However, it seems likely that this relatively high incidence was related to the high administered activities per cycle (3.7 GBq/m^2 body surface, namely activities of about 6.4 GBq per cycle in a standard male) and that individuals with preexisting impairment of renal function were not excluded from PRRT. A further consideration is that routine infusion of protective amino acids was not employed in the earlier component of the study [54].

Recently, the results of an analysis of long-term tolerability of PRRT (n = 807) treated with ^{90}Y-octreotide, ^{177}Lu-octreotate or the combination (Lu 34.4%, Y 44.4%, Lu + Y 19.5%) provided additional PRRT toxicity information and illuminated the role (lack of) of clinical parameters. Nephrotoxicity, transient and persistent, occurred in 279 (34.6%) and was severe in 1.5%. ^{90}Y-peptides or the combination of ^{90}Y/^{177}Lu-peptides showed greater nephrotoxicity than ^{177}Lu-peptides alone. However, only 20–27% of the toxicities could be modeled by clinical parameters. Hypertension and anemia were noted to be the most relevant risk factor. It seems probable that individual susceptibility to toxicity may be more reflective of a genetic predisposal to radiation exposure rather than concomitant clinical disease [56].

An accurate assessment of the glomerular filtration rate, as a measure of renal function (Gates' method), was carried out after PRRT (n = 74) with a median of 21 months (range 12–50) follow-up. The evaluation included potential risk factors, such as diabetes mellitus, hypertension and chemotherapy. Results confirmed an alteration in the glomerular filtration rate, with a relative yearly reduction of 1.8 ± 19%. Sixteen patients experienced a more pronounced reduction (>10 ml/min/year). However, toxicity was only present in 1 of them. None of the clinical factors (see above), including the cumulative administered activity, contributed significantly to the decline of renal function [49].

Hematological

From a hematological point of view, PRRT is generally well tolerated. Severe WHO grade 3 or 4 toxicity occurs in <13% after ^{90}Y-octreotide and in 10% after ^{177}Lu-octreotate. Nevertheless, sporadic cases of MDS or even overt acute leukemia have been reported in 1–2% [14]. Although predicted absorbed doses are lower than the conventional threshold for harm, both acute and permanent bone marrow toxicity remains a cause of concern, particularly if repeated isotope administrations occur [26]. Dose-finding phase I studies indicate that the maximum cumulative administrable activity per cycle of ^{90}Y-octreotide, with renal protection, is 5.18 GBq [57]. An additional important observation derived from dosimetric studies is that hyperfractionation can lower the renal and bone marrow dose [55, 58]. No dose-finding studies have been conducted for ^{177}Lu-octreotate. Investigations employing the dose-limiting toxicity method were abandoned since published data identified that 7.4 GBq could be safely used as a maximum activity per cycle [59]. In a phase I–II study, escalating activities of ^{177}Lu-octreotate up to 7.4 GBq/cycle were undertaken in 51 patients. No major acute or delayed renal or hematological toxicity was observed and the cumulative renal and bone marrow absorbed doses were within the designated safety limits [15]. ^{177}Lu-octreotate was better tolerated than ^{90}Y-octreotide, largely due to the physical characteristics of the two radioisotopes.

In data from a cohort with GEP-NETs (n = 33) treated in a salvage study, toxicity results were encouraging in their relative absence. Thus, retreatment with a median 18 GBq of ^{177}Lu-octreotate (2–4 cycles, up to a median cumulative activity of 44.3 GBq, range 30–84) resulted in no severe nephrotoxicity or MDS during the follow-up (37 ± 16 months from initial PRRT and 23 ± 7 months from the start of salvage PRRT) [60].

An analysis of 203 patients treated with 4 intended cycles of 8 GBq, each at 3-month intervals, included the assessment of risk factors such as the presence of bone metastases, chemotherapy or cumulative administered activity. The incidence of MDS was 1.4%. Myelosuppression was almost invariably reversible and the cumulative administered activity and initial cytopenia were the most important risk factors for myelotoxicity [60].

An analysis of a group (n = 807) treated with ^{90}Y-octreotide, ^{177}Lu-octreotate or the combination showed that MDS occurred in 2.35%. This study also noted that 'classical' risk factors, such as chemotherapy, were only associated with toxicity in 30%. The relevant clinical risk factors were identified as platelet toxicity grade and increased duration of PRRT. This led to the speculation that individual susceptibilities to radiation-associated disease remain to be identified [56].

Recent studies demonstrated that ^{177}Lu-octreotate can be safely utilized even in florid bone metastases, with extreme bone replacement. Significant G3/G4 reversible hematological toxicity occurred in 35% (n = 4) of 11 patients. Toxicity either resolved spontaneously (1 case) or was controlled by support therapy (3 cases). A return to baseline values was obtained in 23 months after completion of PRRT [61].

Finally, the issue of a potential increased toxicity of everolimus, when administered after the completion of PRRT, was addressed in a limited GEP-NET study (n = 24). The group pretreated with PRRT had no significant adjunctive toxicity compared to the naive group. Major events were hyperglycemia (20.8%), fatigue (8.3%), thrombocytopenia (8.3%) and elevated alanine transaminase (8.3%) [62].

References

1 Clark OH, et al: NCCN clinical practice guidelines in oncology: neuroendocrine tumors. J Natl Compr Canc Netw 2009;7:712–747.

2 Modlin IM, et al: Gastroenteropancreatic neuroendocrine tumours. Lancet Oncol 2008;9:61–72.

3 Lawrence B, et al: The epidemiology of gastroenteropancreatic neuroendocrine tumors. Endocrinol Metab Clin North Am 2011;40:1–18.

4 Frilling A, et al: Neuroendocrine tumor disease: an evolving landscape. Endocr Relat Cancer 2012;19: R163–R185.

5 Bodei L, et al: Neuroendocrine tumors; in Aktolun C, Goldsmith SJ (eds): Nuclear Oncology. Philadelphia, Wolters Kluwer, 2015.

6 Mallory GW, et al: Brain carcinoid metastases: outcomes and prognostic factors. J Neurosurg 2013;118: 889–895.

7 Frilling A, et al: Recommendations for management of patients with neuroendocrine liver metastases. Lancet Oncol 2014;15:e8–e21.

8 Pavel M, et al: ENETS consensus guidelines for the management of patients with liver and other distant metastases from neuroendocrine neoplasms of foregut, midgut, hindgut, and unknown primary. Neuroendocrinology 2012;95:157–176.

9 Knigge U, Hansen CP: Surgery for GEP-NETs. Best Pract Res Clin Gastroenterol 2012;26:819–831.

10 Weber HC: Medical treatment of neuroendocrine tumours. Curr Opin Endocrinol Diabetes Obes 2013;20:27–31.

11 Doherty G: Surgical treatment of neuroendocrine tumors (including carcinoid). Curr Opin Endocrinol Diabetes Obes 2013;20:32–36.

12 Stevenson R, Libutti SK, Saif MW: Novel agents in gastroenteropancreatic neuroendocrine tumors. Jop 2013;14:152–154.

13 Kwekkeboom DJ, et al: Overview of results of peptide receptor radionuclide therapy with 3 radiolabeled somatostatin analogs. J Nucl Med 2005; 46(suppl 1):62s–66s.

14 Bodei L, et al: Peptide receptor therapies in neuroendocrine tumors. J Endocrinol Invest 2009;32:360–369.

15 Bodei L, et al: Peptide receptor radionuclide therapy with ^{177}Lu-DOTATATE: the IEO phase I-II study. Eur J Nucl Med Mol Imaging 2011;38:2125–2135.

16 Imhof A, et al: Response, survival, and long-term toxicity after therapy with the radiolabeled somatostatin analogue ^{90}Y-DOTA-TOC in metastasized neuroendocrine cancers. J Clin Oncol 2011;29:2416–2423.

17 Bushnell DL Jr, et al: ^{90}Y-edotreotide for metastatic carcinoid refractory to octreotide. J Clin Oncol 2010; 28:1652–1659.

18 Kwekkeboom DJ, et al: Radiolabeled somatostatin analog [^{177}Lu-DOTA^0, Tyr^3]octreotate in patients with endocrine gastroenteropancreatic tumors. J Clin Oncol 2005;23:2754–2762.

19 Khan S, et al: Quality of life in 265 patients with gastroenteropancreatic or bronchial neuroendocrine tumors treated with [^{177}Lu-DOTA^0, Tyr^3]octreotate. J Nucl Med 2011;52:1361–1368.

20 Kwekkeboom DJ, et al: Treatment with the radiolabeled somatostatin analog [^{177}Lu-DOTA^0, Tyr^3]octreotate: toxicity, efficacy, and survival. J Clin Oncol 2008;26:2124–2130.

21 Kwekkeboom DJ, et al: Somatostatin-receptor-based imaging and therapy of gastroenteropancreatic neuroendocrine tumors. Endocr Relat Cancer 2010;17: R53–R73.

22 Bodei L, et al: The joint IAEA, EANM, and SNMMI practical guidance on peptide receptor radionuclide therapy (PRRNT) in neuroendocrine tumours. Eur J Nucl Med Mol Imaging 2014;40:800–816.

23 Valkema R, et al: Phase I study of peptide receptor radionuclide therapy with [In-DTPA]octreotide: the Rotterdam experience. Semin Nucl Med 2002;32: 110–122.

24 Heppeler A, et al: Receptor targeting for tumor localisation and therapy with radiopeptides. Curr Med Chem 2000;7:971–994.

25 Otte A, et al: Yttrium-90-labelled somatostatin-analogue for cancer treatment. Lancet 1998;351:417–418.

26 Bodei L, et al: Receptor radionuclide therapy with ^{90}Y-[DOTA]^0-Tyr^3-octreotide (^{90}Y-DOTATOC) in neuroendocrine tumours. Eur J Nucl Med Mol Imaging 2004;31:1038–1046.

27 De Jong M, et al: Somatostatin receptor-targeted radionuclide therapy of tumors: preclinical and clinical findings. Semin Nucl Med 2002;32:133–140.

28 Kwekkeboom DJ, et al: [^{177}Lu-DOTA^{0}Tyr^{3}]octreotate: comparison with [^{111}In-DTPA^{0}]octreotide in patients. Eur J Nucl Med 2001;28:1319–1325.
29 Ezziddin S, et al: Predictors of long-term outcome in patients with well-differentiated gastroenteropancreatic neuroendocrine tumors after peptide receptor radionuclide therapy with ^{177}Lu-octreotate. J Nucl Med 2014;55:183–190.
30 Kratochwil C, et al: Intraindividual comparison of selective arterial versus venous ^{68}Ga-DOTATOC PET/CT in patients with gastroenteropancreatic neuroendocrine tumors. Clin Cancer Res 2010;16: 2899–2905.
31 Kratochwil C, et al: Hepatic arterial infusion enhances DOTATOC radiopeptide therapy in patients with neuroendocrine liver metastases. Endocr Relat Cancer 2011;18:595–602.
32 Yachida S, et al: Small cell and large cell neuroendocrine carcinomas of the pancreas are genetically similar and distinct from well-differentiated pancreatic neuroendocrine tumors. Am J Surg Pathol 2012;36: 173–184.
33 Cwikla JB, et al: Efficacy of radionuclide treatment DOTATATE Y-90 in patients with progressive metastatic gastroenteropancreatic neuroendocrine carcinomas (GEP-NETs): a phase II study. Ann Oncol 2010;21:787–794.
34 Pfeifer AK, et al: Peptide receptor radionuclide therapy with Y-DOTATOC and ^{177}Lu-DOTATOC in advanced neuroendocrine tumors: results from a Danish cohort treated in Switzerland. Neuroendocrinology 2011;93:189–196.
35 Sansovini M, et al: Treatment with the radiolabelled somatostatin analog Lu-DOTATATE for advanced pancreatic neuroendocrine tumors. Neuroendocrinology 2013;97:347–354.
36 Ezziddin S, et al: Outcome of peptide receptor radionuclide therapy with ^{177}Lu-octreotate in advanced grade 1/2 pancreatic neuroendocrine tumours. Eur J Nucl Med Mol Imaging 2014;41:925–933.
37 Waldherr C, et al: Tumor response and clinical benefit in neuroendocrine tumors after 7.4 GBq ^{90}Y-DOTATOC. J Nucl Med 2002;43:610–616.
38 Valkema R, et al: Survival and response after peptide receptor radionuclide therapy with [^{90}Y-DOTA^{0}, Tyr^{3}]octreotide in patients with advanced gastroenteropancreatic neuroendocrine tumors. Semin Nucl Med 2006;36:147–156.
39 Teunissen JJ, Kwekkeboom DJ, Krenning EP: Quality of life in patients with gastroenteropancreatic tumors treated with [^{177}Lu-DOTA^{0}, Tyr^{3}]octreotate. J Clin Oncol 2004;22:2724–2729.
40 Paganelli G, et al: 177 Lu-DOTA-octreotate radionuclide therapy of advanced gastrointestinal neuroendocrine tumors: results from a phase II study. Eur J Nucl Med Mol Imaging 2014;14:1845–1851.
41 van Essen M, et al: Peptide receptor radionuclide therapy with ^{177}Lu-octreotate in patients with foregut carcinoid tumours of bronchial, gastric and thymic origin. Eur J Nucl Med Mol Imaging 2007;34: 1219–1227.
42 van Essen M, et al: Salvage therapy with ^{177}Lu-octreotate in patients with bronchial and gastroenteropancreatic neuroendocrine tumors. J Nucl Med 2010;51:383–390.
43 van Essen M, et al: Report on short-term side effects of treatments with ^{177}Lu-octreotate in combination with capecitabine in seven patients with gastroenteropancreatic neuroendocrine tumours. Eur J Nucl Med Mol Imaging 2008;35:743–748.
44 Claringbold PG, et al: Phase II study of radiopeptide ^{177}Lu-octreotate and capecitabine therapy of progressive disseminated neuroendocrine tumours. Eur J Nucl Med Mol Imaging 2011;38:302–311.
45 Kong G, et al: Assessment of predictors of response and long-term survival of patients with neuroendocrine tumour treated with peptide receptor chemoradionuclide therapy (PRCRT). Eur J Nucl Med Mol Imaging 2014;41:1831–1844.
46 Sabet A, et al: Bone metastases in GEP-NET: response and long-term outcome after PRRT from a follow-up analysis. Am J Nucl Med Mol Imaging 2013;3:437–445.
47 de Jong M, et al: Combination radionuclide therapy using ^{177}Lu- and ^{90}Y-labeled somatostatin analogs. J Nucl Med 2005;46(suppl 1):13s–17s.
48 Kunikowska J, et al: Clinical results of radionuclide therapy of neuroendocrine tumours with ^{90}Y-DOTATATE and tandem ^{90}Y/^{177}Lu-DOTATATE: which is a better therapy option? Eur J Nucl Med Mol Imaging 2011;38:1788–1797.
49 Sabet A, et al: Accurate assessment of long-term nephrotoxicity after peptide receptor radionuclide therapy with ^{177}Lu-octreotate. Eur J Nucl Med Mol Imaging 2014;41:505–510.
50 Dale R: Use of the linear-quadratic radiobiological model for quantifying kidney response in targeted radiotherapy. Cancer Biother Radiopharm 2004;19: 363–370.
51 Barone R, et al: Patient-specific dosimetry in predicting renal toxicity with ^{90}Y-DOTATOC: relevance of kidney volume and dose rate in finding a dose-effect relationship. J Nucl Med 2005;46(suppl 1):99s–106s.
52 Bernard BF, et al: D-Lysine reduction of indium-111 octreotide and yttrium-90 octreotide renal uptake. J Nucl Med 1997;38:1929–1933.
53 Valkema R, et al: Long-term follow-up of renal function after peptide receptor radiation therapy with ^{90}Y-DOTA^{0},Tyr^{3}-octreotide and ^{177}Lu-DOTA^{0}, Tyr^{3}-octreotate. J Nucl Med 2005;46(suppl 1):83s–91s.
54 Cybulla M, Weiner SM, Otte A: End-stage renal disease after treatment with ^{90}Y-DOTATOC. Eur J Nucl Med 2001;28:1552–1554.

55 Bodei L, et al: Long-term evaluation of renal toxicity after peptide receptor radionuclide therapy with ^{90}Y-DOTATOC and ^{177}Lu-DOTATATE: the role of associated risk factors. Eur J Nucl Med Mol Imaging 2008;35:1847–1856.
56 Bodei L, et al: Long-term tolerability of PRRT in 807 neuroendocrine tumor patients: the value and limitations of clinical factors. Eur J Nucl Med Mol Imaging, 2015;42:5–19.
57 Bodei L, et al: Receptor-mediated radionuclide therapy with ^{90}Y-DOTATOC in association with amino acid infusion: a phase I study. Eur J Nucl Med Mol Imaging 2003;30:207–216.
58 Cremonesi M, et al: Dosimetry for treatment with radiolabelled somatostatin analogues: a review. Q J Nucl Med Mol Imaging 2010;54:37–51.
59 Kwekkeboom DJ, et al: Treatment of patients with gastro-entero-pancreatic (GEP) tumours with the novel radiolabelled somatostatin analogue [^{177}Lu-DOTA^0, Tyr^3]octreotate. Eur J Nucl Med Mol Imaging 2003;30:417–422.
60 Sabet A, et al: Long-term hematotoxicity after peptide receptor radionuclide therapy with ^{177}Lu-octreotate. J Nucl Med 2013;54:1857–1861.
61 Sabet A, et al: Can peptide receptor radionuclide therapy be safely applied in florid bone metastases? A pilot analysis of late stage osseous involvement. Nuklearmedizin 2014;53:54–59.
62 Kamp K, et al: Safety and efficacy of everolimus in gastrointestinal and pancreatic neuroendocrine tumors after ^{177}Lu-octreotate. Endocr Relat Cancer 2013;20:825–831.

Lisa Bodei
Division of Nuclear Medicine, European Institute of Oncology
via Ripamonti 435
IT–20141 Milan (Italy)
E-Mail lisa.bodei@ieo.it

Papotti M, de Herder WW (eds): Neuroendocrine Tumors: A Multidisciplinary Approach.
Front Horm Res. Basel, Karger, 2015, vol 44, pp 216–238 (DOI: 10.1159/000403593)

Hormone and Receptor Candidates for Target and Biotherapy of Neuroendocrine Tumors

Leo J. Hofland[a] · Timon Vandamme[a, b] · Manuela Albertelli[c] · Diego Ferone[c]

[a]Department of Internal Medicine, Division of Endocrinology, Erasmus Medical Center, Rotterdam, The Netherlands; [b]Department of Oncology, University of Antwerp, Antwerp, Belgium; [c]Section of Endocrinology, Department of Internal Medicine and Medical Specialties and Center of Excellence for Biomedical Research, IRCCS AOU San Martino-IST, University of Genoa, Genoa, Italy

Abstract

Neuroendocrine tumors (NETs) produce various hormones and bioactive substances and are known to express a large variety of peptide hormone receptors. While these hormones and receptors play a role in the pathophysiology of this heterogeneous group of tumors, they also form an important target for treatment and diagnosis. One of the most well-known target receptors in NETs are somatostatin receptors. On the basis of the expression of functional somatostatin receptors on the cell surface of NET cells, somatostatin analogs have already been used for decades to control symptoms related to hormonal overproduction in patients with NETs. Recent placebo-controlled studies have also demonstrated a significant antitumor activity, both in functioning and nonfunctioning NETs. Moreover, other peptide hormone receptors (e.g. receptors for GLP-1, CCK, GRP, secretin and dopamine) can be expressed at a high density in NETs. As such, these classes of receptors may also form potential targets for diagnosis and treatment. Finally, in recent years novel biotherapies targeting several growth factor systems have been introduced in the treatment of patients with NETs and are being explored for their efficacy in this setting, either as monotherapy or in combination treatment. This chapter aims to give an overview on the above topic.

It has been well known for several decades that hormone receptors, mainly G-protein-coupled receptors (GPCRs), play a role in the pathophysiology of neuroendocrine tumors (NETs). In addition, the expression of these GPCRs form the basis for treatment with receptor agonists and they can be used as targets for the diagnosis and treatment with radiolabeled receptor agonists. Without any doubt, somatostatin receptors (SSTR) have formed a cornerstone target for the treatment of NETs with unlabeled and radiolabeled somatostatin analogs (SSAs). On the other hand, recent research has provided evidence for other GPCRs as potential targets for diagnosis, biotherapy and targeted therapy using radiolabeled receptor agonists in NETs. In this chapter, we describe the current knowledge on the expression of hormone receptors, with a special focus on GPCRs, mechanisms of sensitivity and resistance to SSAs, as well as the role of hormone receptors in the diagnosis and treatment of patients with NETs. In addition, the role of combined targeting of NETs by SSAs and other drugs used in the treatment of these tumors is discussed.

Hormone Receptors in Neuroendocrine Tumors

Somatostatin Receptors

Somatostatin (SS) is a polypeptide that exists in two physiologically active forms, respectively, 14- (SS14) and 28-amino acids (SS28) in length. Both isoforms are generated from a single precursor through alternative proteolytic processing. In normal tissues, somatostatin plays an inhibitory role in hormone secretion. It reduces growth hormone (GH), adrenocorticotropic hormone (ACTH), prolactin and thyroid-stimulating hormone (TSH) secretion by the pituitary gland [1, 2]. In the endocrine pancreas, somatostatin inhibits insulin and glucagon secretion [3]. Additionally, it reduces motility and exocrine secretion in the gastrointestinal tract, regulates motor-, cognitive- and sensory functions in the central nervous system, as well as pain transmission in the peripheral nervous system [3, 4]. Both SS14 and SS28 are substrates of rhodopsin-like G-protein-coupled SSTR through a shared receptor-binding domain [5]. SSTR are encoded by five different SSTR genes, named *SSTR1* to *SSTR5* [5]. Although all receptor subtypes are activated by SS14 and SS28 in nanomolar (nM) concentrations, sst_2 seems to have a higher affinity for SS14, whereas sst_5 has a greater affinity for SS28 [6]. Alternative splicing of the *SSTR2* gene leads to two distinct sst_2 receptors, sst_{2A} and sst_{2B}, with different lengths and cytoplasmic carboxy-terminal sequences [7]. Recently, two truncated isoforms of the sst_5 have been discovered. These receptors, lacking one or more of the seven transmembrane domains, are translated from sst_5 mRNA with alternative splicing of noncanonical donor and acceptor splice sites. In human mRNA, variants encoding five (sst_5TMD5) or four (sst_5TMD4) of the sst_5 amino terminal transmembrane domains with distinct C termini have been discovered. These human mRNAs consist of the 5′ coding region of the *SSTR5* gene linked to alternative 3′ open reading frames [8].

Various methods for the in vitro detection of SSTR in tissue have been developed, both for the detection of SSTR mRNA and protein. Methods detecting SSTR mRNA include mRNA quantification through real-time PCR and mRNA in situ hybridization, the latter providing morphological information. However, both are unable to pick up posttranslational changes that could affect the functional protein level [9]. Hence, methods focused on protein detection are preferred. In vitro quantitative SSTR autoradiography allows studying both the quantity and tissue distribution of the receptor protein in a highly binding site-specific manner, and it is considered the gold standard. However, it is a time-consuming technique and only when a sufficient number of SSTR-positive cells are present, reliable detection is possible. Immunohistochemistry is an attractive alternative for the detection of low abundance SSTR-positive cells and provides an excellent spatial resolution. Additionally, it allows SSTR detection in widely available formalin-fixed paraffin-embedded tissue, while for receptor autoradiography fresh frozen tissue is needed. The drawbacks of immunohistochemistry are the lack of possibilities for a reliably quantified expression, the limited availability of highly specific antibodies with good sensitivity for the different SSTR subtypes, and the frequent visualization of an epitope distinct from the binding site.

In normal human tissue, SSTR expression has been found in many tissue types, including the brain, pituitary, pancreas, gut, thyroid, adrenal, kidney and the immune system [for a review, see 10]. Although SSTR receptor subtypes are expressed in a complex tissue-specific pattern, the most abundant SSTR appears to be sst_{2A} [for a review, see 11].

In human NETs, early studies using nonsubtype selective autoradiography showed a high incidence and density of SSTR, particularly in GH- and TSH-secreting pituitary adenomas, pheochromocytomas, paragangliomas and gastroenteropancreatic (GEP) and lung NETs [11]. In GEP-NETs, receptor expression, determined by in vitro autoradiography, is higher in well-differentiated compared to poorly differentiated NETs [12]. Additional studies, using mRNA quantification through RT-qPCR, detected expression of different SSTR subtypes in many NET types, including pituitary adenomas and GEP-NETs [13, 14]. However, the incidence of SSTR subtypes detected through mRNA expression seems to be higher than what can be detected by subtype-specific receptor autoradiography or subtype-specific immunohistochemistry [15]. This apparent contradiction could be due to the extremely high sensitivity of the method, mRNA contamination from adjacent tissues or by mRNA that is not translated into functional protein.

The most prevalent SSTR subtype in NETs is sst_{2A}. Almost all pituitary NETs, including GH- and TSH-producing tumors, express sst_{2A} in large amounts, as determined by receptor autoradiography studies [16]. In GEP-NETs, receptor autoradiography studies found sst_{2A} expression in 80–100% of cases, both in gut NETs and most pancreatic NETs [17]. However, only 50–70% of insulinomas express sst_{2A} [17]. Some NETs may express other SSTR subtypes, such as sst_1, sst_3 and sst_5, either alone or in combination with sst_{2A}. In pituitary adenomas, receptor autoradiography showed that the majority of clinically inactive pituitary adenomas express sst_3 [16]. A significant proportion of the GH-producing adenomas and most ACTH-producing adenomas have sst_5 expression, as determined by mRNA expression [18]. Immunohistochemistry staining has recently shown sst5TMD4 expression in 50% of nonfunctioning pituitary adenomas and 89% of somatotropinomas [19], but it has not yet been evaluated in GEP-NETs. In somatotropinomas, sst5TDM4 expression could be related to aggressive behavior [19]. In most GEP-NETs, SSTR expression is often not limited to one subtype. In addition to

sst_{2A}, sst_1, sst_5 and, to a lesser extent, sst_3 expression has been identified through receptor autoradiography [17]. Insulinomas often express sst_1 or sst_5, either alone or in association with sst_{2A}. In human tumors, sst_4 expression seems very limited [17].

Glucagon-Like Peptide-1 Receptors

Glucagon-like peptide-1 (GLP-1) is an incretin hormone that mediates postprandial insulin secretion through the specific GLP-1 receptor. The GLP-1 receptor is expressed on the pancreatic β-cell. Insulinomas are tumors derived from these β-cells and virtually all highly express GLP-1 receptors, as demonstrated through in vitro GLP-1 receptor autoradiography [17]. Additionally, gastrinomas very frequently show GLP-1 receptor expression using receptor autoradiography, albeit at a lower density compared to insulinomas [17]. Insulinoma detection using conventional imaging techniques, or SSTR targeting scintigraphy, has proven challenging and in vivo molecular imaging techniques using GLP-1-like radioligands have shown a higher sensitivity compared to conventional imaging for the detection of insulinomas in patients [20]. No GLP-1 receptor expression was found in the normal pituitary gland or in pituitary adenomas using receptor autoradiography [21].

Dopamine Receptors

Dopamine is the predominant catecholamine neurotransmitter in the human central nervous system. Additionally, it functions as a modulator of cardiovascular and renal function, gastrointestinal motility and the endocrine system [22]. Dopamine exerts its functions via binding to the G-protein-coupled dopamine receptors (DR) [22]. Up to now, five different DR, divided into two subfamilies, have been characterized: D1-like and D5-like. In pituitary adenomas, DR expression has been demonstrated by immunohistochemistry and receptor autoradiography in GH-secreting, prolactin (PRL)-secreting, ACTH-secreting and nonfunctioning tumors [23–25]. Immunohistochemistry demonstrated DR subtype 2 (D_2) expression in 85% of the well-differentiated GEP-NETs, including islet-cell tumors and tumors of ileal and duodenal origin [26]. This DR expression could have important clinical implications given the frequent coexpression with SSTR and the availability of both DR-specific agonists and SSTR-DR chimeric compounds [27].

Cholecystokinin Receptors

Cholecystokinin (CCK) and gastrin are peptides that act as regulators of various stomach, pancreas and gallbladder functions and as growth factors in the gastrointestinal tract, in addition to their role in as neurotransmitters in the brain. Gastrin and cholecystokinin are substrates of several receptor subtypes, including CCK_1 and CCK_2. The gastrin affinity of CCK_1 is several folds lower than CCK_2 gastrin affinity [28]. CCK receptors are widely expressed in GEP-NETs but have not been found in pituitary adenomas. About 50% of the gastrinomas express CCK_1, but not CCK_2 receptors, in receptor autoradiography studies [17]. In ileal carcinoids, receptor autoradiography shows CCK_1 expression in one third of all cases, while CCK_2 is present in more than half of all cases [17]. Several ileal tumors coexpress CCK_1 and CCK_2. In insulinomas, no CCK_1 expression has been found, but almost all show CCK_2 expression using autoradiography [17].

Gastrin-Releasing Peptide Receptors
Gastrin-releasing peptide (GRP) plays a role in the human brain-gut axis and regulates several physiological processes, including the release of other peptide hormones. Additionally, it seems to play a role in cancer proliferation. GRP mediates its effect through GPCRs, with at least four subtypes, including neuromedin B receptor subtype (BB_1), GRP receptor subtype (BB_2), BB_3 and BB_4 [11]. Receptor autoradiography showed BB_1 expression in ileal carcinoids, while BB_2 expression was frequently found in gastrinomas [17]. BB expression is rarely detected in insulinomas [17].

Secretin Receptors
Secretin is a 27-amino acid neuroendocrine peptide distributed primarily in the gastrointestinal tract and central nervous system. Secretin stimulates biliary, pancreatic and small intestinal fluid, as well as electrolyte secretion [29]. In vitro receptor autoradiography and mRNA RT-qPCR show that secretin receptors are highly expressed in most gastrinomas [30]. This high incidence and level of secretin receptor expression provide the biological rationale for the positive secretin provocation test in Zollinger-Ellison syndrome [31]. A secretin receptor splice variant missing exon 3 could silence the functional secretin receptor [32]. However, mRNA expression of the spliced variant does not seem to influence the results of the secretin provocation test [33]. Instead, a positive secreting provocation test correlates to the level of unspliced receptor mRNA [33].

Interferon Receptors
Interferon receptors consist of type I and type II receptors, encoded by different genes and existing in various configurations [34]. Type I receptors are present in low numbers on the surface of all vertebrate cell examined so far [35]. In GEP-NETs, type I interferon receptors have been used as a target for therapy with interferon-α [36, 37]. In vitro studies have shown a strong effect of interferon-β in GEP-NETs [38]. In the pituitary, it has been suggested that interferon-α might play a role in adenomas non-responsive to conventional medical therapies [39].

Mechanisms Influencing Treatment Response and Uptake of Radiolabeled Somatostatin Analogs

Receptor Number
As mentioned above, one of the cornerstones for the medical treatment of NETs is the expression of SSTR at the cell membrane of NET cells. NETs form a very heterogeneous group of tumors and the expression of SSTR (subtypes) is highly variably among

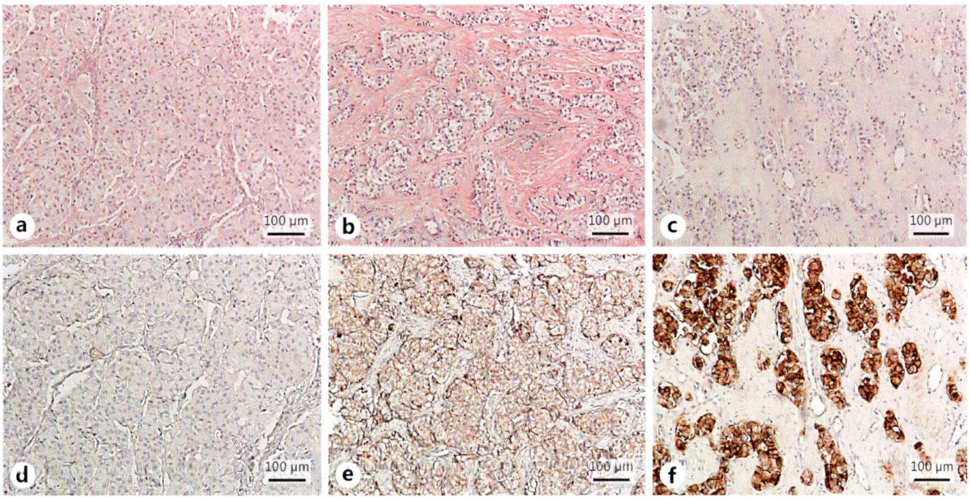

Fig. 1. Variable expression of sst_2 receptors in three pancreatic NETs. **a–c** HE staining. **d–f** Immunohistochemical detection of sst_2 receptors.

as well as within the different types of NETs. Figure 1 shows an example of the variable expression of sst_2 receptors in pancreatic NETs. While in GH-secreting pituitary adenomas a clear relationship between the response to treatment with SSAs and the expression of sst_2 receptors on the tumoral cell membrane is suggested [40], the relationship between sst_2 expression in NETs and treatment response to SSAs is not very well established. In addition, not much is currently known about the potential underlying mechanisms of the variable receptor expression among tumors. Mutations in genes encoding SSTRs (mainly sst_2 and sst_5) have not been found, except for a rare mutation in sst_5 in a single GH-secreting pituitary adenoma [41]. Recent data suggested that epigenetic mechanisms may underlie 'silenced' sst_2 receptor expression, as sst_2 promoter methylation has been associated to a reduced sst_2 expression, and because epigenetic drugs (e.g. DNA methyltransferase inhibitors and histone deacetylase inhibitors) were shown to upregulate tumoral sst_2 expression in various cell models, including NETs [42, 43]. Similar findings were done for D_2 expression in pituitary tumor models [44] in which it was demonstrated that epidrugs restored D_2 expression in GH-secreting pituitary tumor cells, as well as the antitumor activity of dopamine agonists (DA). Whether epidrugs might be a future approach to upregulate sst_2 (and/or D_2) expression in NETs in order to increase the efficacy of treatment with SSAs and peptide receptor-targeted radiotherapy (PRRT) remains a challenging issue for future research.

Feedback Mechanisms

The hormonal environment of SSTR-expressing cells may influence SSTR expression and the response to SS. In pituitary cells, the classical peripheral feedback hormones for the different anterior pituitary cell types are involved in regulating sensitivity to the inhibitory effect of SS on hormone secretions [45]. For NET cells, the role of the hormonal milieu on SSTR expression has been less well investigated. In particular, glucocorticoids (GC) were shown to differentially regulate sst_2 expression in NET cells. de Bruin et al. [46] showed in BON-1 carcinoid and TT medullary thyroid carcinoma cells in vitro that sst_2 expression was strongly downregulated in a dose-dependent manner (IC_{50} values of 0.84 and 0.16 nM, respectively) by treatment with the synthetic glucocorticoid dexamethasone (Dex). In TT cells, Dex-treatment abrogated the calcitonin inhibition by the sst_2-preferring SSA octreotide. Interestingly, the sst_5 and D_2 expression were much more resistant to Dex-treatment. A glucocorticoid-dependent regulation of sst_2 receptors has also been reported in NETs in vivo. In 2 patients with Cushing's syndrome due to ectopic ACTH secretion, the ACTH-secreting bronchial carcinoids were originally not visible by [^{111}In-DTPA^0]octreotide scan (and not appreciated by CT), but became apparent at scan after treatment with the GC receptor antagonist mifepristone [47]. These data suggest a downregulatory effect of GC levels on tumoral sst_2 expression in vivo as well. Additional studies need to demonstrate whether GC lowering or antagonizing therapy may be used to improve the diagnostic accuracy of SSR scintigraphy in patients with ectopic ACTH production of unknown primary origin [47].

Mechanisms of Resistance (Receptor Trafficking and Desensitization)

In recent years, a considerable number of studies have highlighted the role of molecular determinants of resistance to treatment with SSAs in patients with GH-secreting pituitary adenomas. Such determinants include the ratio of coexpression of receptor subtypes (e.g. sst_2 and sst_5 receptors), high levels of sst_5TMD4, low E-cadherin and RKIP levels, as well as low AIP and ZAC-1 expression [40]. In addition, it has been recently demonstrated that a low expression of intracellular regulators of cell surface SSTR expression, the so-called β-arrestins (in particular β-arrestin 1; fig. 2), which are involved in uncoupling of GPCR signaling (desensitization) and in driving agonist-induced receptor internalization (lowering of cell surface receptor number), is associated with the an enhanced response of acromegalic patients to treatment with SSAs. Interestingly, while an escape from treatment with SSAs is rarely observed in acromegalic patients, some SSA-responsive patients with NETs may escape from prolonged treatment and become resistant. The role of the above-mentioned molecular determinants causing resistance to SSAs in NETs patients remains, however, an open challenging question for future research. In this context, recent observations by Waser et al. [48] provided evidence for a considerable heterogeneity in the subcellular distribution of phosphorylated sst_2 receptors among gastrointestinal NETs from patients treated with octreotide. Activation of SSTR by agonist binding is rapidly followed by receptor phosphorylation, representing a critical step for subsequent receptor internalization. Waser et al. [48] showed that, in contrast to octreotide treatment naive NETs that displayed only nonphosphorylated cell surface sst_2 expression, tumors of patients that were treated with octreotide contained mainly phosphorylated sst_2 re-

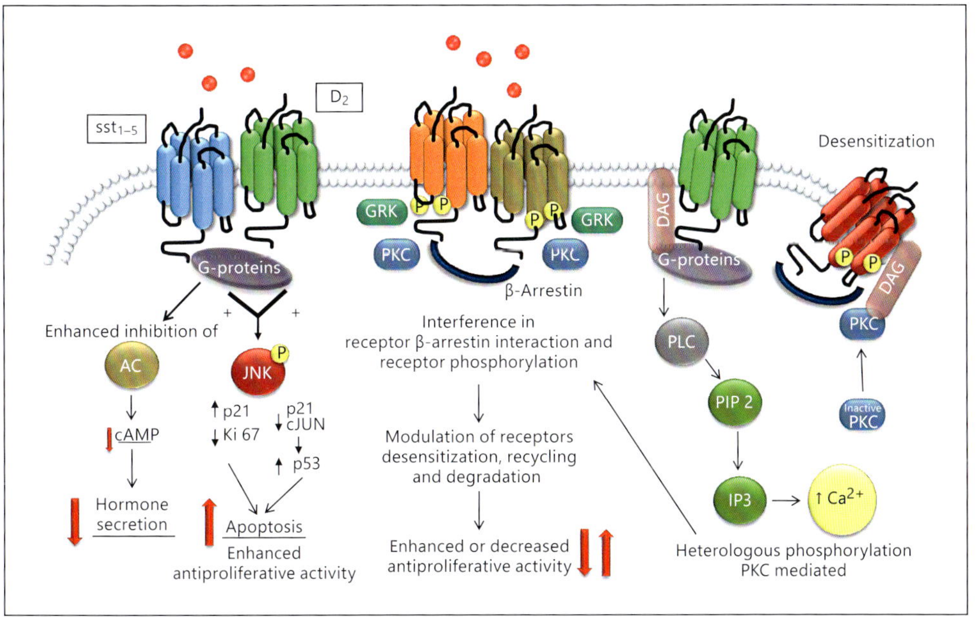

Fig. 2. Schematic representation of possible interactions between SSTR and DR. Adapted from Ferone et al. [74] and Gatto and Hofland [27]. JNK = c-Jun N-terminal kinase; PKC = protein kinase C; PLC = phospholipase C; DAG = diacyl-glycerol; PIP_2 = phosphatidylinositol bisphosphate; IP3 = inositol trisphosphate.

ceptors that were internalized to a highly variable extent. The authors hypothesized that assessing the localization and activation state of sst_2 receptors in tissue samples from sensitive and resistant NET patients may help to better understand resistance to SSA treatment [48].

Role of Hormone Receptors in the Diagnosis of Neuroendocrine Tumors

Although often described as rare, the incidence of NETs has shown a marked increase over the past 3 decades [49, 50]. The Surveillance, Epidemiology and End Result Registry (SEERR) has shown that NET incidence in the USA increased 5-fold from 1973 to 2004 (from 1 to 5 per 100,000 individuals) [50]. NET prevalence (35 in 100,000 in 2004), by contrast, is much higher than NET incidence because of the long-ranging survival of the majority of patients. In fact, considering all GEP-NETs together, these tumors represent the second most prevalent neoplasm of the gastrointestinal tract, following colon adenocarcinoma [50]. At present, the improvement of clinical awareness, diagnostic tools and the setting of an adequate histopathological classification have increased the number of diagnosed cases, although NET diagnosis remains difficult, and is often delayed. As a result, metastatic disease is common at presentation and has been reported in 44–85% in specialized centers [51]. The localization of a NET and the assessment of the extent of the disease are crucial for clinical and therapeutic management of these neoplasms [52]. Currently, commonly used diagnostic techniques include conventional radiology with transabdominal ultrasound, computed tomography (CT), magnetic resonance imaging (MRI) and selective angiography with hormonal sampling.

Very often detection of NETs and the staging of patients by conventional imaging procedures requires integration with functional imaging. In this context, the possibility to target SSTRs by nuclear medicine techniques is crucial, and this approach has vastly improved accuracy in the diagnosing of NETs, mainly by the use of radiolabelled SSAs.

In fact, the demonstration of amine-uptake mechanisms and the high density of membrane peptide hormone receptors on primary NETs, and even on their metastases, is important for both the diagnosis and monitoring of these patients using specific radionuclides [52]. The latter provide a diagnostic modality in which radiolabelled amines or peptide analogs, linked to suitable ligands, are utilized for the identification and localization of NETs [52]. NETs and their metastases can be visualized in vivo using a γ-camera after the injection of various radionuclides, such as ^{123}I-metaiodobenzylguanidine (MIBG) and ^{111}In-pentetreotide [53]. In addition, as indicated above, other small peptide hormone receptors that are expressed on the cell membrane of NET include receptors for vasoactive intestinal peptide (VIP), GLP-1, bombesin, CCK, gastrin and/or substance P, which can be used as markers for in vivo tumor visualization [54, 55].

Currently, functional imaging, with widely available techniques, such as [^{111}In-DTPA^0]octreotide (OctreoScan®) or, more recently, SSTR targeting PET with ^{68}Ga-octreotide, as well as experimental methods available only in some specialized centers, such as ^{99m}Tc-EDDA/HYNIC-Tyr^3-octreotide scintigraphy, or PET with ^{18}F-levo-DOPA, ^{11}C-5-hydroxytryptophan or ^{86}Y-DOTATOC, have shown a critical role in the management of patients harboring these neoplasms [56–58].

The most commonly used SSA, octreotide, was initially conjugated with DTPA (diethylenetriaminepentaacetic acid), but more recently with DOTA (1,4,7,10-tetraa zacyclododecane-1,4,7,10-tetra-acetic acid) allowing a coupling of SSAs with various radioisotopes, mainly ^{111}In [52, 59]. Scintigraphy with [^{111}In-DTPA^0]octreotide seems superior to ^{111}In-lanreotide and has a detection rate of 67–100% for all NETs. Therefore, it can be used for the diagnosis, staging and follow-up of patients with NETs. ^{111}In-DTPA-octreotate, another developed SSA, demonstrated higher tumor uptake than [^{111}In-DTPA^0]octreotide, whereas kidney uptake remained similar. Finally, the superimposition of [^{111}In-DTPA^0]octreotide single photon emission computerized tomography (SPECT) with CT/MRI slices (anatomical-functional image fusion) has shown improved localization and characterization of tumors in patients with NETs, and proved crucial during both diagnostics and follow-up [57, 60–62].

Most clinically used radiolabeled SSAs are agonists that bind with a preferential high affinity to sst_2. Although most NETs do express sst_2, the distribution and density of these receptors is often variable and sometimes too low for effective SSTR targeting [17]. This is likely the reason for the wide sensitivity range (60–100%) of [^{111}In-DTPA^{0}]octreotide scintigraphy and SPECT in the detection of NETs [61]. One possible approach to overcome this problem is the use of radiolabeled tracers with affinity to more than one SSTR subtype. Gastrinomas, ileal carcinoids and VIPomas express sst$_2$ or sst$_5$ with an incidence of almost 100%. [DOTA, 1-Nal3]-octreotide (DOTANOC) is a peptide that allows the targeting of a broader range of SSTR, including sst$_2$, sst$_3$ and sst$_5$ [63].

Furthermore, ^{68}Ga-based radiopharmaceuticals, such as ^{68}Ga-DOTANOC, have shown higher binding affinities to sst$_2$ and sst$_5$ than the respective lutetium and indium derivatives. The higher binding affinity resulted in a significantly higher tumor uptake in a rat tumor model [64]. This finding is relevant because metallic ^{68}Ga is a positron emitter with a half life of 68 min that is ideal for molecular PET imaging. Recently, SSTR PET using ^{68}Ga-DOTATOC or ^{68}Ga-DOTATATE has shown promising results in patients, with a higher lesion detection rate than those achieved with ^{111}In-DTPA-octreotide SPECT [65, 66]. More importantly, SSTR PET changed the clinical management in most patients with negative or inconclusive findings on ^{111}In-DTPA-octreotide scintigraphy [66]. Currently, ^{68}Ga-DOTATOC, ^{68}Ga-DOTATATE and ^{68}Ga-DOTANOC are the most established SSTR PET tracers [67]. Comparative studies with ^{68}Ga-DOTATOC and ^{68}Ga-DOTATATE in the same patient have revealed comparable diagnostic accuracy for the detection of NET lesions [64].

However, in a recent study by Wild et al. [64], a comparison between ^{68}Ga-DOTANOC and ^{68}Ga-DOTATATE PET/CT in the same patients with GEP-NETs was performed with conflicting results. The authors evaluated 18 patients with both methods and concluded that the sst$_2$, sst$_3$ and sst$_5$-preferring radiotracer ^{68}Ga-DOTANOC detected significantly more lesions than the sst$_2$-preferring radiotracer ^{68}Ga-DOTATATE in their patient cohort. Because of the small size of this study population, additional and larger trials are urgently needed to confirm whether these results are of clinical relevance and would justify the widespread adoption of ^{68}Ga-DOTANOC over ^{68}Ga-DOTATATE [64].

In summary, [^{111}In-DTPA^{0}]octreotide scintigraphy/SPECT has represented a gold standard modality for NETs management. However, the recent availability of ^{68}Ga-DOTATOC PET/CT may greatly improve the work-up of patients with NETs. An exemplary ^{68}Ga-DOTATOC PET/CT scan is depicted in figure 3.

Clinical Experience of Targeting Hormone Receptors in Neuroendocrine Tumors

The presence of peptide hormone receptors on NET cells has an important therapeutic implication, favoring the use of such receptors as a target for biological drugs or targeted agents. With respect to therapy, as first-line treatment, localized tumors

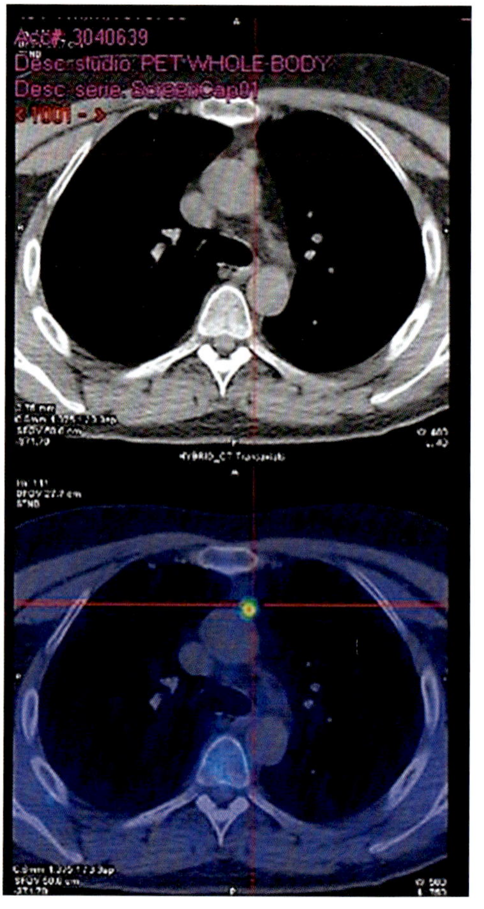

Fig. 3. PET/CT ^{68}Ga DOTATATE: a previously unknown primary visualized by PET with gallium DOTA peptide in a patient with Cushing's syndrome. The primary tumor was an atypical thymic carcinoid.

showing only regional spread require surgery with either radical or cytoreductive intent, probably able to relieve symptoms even of metastatic and/or high-grade NETs [51]. Surgery is still the only curative therapy for NETs, although it can be effective in a minority of patients (about 15–20%). This is due to the very high prevalence of metastatic disease already at the time of diagnosis (40–85% of diagnosed NETs, according to different studies in the literature, as previously stated) [51]. In the case of metastatic NETs, medical treatment is recommended, and very much needed, although a real adjuvant and/or neoadjuvant setting has still not been explored and defined by randomized trials. The current medical treatment for locally advanced or metastatic G1/G2 NETs includes SSAs, interferon-α, radionuclide- (^{90}Y or ^{177}Lu) coupled SSAs and, more recently, targeted therapies [51]. Cytotoxic chemotherapy has mainly been used in patients with highly proliferating NETs (G3), and in particular some pancreatic and lung NETs [51]. Complementary locoregional or ablative therapies are used to treat liver metastases. In patients with NETs the control of clinical symptoms and the stabilization of the disease are the primary goal of a large part of currently available therapies [51]. Considering the very high rate of patients with synchronous metastases at diagnosis, and, therefore, unsuitable for surgery, as well as the typical indolent growth of these tumors allowing long survival even in advanced stages of disease, it has become very important to find more effective medical therapies. In this context, targeting of hormone receptors with biotherapies and the development of targeted therapies for NETs are of extreme interest for the effectiveness so far demonstrated in this particular category of neoplasms and for the general good tolerability profile of these drugs, compared, for example, with classical chemotherapy regimens [51].

Somatostatin Analogs
Neuroendocrine cells are typically regulated by numerous hormones, acting via specific receptors on the cell membrane surface. A number of these receptors are 7-transmembrane domain GPCRs. As indicated above, the most exploited and known ligand-receptor system in clinical practice, including nuclear medicine, is the SS/SSTR. The presence of a suitable density of SSTRs allows the treatment of tumor hypersecretion and of primary and metastatic lesion growth by SS, its analogs and peptide receptor-targeted therapy, owing to postreceptor signaling, triggered by the receptor-ligand internalization [68].

SSTR activation results in the regulation of different intracellular effectors, mediating the antiproliferative and antisecretory effects of SS. In particular, all SSTRs can inhibit adenylyl cyclase activity, to lower intracellular cAMP levels, and modulate ion currents, activating K^+ channels and inhibiting voltage-gated Ca^{2+} channels to control hormone and neurotransmitter release negatively [69]. Furthermore, the modulation of mitogen-activated protein (MAP) kinase activity and phosphotyrosine phosphatases (PTPs), including SHP1, SHP2 and density-enhanced phosphatase-1 (also known as PTPh) [70], are considered the key factors for the antiproliferative effects of SS in several tumor cells [51]. In particular, SS-activated PTPs directly dephosphorylate activating tyrosine either on growth factor receptors (epidermal growth factor, insulin-like growth factor 1, etc.) or on extracellular signal-regulated kinase 1/2, to inhibit the MAP kinase pathway [51]. Antiproliferative activity of SS is also mediated by indirect mechanisms, such as a decrease in the production of GH, growth factors (epidermal growth factor, basic fibroblast growth factor, insulin-like growth factor 1), proangiogenic factors (vascular endothelial growth factor, platelet-derived growth factor) and immunomodulation [71]. Finally, a direct antiangiogenic activity of SS was also demonstrated to be mediated by a direct SSTR-mediated inhibition of nitric oxide synthesis in tumoral endothelial cells [72]. SS has been exploited for endocrine cancer treatment by developing clinically suitable SSAs overcoming the very short half-life of natural SS and the postinfusion rebound hypersecretion of hormones, thus improving the pharmacological efficacy. Octreotide was the first 8-amino acid SSA clinically approved, which was then followed by lanreotide [51]. Both compounds bind primarily to sst_2, and with a lower affinity to sst_5. More recently, the cyclohexapeptide pasireotide, with high affinity for all SSTRs except sst_4, has been developed

[73]. Evolution of SSAs also includes long-acting depot formulations [octreotide long-acting repeatable (LAR), lanreotide prolonged-release, lanreotide autogel, pasireotide LAR] [51].

In the NETs context, SSAs activate intracellular pathways to induce antisecretive and antiproliferative effects [71, 74]. The prevalent signaling depends on the cell-specific distribution of the SSTR subtypes and on the cell signaling molecules involved, as well as on SSTR internalization, desensitization and/or receptor crosstalk [75]. Indeed, different SSAs can induce diverse conformations of the receptor-ligand complex, preferentially activating one pathway with respect to another, and can increase or limit receptor endocytosis [69]. Finally, the expression pattern of SSTRs and their activity in response to therapy with different analogs can be influenced by some intracellular components, such as proteins involved in desensitization and in vesicular trafficking of the internalized receptor (e.g. β-arrestins) [27, 76]. However, in a discrete percentage of cases a therapeutic escape occurs, probably caused by desensitization related to receptor phosphorylation, trafficking and internalization [51].

The 'escape from response' phenomenon, or tachyphylaxis to treatment, is seen in lung or GEP-NETs, either during the short- or the long-term, following initiation of treatment [45]. In this context, although final evidence is lacking, receptor desensitization and degradation (leading to receptor downregulation) may be involved in an 'early' escape (weeks to months) to SSA treatment [45]. On the other hand, cellular events, such as the overgrowth of SSTR-negative clones, mutations in SSTR genes and/or tumor dedifferentiation, frequently observed in cancer natural history, are more likely related to the 'late' escape to SSA (years) observed in patients with NETs [45, 76].

In the beginning of 1980s, the octapeptide analog octreotide was synthesized. Presently, octreotide, together with lanreotide, is the analog approved for therapeutic clinical use. Both these analogs are mainly sst_2-preferring agents, therefore showing high affinity for this receptor, moderately high affinity for sst_5 and intermediate affinity for sst_3 [77].

These 'classical' clinically available SSAs, octreotide and lanreotide, at standard dosages, have been demonstrated to improve the symptoms related to functioning NETs in 64% of patients, with a biochemical response in 66% of cases [51, 78]. Only in about 10% of cases is there a significant reduction of tumor mass, while tumor stabilization occurs in 35–50% of patients [51, 78]. In 2009 a first double-blind, placebo-controlled randomized phase 3 study (octreotide LAR vs. placebo) in patients with well-differentiated metastatic midgut NETs demonstrated that octreotide more than doubled the time to tumor progression compared with placebo (progression-free survival, PFS, in treatment arm, 14.3 months, compared with placebo, 6 months), in both functioning and nonfunctioning NETs [79]. In greater detail, patients with low-grade (Ki-67 <2%) and low hepatic tumor load NETs (<10%), even if nonfunctioning, are likely to benefit from octreotide treatment as the first-line medical therapy [79]. Recently, further data to support the antiproliferative efficacy of SSAs were demonstrated by the CLARINET study [80]. Data from this large randomized trial with lanreotide autogel in metastatic GEP-NETs have shown a clear and significant benefit in terms of prolongation of PFS in patients treated with lanreotide (median PFS not reached) compared with those in the placebo arm (median PFS 18 months, $p < 0.001$) [80]. The study was conducted in patients with advanced, well-differentiated or moderately differentiated, nonfunctioning, SSTR-positive NETs of grade 1 or 2 (a tumor proliferation index, based on staining for the Ki-67 antigen, <10%). The tumors originated in the pancreas, midgut and hindgut, or were of unknown origin. It is interesting to note that the benefit in terms of prolongation of PFS was reached even though the enrolled patient population was in the vast majority (96%) in stable disease, and in 33% of cases had a hepatic tumor volume greater than 25% [80].

In this trial, lanreotide treatment was effective and favorable in all subgroups of patients even if the enrolled population had an indolent disease [80]. Although the two studies, PROMID and CLARINET, are not directly comparable due to many differences in the features of treated patients and in the study designs, as well as the methods of evaluation of the two studies, both have provided compelling evidence that SSAs can inhibit tumor growth in patients with metastatic well-differentiated NETs of the GEP tract. The improvement in PFS and clinical benefit has been demonstrated in both NETs populations, the more 'aggressive' one (PROMID, PFS placebo arm 6 months) and the more 'indolent' (CLARINET, PFS placebo arm 18 months).

Because of these studies, the National Comprehensive Cancer Network (NCCN) international guidelines introduced octreotide (in 2009–2010) and lanreotide (in 2015) in the therapeutic algorithm for functioning or nonfunctioning, metastatic or locally advanced NETs, both in asymptomatic patients with low and symptomatic patients with significant tumor burden.

To overcome tachyphylaxis or resistance to SSAs, a new analog, pasireotide, has been synthesized. While both octreotide and lanreotide primarily target sst_2, pasireotide targets four of the five SSTRs and, theoretically, it represents a more potent antiproliferative agent [51, 73].

Because of its pan-SSTR-binding profile, pasireotide has been tested in a phase 2 study in advanced GEP-NETs, showing symptom improvement in patients refractory or resistant to octreotide LAR [81]. However, so far only an in vitro study has shown similar antitumor efficacy of octreotide and pasireotide in primary cultures derived from human NETs [82].

In addition, a phase 3 study using pasireotide LAR versus a high-dose of octreotide LAR in patients with refractory carcinoid syndrome to standard treatments has shown that pasireotide treatment did not achieve the primary endpoint of improvement in carcinoid syndrome [83]. Nevertheless, these results showed that pasireotide treatment was associated with a statistically significant prolongation in PFS (exploratory endpoint) compared to octreotide [83]. Thereafter, another open-label, single-arm, phase 2 study was conducted to investigate the antitumor activity of pasireotide LAR in treatment-naive patients with metastatic grade 1 or grade 2 pancreatic and extrapancreatic NETs [83].

In this study, the authors also assessed the correlation between SSTR immunoreactivity and clinical outcomes. Twenty-nine patients were treated with pasireotide LAR 60 mg every 4 weeks and 28 were evaluable for response. Prior systemic therapy, including octreotide and lanreotide, was not permitted. The primary endpoint was PFS. Secondary endpoints included overall survival (OS), overall radiographic response rate (ORR) and safety. The median PFS was 11 months. The most favorable effect was observed in patients with low hepatic tumor burden, normal baseline chromogranin A levels and high tumoral sst_5 expression, evaluated by immunohistochemistry. Median OS has not been reached; the 30-month OS rate was 70%. The best radiographic response was partial response in 1 patient (4%), stable disease in 17 patients (60%) and progressive disease in 10 patients (36%). The treatment was associated with a 79% rate of hyperglycemia, including 14% grade 3 hyperglycemia [83]. Although pasireotide, in this study, appears to be an effective antiproliferative agent in advanced NETs, the high incidence of hyperglycemia raises concerns regarding its suitability as a first-line systemic agent in unselected patients [83]. The authors concluded that their results suggest sst_5 expression as a potentially predictive biomarker for response [83].

In summary, to date, pasireotide has found its development primarily in Cushing's disease and in acromegaly [84, 85], while confirmatory results are still to be awaited in NETs. Two trials (a phase 1 and a phase 2), named COOPERATE studies, are currently investigating the effects of pasireotide in combination with everolimus (mTOR inhibitor) in advanced NETs, including pancreatic NETs, so future results might more strongly support its antitumor activity. Moreover, another trial (the LUNA trial) designed especially for thoracic NETs is evaluating the efficacy of pasireotide and everolimus in monotherapy or in combination.

Targeting Other Hormone Receptors: DR and Combined Therapy with Dopaminergic Agents and SSAs

Another way to overcome treatment resistance could be represented by combined therapies acting through the activation of other membrane receptors. In fact, although sst_2 is the most important and most frequently expressed receptor subtype in NETs, as already mentioned, other SSTR subtypes, such as sst_1, sst_3 and sst_5, as well as DRs, in particular D_2, have been proven to be equally important in the control of neuroendocrine cell functions. In a study by O'Toole et al. [86] it was demonstrated that NETs of both intestinal and pancreatic origin may coexpress not only different subtypes of SSTRs, but also high levels of D_2. In the 35 GEP tumors analyzed by real-time PCR and compared to pituitary adenomas, sst_2 and D_2 were coexpressed in 100% of cases and sst_5 in 89%. In a more recent study by Srirajaskanthan et al. [87], the receptor profile of 56 NETs was characterized by immunohistochemistry and, consistently with previous experience, the authors found that D_2 was coexpressed with sst_2 and sst_5 in the majority of low- and intermediate-grade tumors. Both sst_2 and sst_5 were expressed in 100% of low-grade, 94.4% of intermediate-grade and 66.7% of high-grade NETs, whereas D_2 was expressed in 93.1% of low-grade, 77.8% of intermediate-grade and 44.4% of high-grade tumors. Coexpression of all three receptors was found in 93.1% of low-grade tumors. These interesting results have opened the possibility of examining new subtype-specific, bispecific, universal ligands and hybrid compounds which may simultaneously recognize, with high-affinity binding activity, more than one SSTR or both SSTRs and D_2. Despite the very promising preclinical results as well as the data from phase 1 studies, the higher antisecretory and antiproliferative efficacy of chimeric compounds, binding both SSTRs and D_2 has not yet been fully elucidated. At present, there is the lack of an established explanation for the unique activity of these novel hybrid molecules [88]. Possible explanations for the greater potency in suppressing hormone release include their higher binding affinity for sst_2 and their ability to simultaneously bind and activate multiple receptors, which increases the chance that once the ligand is released from one receptor it will rapidly occupy another receptor [88]. The specific receptor distribution on tumor cells is certainly one of the constitutive key points of cell response to both SSAs and DA [27, 74]. Moreover, recent evidence indicates that chimeric molecules would act differently in various tissues tested, and that the effect could differ according to the cell type. In fact, a differential cytotoxicity of chimeric compounds has been observed in vitro in bronchopulmonary and small neuroendocrine cell lines [89]. The responses of each individual cell line suggested that NETs from diverse districts, arising from different neuroendocrine cells, might require cell-specific antiproliferative agents, based on the unique receptor profile of individual lesions [89]. Recently, a functional interface of DRs and SSTRs has been suggested to occur via receptor dimerization. In particular, it has been demonstrated that members of both SSTR and DR superfamilies, when coexpressed in the same cell and in the presence of appropriate ligands, may interact at the membrane level forming homo- and heterodimers [90]. These homo- and heterodimers may constitute a novel receptor, which can activate alternative pathways, possibly enhancing ligand interaction and potentiating signal transduction [74, 89]. Currently, the properties of the dimeric form of these receptors and their therapeutic relevance are far from being fully established. The formation of receptor heterodimers has been observed between unrelated members of different GPCR families, between sst_2 and D_2 and between sst_5 and D_2, but we do not know if this evidence will provide any new insight as to the action of chimeric compounds [88]. Further studies are warranted to clarify the physiological and/or pathological consequences of homo- and heterodimerization in vivo, and to determine whether it will be possible to exploit these processes to optimize available therapeutic options or to develop new drugs with unique properties [88]. With respect to the combined treatment in a real clinical setting (to overcome the resistance to single-agent treatment), the use of a combination with an SSA and a DA has only been explored in a few cases so far [91].

'Hot' SSAs

Tumors overexpressing SSTRs are also candidates for radionuclide therapy, and typically include pituitary adenomas, gastrointestinal and pancreatic NETs, paragangliomas, pheochromocytomas, small cell lung cancers, medullary thyroid carcinomas, breast cancers and malignant lymphomas [52]. Initially, the SS-28 was first labelled with ^{123}I, showing in vivo the rapid cleavage and metabolism that allowed poor visualizing and, therefore, treating of tumors [52].

Soon after octreotide synthesis, the FDA approved ^{111}In-labelled octreotide in 1994 as a diagnostic agent for scintigraphy of patients with NETs. Once octreotide was radiolabelled for diagnostic imaging, in order to localize tumor lesions overexpressing SSTRs [61], the next logical step was to develop PRRT [52]. The theoretical basis of such therapy is principally to convey radioactivity inside the tumor cell, owing to the internalization of the SSTR and radiolabelled analog complex.

Tumors candidate for PRRT with radiolabelled SSAs are sst_2-expressing NETs, as already mentioned, and, at least theoretically, any other tumor histotype known and documented as overexpressing sst_2. Among the inclusion criteria, a high expression of functioning, internalizing SSTRs is critical for an efficient therapy [52]. SSTR scintigraphy, or nowadays PET, is presently the most accurate method to check for the presence of SSTR overexpression. These nuclear medicine techniques have the indications for localizing, staging and following-up patients with NETs; however, the ability to select patients to be submitted to 'cold' or radiolabelled SSAs is the most peculiar [52]. It is important to exclude possible false positives, such as gallbladder accumulation, physiologic uptake in accessory spleens, the presence of recent surgical scars, and any other cause of granulomatous/lymphoid infiltrate that may mimic a tumor lesion. In addition, possible cases of false negatives must be excluded, and, particularly, very small lesions under the resolution power of the methods, recent chemotherapy or dedifferentiated disease. PRRT consists of the systemic administration of the radiopeptide, such as ^{90}Y-DOTATOC or ^{177}Lu-DOTATATE, which are the most used, divided in sequential cycles, administered 6–9 weeks apart, up to a cumulative activity that is calculated based on renal irradiation [52].

PRRT is a promising relatively new treatment modality for inoperable or metastasized GEP-NET patients [92]. The objective response (complete and partial responses) obtained after treatment with ^{90}Y-DOTATOC seems not to differ from that obtained after treatment with ^{177}Lu-octreotate [92]. Most studies reported objective response rates in 20–35% of patients, and the value of PFS and OS (from 16 to 33 months, and from 22 to 46 months, respectively) that resulted favorable with that for SSAs, chemotherapy or new, 'targeted' therapies [92]. New applications of PRRT may include the neoadjuvant use of PRRT for pancreatic NETs. The few case reports available in the literature have described the neoadjuvant use of PRRT in patients with pancreatic NETs who could be operated on successfully after PRRT [92]. As surgery is the only curative option for patients with GEP-NETs, this neoadjuvant treatment seems very promising [92].

Although tumor response rates after initial treatment with PRRT are encouraging, a complete response is rare and eventually the residual tumor(s) will progress again. Retreatment with extra cycles of PRRT as 'salvage therapy' may be considered when better alternatives are not available [92]. It has been reported that 'salvage therapy' with two additional cycles of ^{177}Lu-OCTREOTATE does not lead to serious hematological or nephrotoxic side effects. However, the tumor response rate was lower compared with primary treatment [92].

Although PRRT has already been performed for more than 20 years and several papers have been published, there are not yet available randomized controlled trials comparing PRRT to other treatments (that have a proven benefit when tested in randomized trials in NETs) or placebo, and its positioning in the therapeutic algorithm of NETs remains a strongly debated issue. A randomized study comparing PRRT with ^{177}Lu-OCTREOTATE to high-dose octreotide LAR in patients with progressive metastatic midgut carcinoids was recently initiated in Europe and the USA. However, this study will probably lead to a difficult interpretation of results because the treatment compared to PRRT is not a 'standard' treatment yet, which itself represents a new therapy, of which we ignore the potential benefit, at least at the moment. A study comparing PRRT to sunitinib or everolimus in patients with pancreatic NETs is expected to follow soon.

Interferon

The use of interferon-α, approved for NETs by the European Medicines Agency (EMA), is also well established, although to a lesser extent than SSAs, and was introduced in clinical practice on the basis of the tumor growth inhibition described in preliminary studies [51]. The antitumor effects of interferon-α in NETs are probably caused by multiple complementary mechanisms, including the activation of the Janus kinase/signal transducers and activators of transcription (JAK/STAT) pathways, induction of apoptosis, inhibition of angiogenesis and immunomodulation, leading to the inhibition of secretion and cell proliferation [51]. In 2003, Faiss et al. [93] conducted a prospective, randomized, multicenter study in a group of 80 patients affected by metastatic GEP-NETs treated with lanreotide, interferon-α and with the combination of both drugs. During 12 months of therapy, stable disease was observed in 19 patients (7 in lanreotide, 7 in interferon-α and 5 who received the combination), whereas tumor progression occurred in 14 of 25 patients (lanreotide), 15 of 27 patients (interferon-α) and 14 of 28 patients (combination arm). Side effects leading to an interruption of treatment were more frequent in the combination group than in the monotherapy arms [93]. These results showed for the first time that SSA, interferon-α, or the combination of the two, had comparable antiproliferative effects in the treatment of metastatic GEP-NETs. Response rates were lower compared with those published in previous, nonrandomized studies. In 2005, another randomized trial investigated the effect of octreotide plus interferon-α versus octreotide monotherapy in 105 patients with progressive metastatic foregut (mainly pancreatic) and midgut tumors [94]. Combination treatment was not superior to monotherapy concerning PFS and long-term survival. Patients responding to treatment and those with slow spontaneous tumor growth had a survival advantage [94]. Recently, a randomized multicenter phase 3 trial, which compared chemotherapy and interferon-α in patients with metastatic mixed NETs, reported a PFS of 14 months in interferon-α-treated patients [95]. Despite a trend in favor of interferon, there was no difference in PFS and OS in advanced metastatic carcinoid tumors and the therapeutic effect of both treatments was mild [95]. Presently, interferon-α in combination with octreotide (compared to bevacizumab plus octreotide) is under clinical evaluation. However, common interferon-α adverse effects (in particular fatigue and flu-like syndrome) frequently prevent valuable treatments [51]. For this reason, in 2006, Pavel et al. [96] aimed to assess the efficacy and tolerability of pegylated (PEG) interferon on the management of patients with well-differentiated GEP-NETs. The effect of PEG-interferon-α2b was studied in 17 patients after first-line octreotide treatment. Interferon-α was added when patients showed a tumor progression. Six patients were switched from conventional interferon-α and 11 patients were interferon naive. A tumor response, including stabilization of disease, occurred in 13 of 17 patients. Tolerability of PEG-interferon-α2b was much better than that of interferon-α. Fatigue occurred in 59% of all patients, but was mild in terms of severity [96]. The authors concluded that better tolerability of PEG-interferon-α2b improved patient compliance, justifying its use in patients who do not tolerate conventional α-interferon treatment. However, since its safety profile is definitely less favorable than SSAs, interferon-α is widely considered as a second-line treatment after failure of SSA therapy.

References

1 Brazeau P, Vale W, Burgus R, Ling N, Butcher M, Rivier J, Guillemin R: Hypothalamic polypeptide that inhibits the secretion of immunoreactive pituitary growth hormone. Science 1973;179:77–79.

2 Guillemin R: Hypothalamic hormones a.k.a. hypothalamic releasing factors. J Endocrinol 2005;184: 11–28.

3 Van Op den Bosch J, Adriaensen D, van Nassauw L, Timmermans JP: The role(s) of somatostatin, structurally related peptides and somatostatin receptors in the gastrointestinal tract: a review. Regul Pept 2009;156:1–8.

4 Stengel A, Rivier J, Tache Y: Central actions of somatostatin-28 and oligosomatostatin agonists to prevent components of the endocrine, autonomic and visceral responses to stress through interaction with different somatostatin receptor subtypes. Curr Pharm Des 2013;19:98–105.

5 Hoyer D, Bell GI, Berelowitz M, Epelbaum J, Feniuk W, Humphrey PP, O'Carroll AM, Patel YC, Schonbrunn A, Taylor JE, et al: Classification and nomenclature of somatostatin receptors. Trends Pharmacol Sci 1995;16:86–88.

6 Reisine T, Bell GI: Molecular biology of somatostatin receptors. Endocr Rev 1995;16:427–442.

7 Vanetti M, Kouba M, Wang X, Vogt G, Hollt V: Cloning and expression of a novel mouse somatostatin receptor (sstr2b). FEBS Lett 1992;311:290–294.

8 Cordoba-Chacon J, Gahete MD, Duran-Prado M, Luque RM, Castano JP: Truncated somatostatin receptors as new players in somatostatin-cortistatin pathophysiology. Ann NY Acad Sci 2011;1220:6–15.

9 Fisher WE, Doran TA, Muscarella P 2nd, Boros LG, Ellison EC, Schirmer WJ: Expression of somatostatin receptor subtype 1–5 genes in human pancreatic cancer. J Natl Cancer Inst 1998;90:322–324.

10 Csaba Z, Dournaud P: Cellular biology of somatostatin receptors. Neuropeptides 2001;35:1–23.

11 Reubi JC: Peptide receptors as molecular targets for cancer diagnosis and therapy. Endocr Rev 2003;24:389–427.
12 Reubi JC, Kvols LK, Waser B, Nagorney DM, Heitz PU, Charboneau JW, Reading CC, Moertel C: Detection of somatostatin receptors in surgical and percutaneous needle biopsy samples of carcinoids and islet cell carcinomas. Cancer Res 1990;50:5969–5977.
13 Miller GM, Alexander JM, Bikkal HA, Katznelson L, Zervas NT, Klibanski A: Somatostatin receptor subtype gene expression in pituitary adenomas. J Clin Endocrinol Metab 1995;80:1386–1392.
14 Jais P, Terris B, Ruszniewski P, LeRomancer M, Reyl-Desmars F, Vissuzaine C, Cadiot G, Mignon M, Lewin MJ: Somatostatin receptor subtype gene expression in human endocrine gastroentero-pancreatic tumours. Eur J Clin Invest 1997;27:639–644.
15 Schaer JC, Waser B, Mengod G, Reubi JC: Somatostatin receptor subtypes sst_1, sst_2, sst_3 and sst_5 expression in human pituitary, gastroentero-pancreatic and mammary tumors: comparison of mRNA analysis with receptor autoradiography. Int J Cancer 1997;70:530–537.
16 Reubi JC, Waser B, Schaer JC, Laissue JA: Somatostatin receptor sst_1-sst_5 expression in normal and neoplastic human tissues using receptor autoradiography with subtype-selective ligands. Eur J Nucl Med 2001;28:836–846.
17 Reubi JC, Waser B: Concomitant expression of several peptide receptors in neuroendocrine tumours: molecular basis for in vivo multireceptor tumour targeting. Eur J Nucl Med Mol Imaging 2003;30:781–793.
18 Hofland LJ: Somatostatin and somatostatin receptors in Cushing's disease. Mol Cell Endocrinol 2008;286:199–205.
19 Luque RM, Ibanez-Costa A, Neto LV, Taboada GF, Hormaechea-Agulla D, Kasuki L, Venegas-Moreno E, Moreno-Carazo A, Galvez MA, Soto-Moreno A, Kineman RD, Culler MD, Gahete MD, Gadelha MR, Castano JP: Truncated somatostatin receptor variant sst5TMD4 confers aggressive features (proliferation, invasion and reduced octreotide response) to somatotropinomas. Cancer Lett 2015;359:299–306.
20 Christ E, Wild D, Ederer S, Behe M, Nicolas G, Caplin ME, Brandle M, Clerici T, Fischli S, Stettler C, Ell PJ, Seufert J, Gloor B, Perren A, Reubi JC, Forrer F: Glucagon-like peptide-1 receptor imaging for the localisation of insulinomas: a prospective multicentre imaging study. Lancet Diabetes Endocrinol 2013;1:115–122.
21 Korner M, Stockli M, Waser B, Reubi JC: GLP-1 receptor expression in human tumors and human normal tissues: potential for in vivo targeting. J Nucl Med 2007;48:736–743.
22 Missale C, Nash SR, Robinson SW, Jaber M, Caron MG: Dopamine receptors: from structure to function. Physiol Rev 1998;78:189–225.
23 Pivonello R, Ferone D, de Herder WW, Kros JM, De Caro ML, Arvigo M, Annunziato L, Lombardi G, Colao A, Hofland LJ, Lamberts SW: Dopamine receptor expression and function in corticotroph pituitary tumors. J Clin Endocrinol Metab 2004;89:2452–2462.
24 Ferone D, de Herder WW, Pivonello R, Kros JM, van Koetsveld PM, de Jong T, Minuto F, Colao A, Lamberts SW, Hofland LJ: Correlation of in vitro and in vivo somatotropic adenoma responsiveness to somatostatin analogs and dopamine agonists with immunohistochemical evaluation of somatostatin and dopamine receptors and electron microscopy. J Clin Endocrinol Metab 2008;93:1412–1417.
25 Saveanu A, Jaquet P, Brue T, Barlier A: Relevance of coexpression of somatostatin and dopamine D2 receptors in pituitary adenomas. Mol Cell Endocrinol 2008;286:206–213.
26 Grossrubatscher E, Veronese S, Ciaramella PD, Pugliese R, Boniardi M, De Carlis L, Torre M, Ravini M, Gambacorta M, Loli P: High expression of dopamine receptor subtype 2 in a large series of neuroendocrine tumors. Cancer Biol Ther 2008;7:1970–1978.
27 Gatto F, Hofland LJ: The role of somatostatin and dopamine D2 receptors in endocrine tumors. Endocr Relat Cancer 2011;18:R233–R251.
28 Rozengurt E, Walsh JH: Gastrin, CCK, signaling, and cancer. Annu Rev Physiol 2001;63:49–76.
29 Patel DR, Kong Y, Sreedharan SP: Molecular cloning and expression of a human secretin receptor. Mol Pharmacol 1995;47:467–473.
30 Korner M, Hayes GM, Rehmann R, Zimmermann A, Friess H, Miller LJ, Reubi JC: Secretin receptors in normal and diseased human pancreas: marked reduction of receptor binding in ductal neoplasia. Am J Pathol 2005;167:959–968.
31 Frucht H, Howard JM, Slaff JI, Wank SA, McCarthy DM, Maton PN, Vinayek R, Gardner JD, Jensen RT: Secretin and calcium provocative tests in the Zollinger-Ellison syndrome: a prospective study. Ann Intern Med 1989;111:713–722.
32 Ding WQ, Cheng ZJ, McElhiney J, Kuntz SM, Miller LJ: Silencing of secretin receptor function by dimerization with a misspliced variant secretin receptor in ductal pancreatic adenocarcinoma. Cancer Res 2002;62:5223–5229.
33 Long SH, Berna MJ, Thill M, Pace A, Pradhan TK, Hoffmann KM, Serrano J, Jensen RT: Secretin-receptor and secretin-receptor-variant expression in gastrinomas: correlation with clinical and tumoral features and secretin and calcium provocative test results. J Clin Endocrinol Metabol 2007;92:4394–4402.
34 de Weerd NA, Samarajiwa SA, Hertzog PJ: Type I interferon receptors: biochemistry and biological functions. J Biol Chem 2007;282:20053–20057.

35 De Maeyer E, De Maeyer-Guignard J: Type I interferons. Int Rev Immunol 1998;17:53–73.
36 Oberg K, Eriksson B: The role of interferons in the management of carcinoid tumors. Acta Oncol 1991;30:519–522.
37 Eriksson B, Oberg K: An update of the medical treatment of malignant endocrine pancreatic tumors. Acta Oncol 1993;32:203–208.
38 Vitale G, de Herder WW, van Koetsveld PM, Waaijers M, Schoordijk W, Croze E, Colao A, Lamberts SW, Hofland LJ: IFN-β is a highly potent inhibitor of gastroenteropancreatic neuroendocrine tumor cell growth in vitro. Cancer Res 2006;66:554–562.
39 Vitale G, Caraglia M, van Koetsveld PM, Maroni P, Marra M, Colao A, Lamberts SW, Cavagnini F, Hofland LJ: Potential role of type I interferons in the treatment of pituitary adenomas. Rev Endocr Metab Disord 2009;10:125–133.
40 Gadelha MR, Kasuki L, Korbonits M: Novel pathway for somatostatin analogs in patients with acromegaly. Trends Endocrinol Metab 2013;24:238–246.
41 Lania A, Mantovani G, Spada A: Genetic abnormalities of somatostatin receptors in pituitary tumors. Mol Cell Endocrinol 2008;286:180–186.
42 Torrisani J, Hanoun N, Laurell H, Lopez F, Maoret JJ, Souque A, Susini C, Cordelier P, Buscail L: Identification of an upstream promoter of the human somatostatin receptor, hSSTR2, which is controlled by epigenetic modifications. Endocrinology 2008;149:3137–3147.
43 Veenstra MJ, de Herder WW, Feelders RA, Hofland LJ: Targeting the somatostatin receptor in pituitary and neuroendocrine tumors. Expert Opin Ther Targets 2013;17:1329–1343.
44 Al-Azzawi H, Yacqub-Usman K, Richardson A, Hofland LJ, Clayton RN, Farrell WE: Reversal of endogenous dopamine receptor silencing in pituitary cells augments receptor-mediated apoptosis. Endocrinology 2011;152:364–373.
45 Hofland LJ, Lamberts SW: The pathophysiological consequences of somatostatin receptor internalization and resistance. Endocr Rev 2003;24:28–47.
46 de Bruin C, Feelders RA, Waaijers AM, van Koetsveld PM, Sprij-Mooij DM, Lamberts SW, Hofland LJ: Differential regulation of human dopamine D2 and somatostatin receptor subtype expression by glucocorticoids in vitro. J Mol Endocrinol 2009;42:47–56.
47 de Bruin C, Hofland LJ, Nieman LK, van Koetsveld PM, Waaijers AM, Sprij-Mooij DM, van Essen M, Lamberts SW, de Herder WW, Feelders RA: Mifepristone effects on tumor somatostatin receptor expression in two patients with Cushing's syndrome due to ectopic adrenocorticotropin secretion. J Clin Endocrinol Metabol 2012;97:455–462.
48 Waser B, Cescato R, Liu Q, Kao YJ, Korner M, Christ E, Schonbrunn A, Reubi JC: Phosphorylation of sst2 receptors in neuroendocrine tumors after octreotide treatment of patients. Am J Pathol 2012;180:1942–1949.
49 Modlin IM, Moss SF, Gustafsson BI, Lawrence B, Schimmack S, Kidd M: The archaic distinction between functioning and nonfunctioning neuroendocrine neoplasms is no longer clinically relevant. Langenbecks Arch Surg 2011;396:1145–1156.
50 Yao JC, Hassan M, Phan A, Dagohoy C, Leary C, Mares JE, Abdalla EK, Fleming JB, Vauthey JN, Rashid A, Evans DB: One hundred years after 'carcinoid': epidemiology of and prognostic factors for neuroendocrine tumors in 35,825 cases in the United States. J Clin Oncol 2008;26:3063–3072.
51 Barbieri F, Albertelli M, Grillo F, Mohamed A, Saveanu A, Barlier A, Ferone D, Florio T: Neuroendocrine tumors: insights into innovative therapeutic options and rational development of targeted therapies. Drug Discov Today 2014;19:458–468.
52 Bodei L, Ferone D, Grana CM, Cremonesi M, Signore A, Dierckx RA, Paganelli G: Peptide receptor therapies in neuroendocrine tumors. J Endocrinol Invest 2009;32:360–369.
53 Kaltsas GA, Mukherjee JJ, Grossman AB: The value of radiolabelled MIBG and octreotide in the diagnosis and management of neuroendocrine tumours. Ann Oncol 2001;12(suppl 2):S47–S50.
54 Virgolini I, Raderer M, Kurtaran A, Angelberger P, Banyai S, Yang Q, Li S, Banyai M, Pidlich J, Niederle B, Scheithauer W, Valent P: Vasoactive intestinal peptide-receptor imaging for the localization of intestinal adenocarcinomas and endocrine tumors. N Engl J Med 1994;331:1116–1121.
55 de Jong M, Kwekkeboom D, Valkema R, Krenning EP: Radiolabelled peptides for tumour therapy: current status and future directions – plenary lecture at the EANM 2002. Eur J Nucl Med Mol Imaging 2003;30:463–469.
56 Orlefors H, Sundin A, Garske U, Juhlin C, Oberg K, Skogseid B, Langstrom B, Bergstrom M, Eriksson B: Whole-body ^{11}C-5-hydroxytryptophan positron emission tomography as a universal imaging technique for neuroendocrine tumors: comparison with somatostatin receptor scintigraphy and computed tomography. J Clin Endocrinol Metabol 2005;90:3392–3400.
57 Kaltsas G, Rockall A, Papadogias D, Reznek R, Grossman AB: Recent advances in radiological and radionuclide imaging and therapy of neuroendocrine tumours. Eur J Endocrinol 2004;151:15–27.
58 Pettinato C, Sarnelli A, Di Donna M, Civollani S, Nanni C, Montini G, Di Pierro D, Ferrari M, Marengo M, Bergamini C: ^{68}Ga-DOTANOC: biodistribution and dosimetry in patients affected by neuroendocrine tumors. Eur J Nucl Med Mol Imaging 2008;35:72–79.

59 Reubi JC, Lamberts SJ, Krenning EP: Receptor imaging of human diseases using radiolabeled peptides. J Recept Signal Transduct Res 1995;15:379–392.

60 de Jong M, Valkema R, Jamar F, Kvols LK, Kwekkeboom DJ, Breeman WA, Bakker WH, Smith C, Pauwels S, Krenning EP: Somatostatin receptor-targeted radionuclide therapy of tumors: preclinical and clinical findings. Semin Nucl Med 2002;32:133–140.

61 Krenning EP, Kwekkeboom DJ, Bakker WH, Breeman WA, Kooij PP, Oei HY, van Hagen M, Postema PT, de Jong M, Reubi JC, et al: Somatostatin receptor scintigraphy with [111in-DTPA-D-Phe1]- and [123i-Tyr3]-octreotide: the Rotterdam experience with more than 1,000 patients. Eur J Nucl Med 1993; 20:716–731.

62 Pfannenberg AC, Eschmann SM, Horger M, Lamberts R, Vonthein R, Claussen CD, Bares R: Benefit of anatomical-functional image fusion in the diagnostic work-up of neuroendocrine neoplasms. Eur J Nucl Med Mol Imaging 2003;30:835–843.

63 Wild D, Macke HR, Waser B, Reubi JC, Ginj M, Rasch H, Muller-Brand J, Hofmann M:^{68}Ga-DOTANOC: a first compound for pet imaging with high affinity for somatostatin receptor subtypes 2 and 5. Eur J Nucl Med Mol Imaging 2005;32:724.

64 Wild D, Bomanji JB, Benkert P, Maecke H, Ell PJ, Reubi JC, Caplin ME: Comparison of ^{68}Ga-DOTANOC and ^{68}Ga-DOTANATE PET/CT within patients with gastroenteropancreatic neuroendocrine tumors. J Nucl Med 2013;54:364–372.

65 Gabriel M, Decristoforo C, Kendler D, Dobrozemsky G, Heute D, Uprimny C, Kovacs P, von Guggenberg E, Bale R, Virgolini IJ: ^{68}Ga-DOTA-Tyr3-octreotide PET in neuroendocrine tumors: comparison with somatostatin receptor scintigraphy and CT. J Nucl Med 2007;48:508–518.

66 Srirajaskanthan R, Kayani I, Quigley AM, Soh J, Caplin ME, Bomanji J: The role of ^{68}Ga-dotatate PET in patients with neuroendocrine tumors and negative or equivocal findings on ^{111}In-DTPA-octreotide scintigraphy. J Nucl Med 2010;51:875–882.

67 Ambrosini V, Tomassetti P, Franchi R, Fanti S: Imaging of NETs with pet radiopharmaceuticals. Q J Nucl Med Mol Imaging 2010;54:16–23.

68 Lamberts SW, van der Lely AJ, de Herder WW, Hofland LJ: Octreotide. N Engl J Med 1996;334:246–254.

69 Barbieri F, Bajetto A, Pattarozzi A, Gatti M, Wurth R, Thellung S, Corsaro A, Villa V, Nizzari M, Florio T: Peptide receptor targeting in cancer: the somatostatin paradigm. Int J Pept 2013;2013:926295.

70 Florio T: Somatostatin/somatostatin receptor signalling: phosphotyrosine phosphatases. Mol Cell Endocrinol 2008;286:40–48.

71 Florio T: Molecular mechanisms of the antiproliferative activity of somatostatin receptors (SSTRs) in neuroendocrine tumors. Front Biosci 2008;13:822–840.

72 Florio T, Morini M, Villa V, Arena S, Corsaro A, Thellung S, Culler MD, Pfeffer U, Noonan DM, Schettini G, Albini A: Somatostatin inhibits tumor angiogenesis and growth via somatostatin receptor-3-mediated regulation of endothelial nitric oxide synthase and mitogen-activated protein kinase activities. Endocrinology 2003;144:1574–1584.

73 Bruns C, Lewis I, Briner U, Meno-Tetang G, Weckbecker G: SOM230: a novel somatostatin peptidomimetic with broad somatotropin release inhibiting factor (SRIF) receptor binding and a unique antisecretory profile. Eur J Endocrinol 2002;146:707–716.

74 Ferone D, Gatto F, Arvigo M, Resmini E, Boschetti M, Teti C, Esposito D, Minuto F: The clinical-molecular interface of somatostatin, dopamine and their receptors in pituitary pathophysiology. J Mol Endocrinol 2009;42:361–370.

75 Schonbrunn A: Selective agonism in somatostatin receptor signaling and regulation. Mol Cell Endocrinol 2008;286:35–39.

76 Tulipano G, Schulz S: Novel insights in somatostatin receptor physiology. Eur J Endocrinol 2007; 156(suppl 1):S3–S11.

77 Reubi JC, Schar JC, Waser B, Wenger S, Heppeler A, Schmitt JS, Macke HR: Affinity profiles for human somatostatin receptor subtypes sst_1-sst_5 of somatostatin radiotracers selected for scintigraphic and radiotherapeutic use. Eur J Nucl Med 2000;27:273–282.

78 Colao A, Faggiano A, Pivonello R: Somatostatin analogues: treatment of pituitary and neuroendocrine tumors. Prog Brain Res 2010;182:281–294.

79 Rinke A, Muller HH, Schade-Brittinger C, Klose KJ, Barth P, Wied M, Mayer C, Aminossadati B, Pape UF, Blaker M, Harder J, Arnold C, Gress T, Arnold R: Placebo-controlled, double-blind, prospective, randomized study on the effect of octreotide LAR in the control of tumor growth in patients with metastatic neuroendocrine midgut tumors: a report from the PROMID study group. J Clin Oncol 2009;27: 4656–4663.

80 Caplin ME, Pavel M, Cwikla JB, Phan AT, Raderer M, Sedlackova E, Cadiot G, Wolin EM, Capdevila J, Wall L, Rindi G, Langley A, Martinez S, Blumberg J, Ruszniewski P, CLARINET Investigators: Lanreotide in metastatic enteropancreatic neuroendocrine tumors. N Engl J Med 2014;371:224–233.

81 Kvols LK, Oberg KE, O'Dorisio TM, Mohideen P, de Herder WW, Arnold R, Hu K, Zhang Y, Hughes G, Anthony L, Wiedenmann B: Pasireotide (SOM230) shows efficacy and tolerability in the treatment of patients with advanced neuroendocrine tumors refractory or resistant to octreotide LAR: results from a phase II study. Endocr Relat Cancer 2012;19:657–666.

82 Mohamed A, Blanchard MP, Albertelli M, Barbieri F, Brue T, Niccoli P, Delpero JR, Monges G, Garcia S, Ferone D, Florio T, Enjalbert A, Moutardier V, Schonbrunn A, Gerard C, Barlier A, Saveanu A: Pasireotide and octreotide antiproliferative effects and sst_2 trafficking in human pancreatic neuroendocrine tumor cultures. Endocr Relat Cancer 2014;21:691–704.

83 Cives M, Kunz PL, Morse B, Coppola D, Schell MJ, Campos T, Nguyen PT, Nandoskar P, Khandelwal V, Strosberg JR: Phase II clinical trial of pasireotide long-acting repeatable in patients with metastatic neuroendocrine tumors. Endocr Relat Cancer 2015; 22:1–9.

84 Colao A, Petersenn S, Newell-Price J, Findling JW, Gu F, Maldonado M, Schoenherr U, Mills D, Salgado LR, Biller BM, et al: A 12-month phase 3 study of pasireotide in Cushing's disease. N Engl J Med 2012; 366:914–924.

85 Colao A, Bronstein MD, Freda P, Gu F, Shen CC, Gadelha M, Fleseriu M, van der Lely AJ, Farrall AJ, Hermosillo Resendiz K, Ruffin M, Chen Y, Sheppard M, Pasireotide CSG: Pasireotide versus octreotide in acromegaly: a head-to-head superiority study. J Clin Endocrinol Metab 2014;99:791–799.

86 O'Toole D, Saveanu A, Couvelard A, Gunz G, Enjalbert A, Jaquet P, Ruszniewski P, Barlier A: The analysis of quantitative expression of somatostatin and dopamine receptors in gastro-entero-pancreatic tumours opens new therapeutic strategies. Eur J Endocrinol 2006;155:849–857.

87 Srirajaskanthan R, Watkins J, Marelli L, Khan K, Caplin ME: Expression of somatostatin and dopamine 2 receptors in neuroendocrine tumours and the potential role for new biotherapies. Neuroendocrinology 2009;89:308–314.

88 Ferone D: Somatostatin and dopamine receptors. Tumori 2010;96:802–805.

89 Kidd M, Drozdov I, Joseph R, Pfragner R, Culler M, Modlin I: Differential cytotoxicity of novel somatostatin and dopamine chimeric compounds on bronchopulmonary and small intestinal neuroendocrine tumor cell lines. Cancer 2008;113:690–700.

90 Rocheville M, Lange DC, Kumar U, Patel SC, Patel RC, Patel YC: Receptors for dopamine and somatostatin: formation of hetero-oligomers with enhanced functional activity. Science 2000;288:154–157.

91 Pivonello R, Ferone D, Lamberts SW, Colao A: Cabergoline plus lanreotide for ectopic cushing's syndrome. N Engl J Med 2005;352:2457–2458.

92 van der Zwan WA, Bodei L, Mueller-Brand J, de Herder WW, Kvols LK, Kwekkeboom DJ: GEP-NETs update: radionuclide therapy in neuroendocrine tumors. Eur J Endocrinol 2015;172:R1–R8.

93 Faiss S, Pape UF, Bohmig M, Dorffel Y, Mansmann U, Golder W, Riecken EO, Wiedenmann B, et al: Prospective, randomized, multicenter trial on the antiproliferative effect of lanreotide, interferon alfa, and their combination for therapy of metastatic neuroendocrine gastroenteropancreatic tumors – The International Lanreotide and Interferon Alfa Study Group. J Clin Oncol 2003;21:2689–2696.

94 Arnold R, Rinke A, Klose KJ, Muller HH, Wied M, Zamzow K, Schmidt C, Schade-Brittinger C, Barth P, Moll R, Koller M, Unterhalt M, Hiddemann W, Schmidt-Lauber M, Pavel M, Arnold CN: Octreotide versus octreotide plus interferon-alpha in endocrine gastroenteropancreatic tumors: a randomized trial. Clin Gastroenterol Hepatol 2005;3:761–771.

95 Dahan L, Bonnetain F, Rougier P, Raoul JL, Gamelin E, Etienne PL, Cadiot G, Mitry E, Smith D, Cvitkovic F, Coudert B, Ricard F, Bedenne L, Seitz JF, Federation Francophone de Cancerologie D, Digestive Tumors Group of the Federation Nationale des Centres de Lutte Contre le C: Phase III trial of chemotherapy using 5-fluorouracil and streptozotocin compared with interferon alpha for advanced carcinoid tumors: FNCLCC-FFCD 9710. Endocr Relat Cancer 2009;16:1351–1361.

96 Pavel ME, Baum U, Hahn EG, Schuppan D, Lohmann T: Efficacy and tolerability of pegylated IFN-α in patients with neuroendocrine gastroenteropancreatic carcinomas. J Interferon Cytokine Res 2006;26: 8–13.

Leo J. Hofland
Department of Internal Medicine, Division of Endocrinology, Room Ee-530b, Erasmus MC
Dr. Molewaterplein 50
NL–3015 GE Rotterdam (The Netherlands)
E-Mail l.hofland@erasmusmc.nl

Papotti M, de Herder WW (eds): Neuroendocrine Tumors: A Multidisciplinary Approach.
Front Horm Res. Basel, Karger, 2015, vol 44, pp 239–247 (DOI: 10.1159/000403785)

The Role of Chemotherapy in Well-Differentiated Gastroenteropancreatic Neuroendocrine Tumors

Jonathan Strosberg[a] · Jamie Goldman[b] · Frederico Costa[c] · Marianne Pavel[d]

[a]Moffitt Cancer Center and Research Institute, and [b]University of South Florida, Tampa, Fla., USA; [c]Centro de Oncologia, Hospital Sírio Libanês, São Paulo, Brazil; [d]Charité University Medicine Berlin, Berlin, Germany

Abstract

Even though the neuroendocrine tumor (NET) field has entered the era of 'targeted therapy', the role of cytotoxic chemotherapy continues to be debated. High response rates, ranging from 30 to 70% depending on the line of therapy, are consistently observed in the treatment of pancreatic NETs, with lesser evidence of activity in other foregut tumors. Activity in midgut carcinoid tumors appears to be negligible. Unfortunately, placebo-controlled randomized controlled trials using modern response criteria are lacking: the bulk of the literature consists of small phase II trials and retrospective series. There are also no completed trials comparing modern chemotherapy regimens, and therefore little data exist to favor the use of streptozocin- versus temozolomide- versus oxaliplatin-based therapies. Due to the absence of high-level evidence, it is difficult to generate data-based guidelines on the appropriate sequencing of cytotoxic drugs versus targeted agents. Although conventional wisdom holds that targeted agents such as everolimus or sunitinib are more tolerable than cytotoxic drugs, there is no evidence to support this perception. As a general principle, chemotherapy may be more appropriate as early-line therapy in patients with bulky and/or symptomatic and/or rapidly progressive tumors, particularly of pancreatic origin. In patients with low-volume disease or slow-growing tumors, noncytotoxic drugs may be preferable in early lines of therapy, reserving chemotherapy for the salvage setting. Validation of predictive factors is imperative in order to appropriately match patients with optimal treatment. Methyl-guanine-methyl-transferase (MGMT) deficiency is likely to be a positive predictive factor for alkylating agents, but needs to be evaluated prospectively. It is also unclear whether immunostaining for MGMT expression, which can be somewhat subjective, is superior to PCR-based techniques, which assess MGMT methylation status. Other basic predictive factors, such as ki-67 index, need to be evaluated in prospective clinical trials. It will also be important to evaluate whether newly discovered mutations in pancreatic NETs, such as DAXX/ATRX, are associated with response to chemotherapy.

Gastroenteropancreatic neuroendocrine tumors (GEP-NETs) are clinically and biologically heterogeneous. They are often subdivided into two categories: carcinoid tumors of the gastrointestinal tract and pancreatic NETs. It is increasingly clear that pancreatic NETs are biologically distinct from carcinoid tumors and are typically associated with specific mutations in genes linked to either the PI3Kinase/mTOR pathway (i.e. PTEN, TSC) or genes associated with epigenetic chromatin modeling (i.e. DAXX/ATRX, MEN1) [1]. The genetic landscape of carcinoid tumors is less well understood, but appears to involve allelic deletions and insertions with few identifiable point mutations [2].

On average, pancreatic NETs are substantially more sensitive to cytotoxic drugs, particularly alkylating agents, compared to carcinoid tumors which tend to be fairly resistant to chemotherapy. The precise reasons for these differences in chemosensitivity are uncertain, but may be related to factors such as differential expression of DNA repair enzymes, chromosomal instability, and cell-cycle kinetics. It is less clear whether chemosensitivity rates differ between various primary gastrointestinal sites; however, it is likely that midgut NETs, which tend to be slow growing, are more chemoresistant than other primary sites. This chapter reviews data on cytotoxic chemotherapy in well-differentiated GEP-NETs, including combinations of cytotoxic drugs with targeted agents (table 1).

Streptozocin Combinations

Streptozocin (STZ), a nitrosurea drug derived from *Streptomyces achromogenes*, was one of the first cytotoxic drugs tested in pancreatic NETs and is specifically toxic to pancreatic β-cells [3]. Side effects include nausea, vomiting, myelosuppression and nephrotoxicity. Based on promising phase II data, two randomized controlled trials were launched by the Eastern Cooperative Oncology Group (ECOG) in the 1970s and 1980s. The first of these studies randomly assigned 84 patients to receive streptozocin alone versus STZ combined with 5-fluorouracil (5-FU) [4]. The study reported a response rate of 63% with STZ plus 5-FU versus 36% with STZ monotherapy. The second study randomly assigned 105 patients to three arms: STZ with 5-FU, STZ with doxorubicin (DOX), or chlorozotocin [5]. The superior arm in this study was found to be STZ/DOX which was associated with a response rate of 69% (compared to 45% with STZ/5-FU and 30% with chlorozotocin). Interestingly, the combination of STZ/DOX was also associated with a statistically significant improvement in overall survival (2.2 vs. 1.4 years with STZ/5-FU, $p = 0.004$), although it is important to emphasize that the study was not powered to evaluate survival differences.

The high response rates reported in these early studies have been subsequently challenged due to their lack of rigorous radiographic response criteria. Indeed, nonradiographic criteria, such as changes in liver size on physical exam, were often used to assess response. Two small retrospective series were published questioning the high

and 1 who had liver metastases of unknown primary. The median PFS was 13.7 months. A retrospective study of 24 NET patients, primarily pancreatic, treated with CAPE/OX at two Brazilian centers reported a response rate of 29% and PFS of 9.8 months [27].

Predictors of Response to Chemotherapy

The anticancer activity of alkylating agents such as TEM and streptozocin is counteracted by the DNA-repair enzyme O^6-MGMT which removes a mutagenic alkyl group from O^6-guanine and transfers it to an active cysteine. It has been demonstrated that loss of MGMT expression in high-grade gliomas predicts for improved survival with TEM therapy. MGMT deficiency can be assessed through several methods: immunohistochemical (IHC) analysis of protein expression, or analysis of MGMT promoter methylation via quantitative methylation-specific PCR or pyrosequencing.

Kulke et al. [28] investigated MGMT deficiency using IHC in 97 archival GEP-NET specimens. The study found that 19 of 37 pancreatic NETs (51%) and 0 of 60 carcinoid tumor specimens were MGMT deficient, potentially explaining the enhanced chemosensitivity of pancreatic compared to nonpancreatic NETs. Among 21 patients who had received treatment with TEM, 4 of 5 patients with MGMT-deficient tumors responded, versus 0 of 16 MGMT-proficient tumors. These results were corroborated by Hammel et al. [29] who investigated MGMT expression by IHC in 22 patients with GEP-NETs, primarily of pancreatic origin, treated with TEM or CAPE/TEM. A high MGMT score, seen more in small bowel carcinoid tumors than pancreatic NETs, was predictive of an absence of response ($p = 0.02$). Conversely, Ekeblad et al. [16] found no significant correlation between response to TEM and MGMT expression by immunohistochemistry among 23 NET patients analyzed. Fewer data are available on the potential association between MGMT promoter methylation and response to TEM. Schmitt et al. [30] reported no correlation between promoter methylation (by methylation-specific PCR) and protein expression (immunohistochemistry), suggesting that different assays may result in divergent results.

Interestingly, there has been very limited data on the correlation between tumor grade and response to chemotherapy, despite the fact that chemotherapy is generally thought to be more active in high-proliferative tumors. In a study of STZ, cisplatin and 5-FU, Turner et al. [11] noted a significant trend towards an improved response rate with increased mitotic rate and ki-67 proliferative index.

Choice of Chemotherapy in Intermediate- to High-Grade Tumors

The 2010 WHO pathological classification of NETs defines high-grade (G3) tumors as having a ki-67 index above 20%, and implies that there is a concordance between high-grade proliferation and poorly differentiated histology [31]. However, it is increasingly apparent that high-grade neuroendocrine cancers are heterogeneous, and that not all are poorly differentiated [32]. Indeed, many morphologically well-differentiated GEP-NETs, particularly of the pancreas, fall into the high-grade category due to ki-67 indexes in the 20–55% range.

Recent data indicate that the platinum/etoposide regimen, commonly used to treat poorly differentiated and small cell neuroendocrine cancers, is only marginally active in NETs with ki-67 indexes in the 20–55% range [33]. These tumors, which are often well or moderately differentiated, appear to be substantially more sensitive to alkylating agents such as STZ and TEM. Modifications to the WHO classification have been recommended to reflect the heterogeneity of high-grade NETs and to avoid conflation of well-differentiated G3 tumors with poorly differentiated carcinomas which are biologically distinct [34].

In conclusion, cytotoxic drugs should not be considered an anachronism in the modern era of GEP-NET therapy. Future prospective clinical trials should compare cytotoxic drugs to targeted agents in appropriate patient populations, evaluating clinical outcomes and quality-of-life as endpoints.

References

1 Jiao Y, Shi C, Edil BH, et al: DAXX/ATRX, MEN1, and mTOR pathway genes are frequently altered in pancreatic neuroendocrine tumors. Science 2011;331:1199–1203.

2 Banck MS, Kanwar R, Kulkarni AA, et al: The genomic landscape of small intestine neuroendocrine tumors. J Clin Invest 2013;123:2502–2508.

3 Broder LE, Carter SK: Pancreatic islet cell carcinoma. II. Results of therapy with streptozotocin in 52 patients. Ann Intern Med 1973;79:108–118.

4 Moertel CG, Hanley JA, Johnson LA: Streptozocin alone compared with streptozocin plus fluorouracil in the treatment of advanced islet-cell carcinoma. N Engl J Med 1980;303:1189–1194.

5 Moertel CG, Lefkopoulo M, Lipsitz S, Hahn RG, Klaassen D: Streptozocin-doxorubicin, streptozocin-fluorouracil or chlorozotocin in the treatment of advanced islet-cell carcinoma. N Engl J Med 1992;326:519–523.

6 Cheng PN, Saltz LB: Failure to confirm major objective antitumor activity for streptozocin and doxorubicin in the treatment of patients with advanced islet cell carcinoma. Cancer 1999;86:944–948.

7 McCollum AD, Kulke MH, Ryan DP, et al: Lack of efficacy of streptozocin and doxorubicin in patients with advanced pancreatic endocrine tumors. Am J Clin Oncol 2004;27:485–488.

8 Delaunoit T, Ducreux M, Boige V, et al: The doxorubicin-streptozotocin combination for the treatment of advanced well-differentiated pancreatic endocrine carcinoma – a judicious option? Eur J Cancer 2004;40:515–520.

9 Fjallskog ML, Janson ET, Falkmer UG, Vatn MH, Oberg KE, Eriksson BK: Treatment with combined streptozotocin and liposomal doxorubicin in metastatic endocrine pancreatic tumors. Neuroendocrinology 2008;88:53–58.

10 Kouvaraki MA, Ajani JA, Hoff P, et al: Fluorouracil, doxorubicin, and streptozocin in the treatment of patients with locally advanced and metastatic pancreatic endocrine carcinomas. J Clin Oncol 2004;22:4762–4771.

11 Turner NC, Strauss SJ, Sarker D, et al: Chemotherapy with 5-fluorouracil, cisplatin and streptozocin for neuroendocrine tumours. Br J Cancer 2010;102:1106–1112.

12 Ducreux M, Seitz JF, Smith D, et al: Efficacy and safety of bevacizumab combined with chemotherapy in the treatment of patients with metastatic well-differentiated duodeno-pancreatic endocrine tumors (BETTER study). J Clin Oncol 2012;30(suppl):4036.

13 Sun W, Lipsitz S, Catalano P, Mailliard JA, Haller DG: Phase II/III study of doxorubicin with fluorouracil compared with streptozocin with fluorouracil or dacarbazine in the treatment of advanced carcinoid tumors: Eastern Cooperative Oncology Group Study E1281. J Clin Oncol 2005;23:4897–4904.

14 Dahan L, Bonnetain F, Rougier P, et al: Phase III trial of chemotherapy using 5-fluorouracil and streptozotocin compared with interferon alpha for advanced carcinoid tumors: FNCLCC-FFCD 9710. Endocr Relat Cancer 2009;16:1351–1361.

15 Ramanathan RK, Cnaan A, Hahn RG, Carbone PP, Haller DG: Phase II trial of dacarbazine (DTIC) in advanced pancreatic islet cell carcinoma. Study of the Eastern Cooperative Oncology Group-E6282. Ann Oncol 2001;12:1139–1143.

16 Ekeblad S, Sundin A, Janson ET, et al: Temozolomide as monotherapy is effective in treatment of advanced malignant neuroendocrine tumors. Clin Cancer Res 2007;13:2986–2991.

17 Kulke MH, Stuart K, Enzinger PC, et al: Phase II study of temozolomide and thalidomide in patients with metastatic neuroendocrine tumors. J Clin Oncol 2006;24:401–406.

18 Chan JA, Stuart K, Earle CC, et al: Prospective study of bevacizumab plus temozolomide in patients with advanced neuroendocrine tumors. J Clin Oncol 2012;30:2963–2968.

19 Chan JA, Blaszkowsky L, Stuart K, et al: A prospective, phase 1/2 study of everolimus and temozolomide in patients with advanced pancreatic neuroendocrine tumor. Cancer 2013;119:3212–3218.

20 Fine R, Fogelman D, Schreibman S: Effective treatment of neuroendocrine tumors with capecitabine and temozolomide. ASCO Annual Meeting Proceedings. J Clin Oncol 2005;23:4216.

21 Fine RL, Gulati AP, Krantz BA, et al: Capecitabine and temozolomide (CAPTEM) for metastatic, well-differentiated neuroendocrine cancers: the Pancreas Center at Columbia University experience. Cancer Chemother Pharmacol 2013;71:663–670.

22 Strosberg JR, Fine RL, Choi J, et al: First-line chemotherapy with capecitabine and temozolomide in patients with metastatic pancreatic endocrine carcinomas. Cancer 2011;117:268–275.

23 Abbasi S, Kashashna A, Albaba H: Efficacy of capecitabine and temozolomide combination in well-differentiated neuroendocrine tumors: Jordan experience. Pancreas 2014;43:1303–1305.

24 Fine RL, Gulati AP, Tsushima DA, et al: Prospective phase II study of capecitabine and temozolomide (CAPTEM) for progressive, moderately, and well-differentiated metastatic neuroendocrine tumors (abstract). J Clin Oncol 2014;32(suppl 3):179.

25 Bajetta E, Catena L, Procopio G, et al: Are capecitabine and oxaliplatin (XELOX) suitable treatments for progressing low-grade and high-grade neuroendocrine tumours? Cancer Chemother Pharmacol 2007; 59:637–642.

26 Kunz PL, Kuo T, Zhan JM, et al: A phase II study of capecitabine, oxaliplatin, and bevacizumab for metastatic or unresectable neuroendocrine tumors (abstract). J Clin Oncol 2010;28(15 suppl):4104.

27 Ferrarotto R, Testa L, Riechelmann RP, et al: Combination of capecitabine and oxaliplatin is an effective treatment option for advanced neuroendocrine tumors. Rare Tumors 2013;5:e35.

28 Kulke MH, Hornick JL, Frauenhoffer C, et al: O^6-methylguanine DNA methyltransferase deficiency and response to temozolomide-based therapy in patients with neuroendocrine tumors. Clin Cancer Res 2009;15:338–345.

29 Hammel P, Hentic O, Cros J, et al: Methylguanine DNA methyl transferase (MGMT) expression to predict response to temozolomide (TMZ) in patients with digestive neuroendocrine tumors (NETs). J Clin Oncol 2012;30(suppl):abstr 4133.

30 Schmitt AM, Pavel M, Rudolph T, et al: Prognostic and predictive roles of MGMT protein expression and promoter methylation in sporadic pancreatic Neuroendocrine neoplasms. Neuroendocrinology 2014;100:35–34.

31 Bosman F, Carneiro F, Hruban R, Theise N (eds): WHO Classfication of Tumours of the Digestive System. Lyon, IARC, 2010.

32 Velayoudom-Cephise FL, Duvillard P, Foucan L, et al: Are G3 ENETS neuroendocrine neoplasms heterogeneous? Endocr Relat Cancer 2013;20:649–657.

33 Sorbye H, Welin S, Langer SW, et al: Predictive and prognostic factors for treatment and survival in 305 patients with advanced gastrointestinal neuroendocrine carcinoma (WHO G3): the NORDIC NEC study. Ann Oncol 2013;24:152–160.

34 Sorbye H, Strosberg J, Baudin E, Klimstra DS, Yao JC: Gastroenteropancreatic high-grade neuroendocrine carcinoma. Cancer 2014;120:2814–2823.

Jonathan Strosberg
Moffitt Cancer Center and Research Institute
12902 Magnolia Drive
Tampa, FL 33612 (USA)
E-Mail jonathan.strosberg@moffitt.org

Papotti M, de Herder WW (eds): Neuroendocrine Tumors: A Multidisciplinary Approach.
Front Horm Res. Basel, Karger, 2015, vol 44, pp 248–262 (DOI: 10.1159/000403885)

Other Novel Therapies: Biomarkers, microRNAs and microRNA Inhibitors, DNA Methylation, Epigenetics, Immunotherapy and Virotherapy

Valeria Giandomenico[a] · Chrissie Thirlwell[c] · Magnus Essand[b]

Departments of [a]Medical Sciences, Endocrine Oncology, and [b]Immunology, Genetics and Pathology, Clinical Immunology, Rudbeck Laboratory, Uppsala University, Uppsala, Sweden; [c]Cancer Research UK, Medical Genomics Laboratory, UCL Cancer Institute, London, UK

Abstract

Neuroendocrine tumors (NETs) consist of heterogeneous neoplasms. The neuroendocrine cells of the human body are confined to certain organs, such as the thyroid, pancreas and adrenals, or they are dispersed throughout the body in the respiratory tract and in the intestinal mucosa. The cells belong to the diffuse endocrine cell system, share a neuroendocrine phenotype, and accumulate precursor molecules which are then processed into hormones, peptides or amines. The tightly controlled release on stimulation is either to the blood stream or adjacent cells or neurons. Neuroendocrine cells regulate various processes in the human body, such as gastrointestinal secretion, blood pressure and response to stress. NETs present a wide spectrum of malignant diseases from rather benign to very malignant and lethal variants. NETs may occur in any organ, but are mainly detected in the gastroenteropancreatic system and in the lungs. The understanding of NET biology and treatments has changed dramatically during the last decade. Today, the main problems that clinicians and translational scientists face in overcoming these malignancies relate to various aspects within the molecular pathogenesis of NETs. This chapter focuses on the importance of novel biomarkers: microRNA and microRNA inhibitors; DNA methylation and epigenetics, and immunotherapy and virotherapy to develop novel treatments for NETs.

Novel Biomarkers

Our understanding of neuroendocrine tumor (NET) biology and treatments has changed dramatically during the last decade through exploring genetics, molecular pathways, targets and potential novel biomarkers in NETs. Major cellular activities, such as proliferation, differentiation, apoptosis and survival, are tightly controlled by signaling networks which are mainly deregulated in cancer cells. These processes have been going through a real revolution as the novel molecular-targeted therapies have been developed against different malignancies. New findings have shown that to interfere with specific molecular events by using targeted therapy might be a feasible alternative and that these novel treatments may damage normal cells less than previous treatments. The main problems that clinicians and translational scientists face in overcoming gastroenteropancreatic NETs (GEP-NETs) relate to various phenomena within molecular pathogenesis. Thus, an enhanced search for new GEP-NET biomarkers is an unmet need because molecular markers play a critical role in developing personalized therapies. Moreover, it is important to emphasize the best therapeutic approaches so far, which are extensively described in the references [1–3].

NET Therapeutic Targets
Somatostatin receptors (SSTRs) have been the main target for NET medical therapy during the last decades. The first somatostatin analog octreotide was approved by the FDA in 1988. SSTRs are expressed on NET cellular surfaces up to 80%. They belong to a family of five G-protein-coupled receptors (SSTR1–5) and mediate several biological activities, such as the regulation of exocrine and endocrine secretions, cell proliferation and angiogenesis. The reported novel truncated receptor variants suggested their potential role in diagnosis, prognosis and therapeutic targets, and scientific studies are ongoing [4]. Somatostatin analogs, such as octreotide, lanreotide and pasireotide, exert their clinical effects specifically targeting different SSTRs. The signaling pathways used by these receptors are tightly controlled, highly specific, and are complicated by networking with many other molecules. Because somatostatin analogs have recently been shown to improve progression-free survival and control symptoms related to hypersecretion, they became a first-line therapy [5].

NET Predictive Markers and Molecular Pathways
Several molecules recently reached investigation at the preclinical and clinical settings. They are tyrosine kinase receptors (TKRs), their ligands and molecules of the mammalian target of rapamycin (mTOR) molecular pathway. However, they require further investigation to optimize their use in clinics.

TKRs are key regulators of pivotal cellular processes, such as cell growth and neoangiogenesis. Their aberrant expression has been correlated to the development of several malignancies and they have become promising targets for antitumor therapy. TKRs have also led to the identification of potential therapeutic biomarkers in several NETs. TKRs that have pivotal roles in tumor proliferation have been shown to affect gastrointestinal (GI) and pancreatic NETs (pNETs). Thus, findings about the epidermal growth factor receptor over the last decade has prompted a preclinical rationale to perform further investigations by using anti-epidermal growth factor receptor (EGFR) monoclonal antibodies in selected primary ileal NET and pNET patients.

We also emphasize the potential importance of other TKRs, such as mesenchymal-epithelial transition receptor (c-Met) and insulin-like growth factor receptor. Both are overexpressed in malignant tissue and have the capacity to interact with EGFR. These findings supported the idea of developing dual-target therapy involving monoclonal antibodies against more than one TKR [3].

Furthermore, several TKRs cover important roles in neoangiogenesis and have been shown to affect GI-NETs and pNETs. Because angiogenesis is a crucial process in tumor progression and metastasis, blocking angiogenesis has been suggested as an efficient therapeutic approach for many malignancies. The TKRs that are pivotal in this process are the vascular EGFR (VEGFR), the platelet-derived GFR and the fibroblast GFR. Indeed, various molecules against these targets and their ligands have been approved in clinical practice for several malignancies. Moreover, the development of monoclonal antibodies and their application in cancer therapy also opened a window of hope for NETs, which are highly vascularized and characterized by high levels of molecular markers of angiogenesis. Nevertheless, several studies have shown infrequent expression of VEGF and VGFR in midgut carcinoids, also denoted small intestinal NETs. Despite this, preliminary positive data suggested the VEGF pathway might promote tumor growth in pNETs. Furthermore, preclinical data have shown the activity of anti-VEGFR mouse monoclonal antibodies in a mouse pNETs model supports the potential use of these molecules against pNETs as potential drugs. Current discrepancies of the effect of these monoclonal antibodies as potential drugs between GI-NETs and pNETs support further investigation to establish whether and how they can be used in clinics. Taken together, these findings strengthen the need for further study on the effects of tyrosine-kinase inhibitor-specific monoclonal antibodies for NETs therapy [3].

PI3K/AKT/mTOR Pathway and Everolimus

The PI3K/AKT/mTOR pathway is an intracellular pathway that controls most aspects of cancer, such as cell cycle, survival, metabolism, motility and genomic instability. The mTOR is a serine-threonine protein kinase that covers a central role in its pathway and its activation is tightly regulated through positive and negative feedback. Two distinct complexes, mTORC1 and mTORC2, are formed by mTOR and are specifically activated to exert slightly different effects phenomena [4]. Nevertheless, six general classes of agents that target the PI3K/AKT/mTOR network are in clinical trials: (1) pan-class I PI3K inhibitors, (2) isoform-selective PI3K inhibitors, (3) rapamycin analogs (rapalogs), (4) active-site mTOR inhibitors, (5) pan-PI3K-mTOR inhibitors and (6) AKT inhibitors [6].

Everolimus was found to be an elective inhibitor of mTOR after many preclinical and clinical trials. This drug specifically regulates the mTORC1 protein, but not the mTORC2 protein, in a similar way to different mTOR inhibitors. This effect leads to a hyperactivation of the kinase AKT via inhibition on the mTORC1-negative feedback loop, while not inhibiting the mTORC2-positive feedback to AKT. Increased

AKT activity leads to longer survival in some cell types. An important study with advanced extrapancreatic NET/GI-NET patients suggested that everolimus might be active against these malignancies [7]. Nevertheless, the study did not clarify a predefined efficacy end point and clinical trials using everolimus alone and/or in combination with other drugs are ongoing [8, 9].

Taken together, these studies on therapeutic strategies for GEP-NETs development require the following: suitable patient selection; sequencing studies; new drugs to control several molecular pathways, such as novel target inhibitors; serotonin synthesis inhibitors; molecules to inhibit c-MET in VEGFR-resistant tumors; PI3K/AKT/mTOR pathway inhibitors, and combination therapies [10].

microRNAs and microRNA Inhibitors

Many solid and hematological malignancies have poor survival rates with few therapeutic options. The discrepancy between genotype and clinical phenotype motivated scientists to investigate molecular aspects of cancer cells to develop novel targeted therapeutics. During the last 2 decades different components of the genome, denoted microRNAs (miRNAs), have emerged as key regulators of pivotal biological processes. They are short sequences of 18–25 nucleotides and represent a family of noncoding RNAs; they are able to target tens to hundreds of genes simultaneously in the human genome and play an important role of gene control. miRNAs function as a repressor of eukaryotic gene regulation by binding to the 3′-untranslated regions of target miRNAs. The binding triggers cleavage or translational inhibition of the mRNA, depending on the degree of complementarities. Hundreds of miRNAs are present in mammals and regulate the expression of genes of more than 30% of the genome. Thus, they are involved in regulation of different cellular phenomena, such as cell proliferation, apoptosis, differentiation, viral infection and tumorigenesis. Because miRNAs are highly deregulated in cancer cells they have become prognostic biomarkers and therapeutic candidates for use in cancer therapy. Nevertheless, several gaps are left to translate current miRNA understanding to novel therapy development [11].

Patient cancer tissues exhibit miRNA expression signatures different from those in normal tissues. This difference enables the identification of the molecular pathway regulations in both tissues and outlines different molecular pathway regulation in normal and cancer tissues. Genome-wide profiling has depicted specific signatures able to discriminate different types of cancer with a high degree of accuracy. This approach has been suitable in identifying overexpressed and downregulated miRNAs in several malignancies, such as most solid tumors and hematological malignancies [12]. Despite advances in understanding the mechanisms that cause miRNA aberrant regulation, to fully explain the biological role of miRNAs during cancer initiation and development is a challenge. A growing number of potential oncogenic and suppressor miRNAs have been identified and specific miRNA signatures might be used to predict the clinical outcome of pancreatic [13], lung [14, 15] and, more recently, small intestinal NETs [16, 17]. Bioinformatic analysis and advanced molecular biology methods might be used to identify specifically and differentially expressed miRNAs, which may be developed as novel biomarkers and therapeutic molecular targets for GEP-NETs [18, 19].

Despite the recent improvement in our understanding of miRNAs, one substantial remaining task is to translate bench-based findings into clinical practice [20]. Today, there are several strategies to target miRNAs or use them as targeting agents in cancer, such as: inhibition of oncogenic miRNAs by antisense DNA oligonucleotides; antagomirs, locked nucleic acids, RNA sponges, miR-masking; exogenous expression of tumor suppressor miRNAs, and targeting miRNAs by using small molecules [21]. Diverse strategies either to target or replace miRNAs have led to several studies about improving the specific delivery of miRNAs to tumor tissues. At the beginning of these studies recombinant adenoviral- and lentiviral-vectors were proposed to replace the tumor suppressor miRNAs. However, these approaches seem to be toxic because of their association to immune response induction. Thus, recently, development of non-viral dependent alternative approaches, e.g. lipid-based nanoparticles containing miRNAs for proper delivery, is considered more feasible. Synthetic delivery systems are preferable because they elicit less immunogenicity. Currently, these synthetic systems have relatively low efficiency, and long-term studies on their toxicity are lacking [22]. This emphasizes the importance for further studies of a variety of miRNA delivery approaches to ensure new clinical options.

Furthermore, the presence of miRNAs in body fluids, i.e. serum, plasma and urine, might represent a suitable source of noninvasive biomarkers in cancer. Collecting samples of body fluids from patients also limits the difficulties of collecting enough tumor tissues, particularly in rare malignancies such as NETs. Because deregulated miRNA expression is an early event in tumorigenesis, to measure circulating miRNA levels might also be useful for early cancer detection, which might contribute considerably in the development new treatments. miRNAs have a huge impact on gene expression globally; moreover, because they are deregulated in cancer, targeting or replacing miRNAs shows considerable promise for sensitizing cancer cells to therapy agents and for preventing the metastasis. However, most studies have used two-dimensional cell culture systems. These models do not consider the contribution of the tumor microenvironment and oversimplify the therapy regimens used in the clinics. Transgenic mouse models and/or syngenic tumor transplantation models with an intact tumor microenvironment should be used to develop drug-resistant animal models. Furthermore, patient-derived xenografts with a known therapy history might be used to deliver miRNAs into tissues and to study whether miRNAs can sensitize refractory tumors to various therapies. There are currently numerous clinical trials using miRNAs as biomarkers of tumor progression, metastasis and response to chemotherapy or targeted therapy agents (www.clinicaltrials.gov). However, more research should be carried out to establish whether miRNAs are feasible for clinical therapy use [22].

Epigenetics of Neuroendocrine Tumors – DNA Methylation and Histone Modifications

Epigenetics can be defined as a heritable change in gene expression without a change in the underlying DNA sequence. Epigenetic modifications include DNA methylation, histone modifications and miRNAs. To date, DNA methylation is the most studied and best understood epigenetic modification. In recent years, our understanding of the role of DNA methylation in tumorigenesis has evolved markedly due to developments in both array-based and sequencing-based approaches for studying the epigenome. Many human diseases are caused by epigenetic drivers which are already impacting both clinical practice and the introduction of novel therapies. Epigenetic changes play an important role in cancer development [23]. This section will focus on DNA methylation and histone modifications in pNETs and intestinal NETs as miRNAs are covered elsewhere in this chapter.

DNA Methylation in NET Development

Pancreatic NETs

DNA methylation occurs primarily at the 5′-position of the cytosine ring where cytosine is adjacent to guanine in the DNA sequence. These dinucleotides are termed 'CpGs', and there are an estimated 28 million CpGs across the human genome. CpGs are clustered in 'islands' in the promoter regions of approximately 70% of genes; however, DNA methylation occurs in all coding and noncoding regions to some degree. DNA methylation occurs via the DNA methyltransferase (DNMT) family of enzymes. DNMT1 maintains methylation during cellular replication and DNMT3 produces de novo methylation, whereas DNMT2 has no clear role at present [24, 25]. DNA methylation patterns are both tissue specific in normal tissues throughout the body and specific to different tumor types. Therefore, when studying DNA methylation in cancer it is imperative that matched normal tissue is available for analysis. The first studies of DNA methylation in cancer identified global hypomethylation in human cancer cell lines [26]. DNA hypermethylation in CpG islands at promoter regions has been associated with a subsequent loss of expression of tumor suppressor genes such as *VHL, BRCA, RASSF1A* and *CDKN2A(p16INK4a)* [27].

To date, published studies of DNA methylation in NETs include candidate gene-driven approaches and an array-based approach interrogating 27,000 CpGs across the genome in 24 NET samples [28, 29]. In the largest candidate gene-driven study, 11 candidate genes were studied in 48 pNETs, the majority of which (94%) were nonfunctional.

Hypermethylation of the promoter region at the *RASSF1A* tumor suppressor gene was observed in 75% of tumors when compared with normal adjacent tissue. *RASSF1A* promoter methylation was observed in 100% of metastatic pNETs and 71% of nonmetastatic pNETs [30].

Cyclin-dependent kinase inhibitor 2a (CDKN2A)/p16INK4a is a tumor suppressor gene that plays a vital role in cell cycle regulation. Methylation at the *CDKN2A* locus has been demonstrated in 40% of pNETs and is associated with early tumor recurrence and reduced overall survival [28]. It is also observed in the pNET cell line QGP1 [31].

Hypermethylation at the *CDKN2A* promoter has also been identified in up to 63% of gastrinomas independent of the disease stage, location of primary or prognosis. This suggests that methylation at the *CDKN2A* promoter may be an early occurrence in gastrinoma tumorigenesis. Conversely, insulinomas have a low frequency (17%) of hypermethylation at *CDKN2A* [19].

The O^6-methylguanine DNA methyltransferase (MGMT) promoter is methylated in 40% of pNETs. Loss of MGMT assessed by immunohistochemistry corresponds to the response to temozolomide chemotherapy [32].

Intestinal NETs

Using a candidate gene-driven approach in a study of 16 intestinal NETs, Chan et al. [33] identified increased promoter methylation at *MGMT* (25% cases), *THSB1* (44% cases), *p14* (44% cases) and *RARβ* (25% cases). *RASSF1A* has also been found to be hypermethylated in two further candidate gene-driven studies. This occurred in 32% (20/62) of small intestinal NETs [34]. A recent array-based approach studying 10 primary intestinal NETs and matched lymph node metastases identified 2,697 CpG sites to be significantly differentially methylated. The Illumina HumMeth27K array was used in this study which interrogates 27,000 CpG sites located primarily in the promoter regions of genes.

Of the 2,697 CpGs identified, gene ontology analysis found that genes regulating cell growth, apoptosis, proliferation and metastases-related genes demonstrated significantly different levels of DNA methylation when primary tumors and lymph node metastases were compared. *RUNX3*, *TP73*, *CHFR*, *MAPK4*, *CCND1*, *AHRR* and *RB1* were all found to be highly methylated in this study. However, this pilot study requires further validation in a larger cohort.

A CpG island methylator phenotype (CIMP) describes increased methylation at multiple CpG sites across CpG islands. CIMP positivity was seen in 20% of NET cases in a study comprising 71 pNETs and intestinal NETs. This corresponded with those tumors with a ki-67 of >10%; CIMP negativity corresponded with improved overall survival [35].

Histone Modifications in NET Development

Histones form one of the main components of chromatin; they function to package DNA into nucleosomes. Posttranslational histone modifications (comprising methylation, acetylation and phosphorylation) function to regulate transcription by rendering chromatin 'open/permissive' or 'closed/repressive'. This process establishes and maintains chromatin structure, which in turn ensures cellular identity through repression of nonessential genes. Histone modifications are catalyzed by several genes, such as histone deacetylases and acetyltransferases.

To date, there have been few studies on histone modifications occurring in NET development. Published studies include small numbers of tumors and have only been performed on intestinal NETs. In a study of 16 low-grade primary intestinal NETs, H3K4 dimethylation was seen in 93% of tumors, whereas in hepatocellular cancer and pancreatic adenocarcinoma the incidence is much lower [36]. Therefore, modifications at the H3K4 locus have been identified as a potential event in intestinal NET development; however, further studies are required.

Chromatin Remodelers in pNET Development

Exome sequencing of ten sporadic pNETs, followed by Sanger sequencing validation in a cohort of 58 pNETs, identified commonly mutated genes involved in chromatin remodeling [37]. Forty-four percent of tumors were found to harbor inactivating mutations in *MEN1*, whereas 43% harbored mutations in either *ATRX* or *DAXX* (18 and 25%, respectively; death domain-associated protein or alpha thalassemia/mental retardation syndrome X-linked). Mutations in *ATRX* and *DAXX* were mutually exclusive, but overlapped with MEN1 mutations in 16 cases (23.5%).

Prior to this study *ATRX* and *DAXX* had not previously been associated with NET development. *ATRX* had previously been implicated in glioma development. The proteins encoded by *ATRX* and *DAXX* have multiple functions, including chromatin remodeling during heterochromatin assembly at repetitive guanine-rich regions (such as telomeres), where they are required for incorporation of the histone variant H3.3 [38]. In this study, the presence of mutations in *ATRX/DAXX* was associated with improved prognosis; however, the exact opposite was observed in a larger cohort [39]. The main difference between these two confounding studies is that the first study analyzed mainly liver metastases and the second larger study analyzed primary tumors.

Summary

It is clear that epigenetic changes play a key role in NET development. This is particularly relevant for intestinal NETs which are mutationally quiet, with only 8% of tumors harboring mutations in *CDKN1B* [40]. Through ongoing collaborative large-scale array-based and sequencing-based studies, definitive analyses of these tumors are underway. It is hoped that in the future epigenetically targeted therapies may have a role in the clinicians' therapeutic armory when treating NETs, and that novel diagnostic and prognostic epigenetic biomarkers will be identified to improve the management and outcomes for our patients.

Recent Advancements in Cancer Immunotherapy

Cancer immunotherapy, a strategy that harnesses the body's immune system to combat tumors, is currently going through a tremendous revitalization process. A clear indication of this is that the editors of *Science* chose cancer immunotherapy as

'Breakthrough of the Year' for 2013. There are two main approaches that have shown adequate therapeutic benefits for patients with advanced cancer: (1) administration of antibodies that target the patient's own T cells, giving them the power to attack tumor cells, and (2) isolation of the cancer patient's T cells, followed by introduction of a new receptor and then adoptive transfer of the engineered T cells back to the patient.

Monoclonal antibodies (MAbs) directed against tumor-associated antigens expressed by tumor cells and MAbs directed against growth factors of importance for tumor neovascularization have been successfully established as anticancer drugs during the last decade [41]. The potential of therapeutic T cells to be attracted to sites of disease, expand and persist after a single injection remains a major advantage over MAbs.

Immune Checkpoint Antibodies

The immune response of T cells is controlled by equilibrium between costimulatory and inhibitory signals, called immune checkpoints. The checkpoints act much like the brakes on a car. A patient's T cells can therefore be reactivated if antibodies against T cell immune checkpoints are administered. Such antibodies do not directly target tumor cells but release the brake from T cells, giving them the power to attack and eradicate tumor cells [42]. However, because they activate T cells rather unspecifically, a certain degree of autoimmunity is inevitable. Two inhibitory receptor molecules on T cells, CTLA-4 and PD-1, when triggered, provide signals to the T cells to stop exerting lytic activity. Ipilimumab, a fully human anti-CTLA-4 antibody, received US FDA license approval in 2011 for the treatment of metastatic melanoma, and lambrolizumab, a humanized anti-PD-1 antibody, received FDA breakthrough designation in 2013 for the same disease.

Adoptive Transfer of Genetically Engineered T Cells

T cells can be isolated from the blood samples of patients and given a new receptor that recognizes an antigen presented by tumor cells. The genetically transferred receptor is either a new T cell receptor or a chimeric antigen receptor consisting of an antibody fragment for antigen recognition and T cell receptor signaling domains for T cell activation. An adequate number of genetically engineered T cells from a patient can therefore be produced for adoptive transfer back to the patient. Indeed, genetically engineered T cells have recently been successfully used in cancer treatment, especially CD19 chimeric antigen receptor T cells against both chronic and acute B cell leukemia [43]. Highly specific T cells have a clinical advantage compared with conventional therapies because of the specific lysis of antigen-positive cells, leaving other tissues intact.

Therapies with immune checkpoint antibodies and engineered T cells are novel and have not yet reached the field of neuroendocrine cancer and many other solid cancers. The main side effect of anti-CTLA-4 and anti-PD-1 antibodies is colitis, an autoimmune reaction in the gastric tract caused by the reactivated T cells. The fact that many GEP-NET patients have a long life expectancy needs to be considered when balancing potential benefits against the side effects of ipilimumab or lambrolizumab treatments. The main drawbacks with treatment using engineered patient T cells are that very specific antigen targets need to be identified and that the treatment is expensive and requires advanced logistics.

Cancer Vaccination

Therapeutic cancer vaccination can also be used if a tumor-associated antigen is identified, sometimes together with specialized antigen-presenting dendritic cells (DCs), so-called DC vaccines. An alternative is to use tumor cell lysate as a cancer vaccine together with cytokines. These approaches have been evaluated for many tumors, in general with poor results. Cancer vaccination trials for neuroendocrine cancer were reviewed by Bridle [44] in 2011. The overall finding was that neuroendocrine cancer vaccines often fail to induce detectable tumor-specific immune responses in humans. For GEP-NETs, only one paper has reported on vaccination for a single patient within the last 5 years. In that case, vaccination against the ganglioside NGcGM3 (NeuGCGM3) in combination with interferon (IFN)-α was used. With the disease having progressed after treatment with recombinant human IFN-α alone, the patient was immunized five times with NGcGM3 by the intramuscular route at 2-week intervals and then at monthly intervals for more than 12 months. A total of 56 months later, the patient had stable disease. However, given the poor success rate of therapeutic cancer vaccination trials in general, cancer vaccination as a single regimen is not to be recommended for NET patients.

One particular example where vaccination could be beneficial is for a rare form of neuroendocrine skin cancer called Merkel cell carcinoma. The Merkel cell polyomavirus is believed to be the cause of Merkel cell carcinoma and antigens expressed by Merkel cell polyomavirus could in the future be targeted as tumor-associated antigens both in preventive and therapeutic vaccinations.

Other Forms of Immunotherapy

For a recent perspective on the history of immunotherapy and where we stand today, readers are referred to Rosenberg [45]. Traditional immunotherapies based on cytokines such as IFN-α and interleukin (IL)-2 have been evaluated for GEP-NETs. In fact, pegylated IFN-α is now a first-line treatment option in many countries for metastatic small intestinal NETs. IFN-α exerts antitumor effects through various mechanisms, including stimulation of T cells, induction of cell cycle arrest in the G1 and G0 phases, and inhibition of angiogenesis. IL-2 as a single regimen is not used for NETs.

Although IL-2 activates effector T cells, its strong promoting effect on regulatory T cells with immunosuppressive features has reduced the interest in IL-2 treatment during the last decade. High-dose IL-2 treatment is also associated with severe side effects.

Oncolytic Viruses as Immunotherapy

A tumor cell and a virus-infected cell have many similarities and consequently most viruses replicate better in a tumor cell than in a normal cell. This is particularly true for RNA viruses. The notion that viruses can kill tumor cells has been known for more than a century, although coordinated research efforts did not begin until the 1960s. As virus genome sequences have been revealed and become public, our understanding of virus-cell interactions has increased and genetic engineering technologies have advanced, it is today possible to engineer viruses that are highly selective for tumor cells, hence the term oncolytic virus. Upon infection, the engineered virus propagates inside the tumor cell and breaks the cell membrane leading to the release of large amounts of progeny virus, which can infect and then kill neighboring tumor cells. The lytic cell death caused by a virus is perceived as danger by the immune system. It activates professional antigen-presenting cells to take up antigens from the dying tumor cells, migrate to draining lymph nodes, and present peptides from viral and tumor-associated antigens to naive T cells. The T cells become activated; they enter the circulation and travel to the site of the tumor. Therefore, the immune response raised against tumor-associated antigens can last long after the immune system has defeated the virus infection.

The use of oncolytic viruses that preferentially infect, replicate in and destroy tumor cells is an emerging immunotherapeutic approach for cancer. For a recent review on virus-based therapy of NETs readers are referred to Essand [46]. Our group has systematically developed a recombinant oncolytic adenovirus to treat NETs, which is about to enter a clinical trial for GEP-NET patients with liver metastases. Most adenoviruses infect cells by binding to the coxsackie-adenovirus receptor. However, because this molecule is involved in cell-cell interaction its expression is often downregulated on tumor cells. We have therefore added a second route of infection by introducing a cell-penetrating peptide in the virus capsid, and thereby shown increased tumor cell infectivity. In order to make the adenovirus selective for replication in neuroendocrine cells, we have replaced the native viral E1A promoter with the human chromogranin A promoter. The adenovirus E1A gene is directly responsible for virus replication; therefore, this genetic alteration blocks virus replication in all cells that are not of neuroendocrine origin. Furthermore, to reduce potential liver toxicity we have introduced target sequences for liver-specific microRNAs in the virus genome, thereby minimizing the activity of the virus in healthy liver cells [46].

The oncolytic cell death induced by a virus leads to a microbe-associated inflammatory response, which is optimal for antigen presentation by DCs. It also leads to the release of tumor-associated antigens from the dying tumor cells that can be captured by resident DCs. To enhance this effect even further, strategies have been developed to arm oncolytic viruses with a gene that can activate and stimulate an appropriate immune response against the tumor cells. Granulocyte macrophage colony-stimulating factor (GM-CSF) is a cytokine that functions as a white blood cell growth factor. The gene encoding GM-CSF has been successfully introduced into the genome of oncolytic herpes virus, vaccinia virus and adenovirus. Another gene of interest that has been successfully introduced in oncolytic adenovirus is CD40L, a molecule of importance for helper T cell activation. The main function of GM-CSF and CD40L in the context of oncolytic virus therapy is to attract and activate DCs to reveal and present 'hidden' tumor-associated antigens in an optimal context for the activation of T cells. However, it is at present unclear whether GM-CSF and CD40L expression in the context of virus-induced cell death will be sufficient to overcome self-tolerance and lead to potent systemic antitumor responses.

Recent research has focused on a virulence factor from the bacterium *Helicobacter pylori* called *H. pylori* neutrophil-activating protein (HP-NAP) as an immune stimulatory gene for oncolytic adenoviruses with activity in NETs [47]. The main advantage of HP-NAP is that it activates both the innate and adoptive immune system. It is a chemoattractant that recruits neutrophils and activates them to secrete cytokines, release reactive oxygen species, and directly kill tumor cells. Furthermore, HP-NAP can polarize resident tissue DCs at tumor sites to secrete cytokines promoting a so-called Th1-like immune response. It also matures DCs and causes them to migrate to draining lymph nodes where they present tumor antigens to naive T cells. Due to their Th1 polarizing phenotype, the HP-NAP-matured DCs activate cytolytic T cells that can enter the circulation and migrate to the tumor area where they efficiently kill tumor cells.

Combination Treatments

It is likely that we will see more combination therapies where immunotherapy is combined with conventional cancer therapies and where various strategies of immunotherapies are combined with each other. Many trials are currently evaluating the combination of anti-CTLA-4 or anti-PD-1 antibodies with chemotherapies, and it is likely that when oncolytic viruses become more commonly used they will also be combined with antibodies against immune checkpoints to fully activate the immune system against cancer.

Immune Scoring of Tumors to Predict Clinical Outcome

The most commonly used system for classification of the extent of cancer spread is the TNM staging system, where T relates to tumor burden, N indicates whether tumor cells are present in draining lymph nodes and M provides information about distant metastases. The TNM staging system is also used for GEP-NETs. This staging system focuses on tumor-cell characteristics and does not consider the tumor microenvironment. It is today clear that immune cell infiltration in tumors correlates with clinical outcome. Generally speaking, T cell infiltration is a good prognostic sign, whereas macrophage infiltration can be a poor prognostic sign. Multivariable analyses have shown that a so-called immunoscore, i.e. immunohistochemistry staining for CD8+ T cells in the center and invasive margin of the tumor, provides better prognostic information than the TNM system [48, 49]. There is therefore a trend to include the concept of immunoscore as a parameter in the classification of many malignant tumors, and it is important that immunoscore analyses are introduced in pathological examinations of NET surgery samples to investigate whether this information can add prognostic information for NET patients. It is likely that immune scoring will be used in the future to determine which patients are most likely to respond to immunotherapy.

Future Perspectives

In conclusion, as our understanding has increased about the immune system's role in tumor progression and tumor control, it is a fair guess that the use of well-designed immunotherapy trials will increase for many malignancies, including NETs. It is also likely that we will see the introduction of immunoscore in NET diagnostics.

References

1 Oberg K, Casanovas O, Castano JP, Chung D, Delle Fave G, Denefle P, Harris P, Khan MS, Kulke MH, Scarpa A, Tang LH, Wiedenmann B: Molecular pathogenesis of neuroendocrine tumors: implications for current and future therapeutic approaches. Clin Cancer Res 2013;19:2842–2849.

2 Capdevila J, Meeker A, Garcia-Carbonero R, Pietras K, Astudillo A, Casanovas O, Scarpa A: Molecular biology of neuroendocrine tumors: from pathways to biomarkers and targets. Cancer Metastasis Rev 2014;33:345–351.

3 De Dosso S, Grande E, Barriuso J, Castellano D, Tabernero J, Capdevila J: The targeted therapy revolution in neuroendocrine tumors: in search of biomarkers for patient selection and response evaluation. Cancer Metastasis Rev 2013;32:465–477.

4 Castano JP, Sundin A, Maecke HR, Villabona C, Vazquez-Albertino R, Navarro E, Oberg K: Gastrointestinal neuroendocrine tumors (NETs): new diagnostic and therapeutic challenges. Cancer Metastasis Rev 2014;33:353–359.

5 Chalabi M, Duluc C, Caron P, Vezzosi D, Guillermet-Guibert J, Pyronnet S, Bousquet C: Somatostatin analogs: does pharmacology impact antitumor efficacy? Trends Endocrinol Metab 2014;25:115–127.

6 Fruman DA, Rommel C: PI3K and cancer: lessons, challenges and opportunities. Nat Rev Drug Discov 2014;13:140–156.

7 Pavel ME, Hainsworth JD, Baudin E, Peeters M, Horsch D, Winkler RE, Klimovsky J, Lebwohl D, Jehl V, Wolin EM, Oberg K, van Cutsem E, Yao JC: Everolimus plus octreotide long-acting repeatable for the treatment of advanced neuroendocrine tumours associated with carcinoid syndrome (RADIANT-2): a randomised, placebo-controlled, phase 3 study. Lancet 2011;378:2005–2012.

8 Liu E, Marincola P, Oberg K: Everolimus in the treatment of patients with advanced pancreatic neuroendocrine tumors: latest findings and interpretations. Therap Adv Gastroenterol 2013;6:412–419.

9 Grozinsky-Glasberg S, Pavel M: Inhibition of mTOR in carcinoid tumors. Target Oncol 2012;7:189–195.

10 Raymond E, Garcia-Carbonero R, Wiedenmann B, Grande E, Pavel M: Systemic therapeutic strategies for GEP-NETS: what can we expect in the future? Cancer Metastasis Rev 2014;33:367–372.
11 Garzon R, Marcucci G, Croce CM: Targeting microRNAs in cancer: rationale, strategies and challenges. Nat Rev Drug Discov 2010;9:775–789.
12 Di Leva G, Croce CM: miRNA profiling of cancer. Curr Opin Genet Dev 2013;23:3–11.
13 Roldo C, Missiaglia E, Hagan JP, Falconi M, Capelli P, Bersani S, Calin GA, Volinia S, Liu CG, Scarpa A, Croce CM: MicroRNA expression abnormalities in pancreatic endocrine and acinar tumors are associated with distinctive pathologic features and clinical behavior. J Clin Oncol 2006;24:4677–4684.
14 Vannini I, Fanini F, Fabbri M: MicroRNAs as lung cancer biomarkers and key players in lung carcinogenesis. Clin Biochem 2013;46:918–925.
15 Lee HW, Lee EH, Ha SY, Lee CH, Chang HK, Chang S, Kwon KY, Hwang IS, Roh MS, Seo JW: Altered expression of microRNA miR-21, miR-155, and let-7a and their roles in pulmonary neuroendocrine tumors. Pathol Int 2012;62:583–591.
16 Ruebel K, Leontovich AA, Stilling GA, Zhang S, Righi A, Jin L, Lloyd RV: MicroRNA expression in ileal carcinoid tumors: downregulation of microRNA-133a with tumor progression. Mod Pathol 2010;23:367–375.
17 Li SC, Essaghir A, Martijn C, Lloyd RV, Demoulin JB, Oberg K, Giandomenico V: Global microRNA profiling of well-differentiated small intestinal neuroendocrine tumors. Mod Pathol 2013;26:685–696.
18 Santarpia L, Nicoloso M, Calin GA: MicroRNAs: a complex regulatory network drives the acquisition of malignant cell phenotype. Endocr Relat Cancer 2010;17:F51–F75.
19 Karpathakis A, Dibra H, Thirlwell C: Neuroendocrine tumours: cracking the epigenetic code. Endocr Relat Cancer 2013;20:R65–R82.
20 Gavrilov K, Saltzman WM: Therapeutic siRNA: principles, challenges, and strategies. Yale J Biol Med 2012;85:187–200.
21 Iorio MV, Croce CM: microRNA involvement in human cancer. Carcinogenesis 2012;33:1126–1133.
22 Raza U, Zhang JD, Sahin O: MicroRNAs: master regulators of drug resistance, stemness, and metastasis. J Mol Med 2014;92:321–326.
23 Jones PA, Baylin SB: The fundamental role of epigenetic events in cancer. Nat Rev Genet 2002;3:415–428.
24 Okano M, Xie S, Li E: Cloning and characterization of a family of novel mammalian DNA (cytosine-5) methyltransferases. Nat Genet 1998;19:219–220.
25 Okano M, Bell DW, Haber DA, Li E: DNA methyltransferases Dnmt3a and Dnmt3b are essential for de novo methylation and mammalian development. Cell 1999;99:247–257.
26 Feinberg AP, Vogelstein B: Hypomethylation distinguishes genes of some human cancers from their normal counterparts. Nature 1983;301:89–92.
27 Esteller M: Epigenetics in cancer. New Engl J Med 2008;358:1148–1159.
28 House MG, Herman JG, Guo MZ, Hooker CM, Schulick RD, Lillemoe KD, Cameron JL, Hruban RH, Maitra A, Yeo CJ: Aberrant hypermethylation of tumor suppressor genes in pancreatic endocrine neoplasms. Ann Surg 2003;238:423–431, discussion 431–422.
29 Verdugo AD, Crona J, Starker L, Stalberg P, Akerstrom G, Westin G, Hellman P, Bjorklund P: Global DNA methylation patterns through an array-based approach in small intestinal neuroendocrine tumors. Endocr Relat Cancer 2014;21:L5–L7.
30 Malpeli G, Amato E, Dandrea M, Fumagalli C, Debattisti V, Boninsegna L, Pelosi G, Falconi M, Scarpa A: Methylation-associated down-regulation of RASSF1A and up-regulation of RASSF1C in pancreatic endocrine tumors. BMC Cancer 2011;11:351.
31 Lubomierski N, Kersting M, Bert T, Muench K, Wulbrand U, Schuermann M, Bartsch D, Simon B: Tumor suppressor genes in the 9p21 gene cluster are selective targets of inactivation in neuroendocrine gastroenteropancreatic tumors. Cancer Res 2001;61:5905–5910.
32 Kulke MH, Hornick JL, Frauenhoffer C, Hooshmand S, Ryan DP, Enzinger PC, Meyerhardt JA, Clark JW, Stuart K, Fuchs CS, Redston MS: O6-methylguanine DNA methyltransferase deficiency and response to temozolomide-based therapy in patients with neuroendocrine tumors. Clin Cancer Res 2009;15:338–345.
33 Chan AO, Kim SG, Bedeir A, Issa JP, Hamilton SR, Rashid A: CpG island methylation in carcinoid and pancreatic endocrine tumors. Oncogene 2003;22:924–934.
34 Pizzi S, Azzoni C, Bottarelli L, Campanini N, D'Adda T, Pasquali C, Rossi G, Rindi G, Bordi C: RASSF1A promoter methylation and 3p21.3 loss of heterozygosity are features of foregut, but not midgut and hindgut, malignant endocrine tumours. J Pathol 2005;206:409–416.
35 Arnold CN, Sosnowski A, Schmitt-Graff A, Arnold R, Blum HE: Analysis of molecular pathways in sporadic neuroendocrine tumors of the gastro-entero-pancreatic system. Int J Cancer 2007;120:2157–2164.
36 Magerl C, Ellinger J, Braunschweig T, Kremmer E, Koch LK, Holler T, Buttner R, Luscher B, Gutgemann I: H3K4 dimethylation in hepatocellular carcinoma is rare compared with other hepatobiliary and gastrointestinal carcinomas and correlates with expression of the methylase Ash2 and the demethylase LSD1. Hum Pathol 2010;41:181–189.

37 Jiao Y, Shi C, Edil BH, de Wilde RF, Klimstra DS, Maitra A, Schulick RD, Tang LH, Wolfgang CL, Choti MA, Velculescu VE, Diaz LA Jr, Vogelstein B, Kinzler KW, Hruban RH, Papadopoulos N: DAXX/ATRX, MEN1, and mTOR pathway genes are frequently altered in pancreatic neuroendocrine tumors. Science 2011;331:1199–1203.

38 Heaphy CM, de Wilde RF, Jiao Y, Klein AP, Edil BH, Shi C, Bettegowda C, Rodriguez FJ, Eberhart CG, Hebbar S, Offerhaus GJ, McLendon R, Rasheed BA, He Y, Yan H, Bigner DD, Oba-Shinjo SM, Marie SK, Riggins GJ, Kinzler KW, Vogelstein B, Hruban RH, Maitra A, Papadopoulos N, Meeker AK: Altered telomeres in tumors with ATRX and DAXX mutations. Science 2011;333:425.

39 Marinoni I, Kurrer AS, Vassella E, Dettmer M, Rudolph T, Banz V, Hunger F, Pasquinelli S, Speel EJ, Perren A: Loss of DAXX and ATRX are associated with chromosome instability and reduced survival of patients with pancreatic neuroendocrine tumors. Gastroenterology 2014;146:453–460.e5.

40 Francis JM, Kiezun A, Ramos AH, et al: Somatic mutation of CDKN1B in small intestine neuroendocrine tumors. Nat Genet 2013;45:1483–1486.

41 Scott AM, Wolchok JD, Old LJ: Antibody therapy of cancer. Nat Rev Cancer 2012;12:278–287.

42 Pardoll DM: The blockade of immune checkpoints in cancer immunotherapy. Nat Rev Cancer 2012;12:252–264.

43 Kalos M, June CH: Adoptive T cell transfer for cancer immunotherapy in the era of synthetic biology. Immunity 2013;39:49–60.

44 Bridle BW: Neuroendocrine cancer vaccines in clinical trials. Expert Rev Vaccines 2011;10:811–823.

45 Rosenberg SA: Raising the bar: the curative potential of human cancer immunotherapy. Sci Transl Med 2012;4:127ps8.

46 Essand M: Virotherapy of neuroendocrine tumors. Neuroendocrinology 2013;97:26–34.

47 Ramachandran M, Yu D, Wanders A, Essand M, Eriksson F: An infection-enhanced oncolytic adenovirus secreting *H. pylori* neutrophil-activating protein with therapeutic effects on neuroendocrine tumors. Mol Ther 2013;21:2008–2018.

48 Galon J, Mlecnik B, Bindea G, et al: Towards the introduction of the 'Immunoscore' in the classification of malignant tumours. J Pathol 2014;232:199–209.

49 Fridman WH, Pages F, Sautes-Fridman C, Galon J: The immune contexture in human tumours: impact on clinical outcome. Nat Rev Cancer 2012;12:298–306.

Valeria Giandomenico
Medical Sciences, Endocrine Oncology, Centre of Excellence for Endocrine Tumors
Uppsala University Hospital
SE–751 85 Uppsala (Sweden)
E-Mail valeria.giandomenico@medsci.uu.se

Author Index

Subject Index